Culpeper's
Complete Herbal

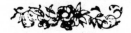

CULPEPER'S
COMPLETE
HERBAL

Nicholas Culpeper

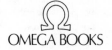

OMEGA BOOKS

'Herbs and plants are medical jewels gracing the woods, fields and lanes, which few eyes see, and few minds understand. Through this want of observation and knowledge the world suffers immense loss.'

LINNAEUS (1707-1778)

This edition published 1985 by Omega Books Ltd,
1 West Street, Ware, Hertfordshire.

ISBN 1 85007 026 1

Printed and bound in England by MacKays of Chatham.

INTRODUCTION.

THE study of Botany is a delightful one. The exercise in collecting plants invigorates the health, and the examination of them, and the discrimination of their kinds, improves the intellectual qualities. Botany also is extensively applied to useful purposes. From the vegetable kingdom man derives a large share of his sustenance, and from the same source he derives agents for the cure of his complaints.

By a knowledge of Botany, the physician is enabled to make improvements in the *materia medica*, and by an acquaintance with the affinities of plants, he is prepared to investigate with advantage, the properties and uses of the native productions of any part of the globe, and to use and apply them as remediable means for the relief of mankind.

There have always been medical men who have gained a knowledge of Botany. But the great mass of practitioners at the present day are as ignorant of the science of Botany as the horses on which they ride. No medical man should consider his education complete without a knowledge of Botany.

It is well observed by an eminent American physician,—"Botanical practice is destined to a continued course of improvement—going on from perfection to perfection, as long as new agents are found, or new developments of the powers of those agents are discovered by the careful practitioner, and the intelligent chemist.　The march of improvement results more and more in the rejection of dangerous minerals, and deleterious substances from among those articles resorted to for the cure of diseases ; and we are confidently looking forward to the period when the liberal influence of *eclectic* (choosing the best) principles, and the developments of an unbigoted, enlightened practice, shall make it manifest that *vegetable* remedies, and those alone, are necessary, proper, and sufficient, to control and obviate the disorders incident to the human frame."

Let Botany be studied by all, and they will be amply rewarded with new ideas, and agreeable and effectual remedies.　For this purpose *Culpeper's Herbal*, and *Dr. Robinson's Herbal*, may be consulted with great advantage.

Gu

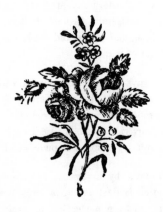

CULPEPER'S
COMPLETE HERBAL.

☞ *Herbs are invaluable, on account of their healing and curative power. Culpeper had a good knowledge of the appearance and virtues of Herbs, and has always been deemed a popular writer. In this Edition some gross errors have been corrected. and the style a little amended.*

AMARA DULCIS

CONSIDERING different shires in this nation give divers names to the same herb, and that the name which it bears in one country is not known in another, I shall set down all the names that I know of each herb. Pardon me for setting that name first which is most common to myself. Besides Amara Dulcis, some call it Mortal, others Bitter-sweet; some Woody Night-shade, and others Felon-wort.

Description.—It grows up with woody stalks, even to a man's height, and sometimes higher. The leaves fall off at the approach of winter, and spring out of the same stalks in spring. The branch is compassed about with a whitish bark, and hath a pith in the middle of it : the main branch brancheth itself into many small ones with claspers, laying hold on what is next to them, as vines do. It bears many leaves : they grow in no regular order. The leaves are longish, though somewhat broad, and pointed at the ends : many of them have two little leaves growing at the end of their foot-stalks ; some have but one, and some none. The leaves are of a pale green colour; the flowers are of a purple colour, or dark blue, like to violets, and they stand many of them together in knots : the berries are green at first, but when they are ripe they are very red ; they taste like the crabs which we in Sussex call Bitter-sweets, viz. sweet at first, and bitter afterwards.

Place. — They grow commonly almost throughout England, in moist and shady places.

Time.—The leaves shoot out about the latter end of March, if the temperature of the air be ordinary ; it flowereth in July, and the seeds are ripe soon after, usually in the next month.

Government and Virtues.—It is under the planet Mercury, and a notable herb, if it be rightly gathered under his influence. It is effectual in preventing witchcraft both in men and beast, as also all sudden diseases. Being tied around about the neck, it is one of the remedies for the vertigo or dizziness in the head ; and that is the reason (as Tragus saith) the people in Germany commonly hang it about their cattle's neck, when they fear any such evil hath betided them : country people commonly use to take the berries of it, and having bruised them, they applied them to felons, and thereby soon rid their fingers of such troublesome guests.

Take notice, it is a Mercurial herb, and therefore of very subtle parts, as indeed all Mercurial plants are ; take a pound of the wood and leaves together, bruise the wood, then put into a pot, and put to it three pints of white wine, put on the pot-lid and shut it close ; let it infuse hot over a gentle fire twelve hours, then strain it, this makes a most excellent drink to open obstructions of the liver and spleen, to help difficulty of breath, bruises and falls, and congealed blood in any part of the body ; it relieves the yellow-jaundice, the dropsy and the black jaundice, and cleanses woman newly brought to bed. You may drink a quarter of a pint of the infusion every morning. It purgeth the body very gently.

ALL-HEAL.

IT is called All-heal, Hercules' all-heal, and Hercules' wound wort, because it is supposed that Hercules learned the herb and its virtues from Chiron, when he learned physic of him. Some call it panay ; others opphane-wort.

Description.—Its root is long, thick, and very full of juice, of a hot biting taste : the leaves are great and large, and winged almost like ash-tree leaves, but are something hairy, each leaf consisting of five or six pairs of such wings set one against the other upon foot-stalks, broad below but narrow towards the end ; one of the leaves is a little deeper at the bottom than the other, of a fair, yellowish, fresh green colour; they are of a bitterish taste being chewed in the mouth. From among these ariseth up a stalk, green in colour, round in form, great and strong in magnitude, five or six feet high, with many joints and some leaves thereat ; towards the top come forth umbles of small yellow flowers, and after these are passed away, you may find whitish, yellow, short flat seeds, bitter also in taste.

Place.—Having given you the description of the herb from the bottom to the top, there are other herbs called by this name ; but because they are strangers in England, I give only the description of this, which is easily to be had in many gardens.

Time.—Although Gerard saith, That they flower from the beginning of May to the end of December, experience teacheth those who keep it in their gardens, that it flowers not till the latter end of the summer, and sheds its seed soon after.

Government and Virtues.—It is under the dominion of Mars, hot, biting, and cholerick ; and remedies what evils Mars afflicts the body of a man with, by sympathy, as vipers' flesh attracts poison, and the loadstone iron. It kills worms, helps the gout, cramps, and convulsions ; provokes urine, and helps all joint aches. It helps all cold griefs of the head, the vertigo, falling sickness, lethargy, winds, colick, obstructions of the liver and spleen, stone in the kidneys and bladder. It provokes the terms, expels the dead birth : it is excellent for the griefs of the sinews, itch, stone, and tooth-ache, the bite of mad dogs and venomous beasts, and purgeth choler very gently.

ALKANET.

BESIDES the common name, is called Orchanet, and Spanish Bugloss, and by apothecaries, Enchusa.

Description.—Of the many sorts of this herb, there is but one known to grow commonly in this nation ; of which one takes this description :—It hath a great and thick root, of a reddish colour ; long, narrow, hairy leaves, green like the leaves of Bugloss, which lie very thick upon the ground ; the stalks rise up compassed round about, thick with leaves, which are less and narrower than the former ; they are tender, and slender, the flowers are hollow, small, and of a reddish colour.

Place.—It grows in Kent, near Rochester, and in many places in the west country, both in Devonshire and Cornwall.

Time.—They flower in July and beginning of August, and the seed is ripe soon after, but the root is in its prime, as carrots and parsnips are, before the herb runs up to stalk.

Government and Virtues.—It is under the dominion of Venus, and one of her darlings, though hard to come by. It heals old ulcers, hot inflammations, burnings by fire and St. Anthony's fire; for these uses make it into an ointment; or make a vinegar of it, as you make vinegar of roses, it helps the morphy and leprosy ; It helps the yellow jaundice, spleen, and gravel in the kindneys. Dioscorides saith, it helps such as are bitten by venomous beasts, whether it be taken inwardly or applied to the wound ; nay, he saith further, if any that hath newly eaten it do but spit into the mouth of a serpent, the serpent instantly dies. Its stays the flux of the belly, kills worms, helps the fits of the mother. Its decoction made in wine, and drank, strengtheus the back, and easeth the pains thereof. It heals bruises and falls, and is a gallant remedy to drive out the small pox and measles, an ointment made of it is excellent for green wounds, pricks, or thrusts.

ADDER'S TONGUE, OR SERPENT'S TONGUE.

Description.—This herb hath but one leaf, which grows with the stalk a finger's length above the ground, being flat and of a fresh green colour ; broad like Water Plantane, but less, without any rib in it ; from the bottom of which leaf on the inside riseth up, ordinarily, one, sometimes two or three slender stalks, the upper part whereof is somewhat bigger, and dented with small dents of a yellowish green colour, like the tongue of an adder serpent, (only this is as useful as they are formidable). The roots continue all the year.

Place.—It grows in moist meadows, and in such like places.

Time.—It is to be found in May or April, for it quickly perisheth with a little heat.

Government and Virtues.—It is under the dominion of the Moon and Cancer, and therefore, if the weakness of the retentive faculty be caused by an evil influence of Saturn in any part of the body governed by the Moon, or under the dominion of Cancer, this herb cures it by sympathy. It cures these diseases after specified, in any part of the body under the influence of Saturn, by antipathy.

It is temperate in respect of heat, but dry in the second degree. The juice of the leaves drank with the distilled water of Horse-tail, is a singular remedy of all manner of wounds in the breast, bowels, or other parts of the body, and is given with good success unto those that are troubled with casting, vomiting, or bleeding at the mouth and nose, or otherwise downwards. The said juice given in the distilled water of oaken buds, is very good for women who have their usual courses, or the whites flowing down too abundantly. It helps sore eyes. Of the leaves infused or boiled in oil, omphacine, or unripe olives, set in the sun for certain days, or the green leaves sufficiently boiled in the said oil, is made an excellent green balsam, not only for green and fresh wounds, but also for old and inveterate ulcers, especially if a little fine clear turpentine be dissolved therein. It also stayeth and refresheth all inflammations that arise upon pains by hurts and wounds.

What parts of the body are under each planet and sign, and also what disease may be found in my astroligical judgment of diseases ; and for the internal work of nature in the body of man, as vital, animal, natural and procreative spirits of man ; the apprehension, judgment, memory ; the external senses,—seeing, hearing, smelling, tasting, and feeling ; the virtues attractive, retentive, digestive, &c.—such parts are benefited by such Herbs.

Lastly. To avoid wetting paper with one thing many times, and also to ease your purses in the price of the book, and withal to make you studious in physic, you have at the latter end of the book, the way of preserving all herbs either in juice, conserve, oil, ointment or plaster, electuary, pills or troches.

AGRIMONY.

Description.—This hath divers long leaves, some greater, some smaller, set upon a stalk, all of them dented about the edges, green above and greyish underneath, and a little hairy withal ; among which riseth up usually but one strong, round, hairy, brown stalk, two or three feet high, with smaller leaves set here and there upon it. At the top hereof grow many small yellow flowers, one above another, in long spikes, after which come round heads of seed, hanging downwards, which will cleave to and stick upon garments, or any thing that shall rub against them. The knot is black, long, and somewhat woody, abiding many years, and shooting afresh every spring; which root, though small, hath a reasonable scent.

Place.—It groweth upon banks, near the sides of hedges.

Time.—It flowereth in July and August, the seed being ripe shortly after.

Government and Virtues.—It is an herb under Jupiter and the sign Cancer ; and strengthens those parts under the planet and sign, and removes diseases in them by sympathy ; and those under Saturn, Mars, and Mercury, by antipathy, if they happen in any part of the body governed by Jupiter, or under the signs Cancer, Sagittary, or Pisces, and therefore must needs be good for the gout, either used outwardly in oil or ointment, or inwardly in an electuary, or syrnp, or concerted juice; for which see the latter end of the work.

It is of a cleansing and cutting faculty, without any manifest heat, moderately drying and binding. It openeth and cleanseth the liver, helpeth the jaundice, and is very beneficial to the bowels, healing all inward wounds, bruises, hurts, and other distempers. The decoction of the herb made with wine, and drank, is good against the biting and stinging of serpents, and helps them that makes foul, troubled, or bloody water, and makes them urinate clear speedily; it also helpeth the colick, cleanseth the breast, and rids away the cough. A draught of the decoction taken warm before the fit, first removes, and in time rids away the tertian, or quartan agues. The leaves and seeds taken in wine stays the bloody flux; outwardly applied, being stamped with old swine's grease, it helpeth old sores, cancers, and inveterate ulcers, and draweth forth thorns and splinters of wood, nails, or any other such thing gotten into the flesh : it helpeth to strengthen the members that be out of joint; and being bruised and applied, or the juice dropped in, it helpeth foul and imposthumed ears.

The distilled water of the herb is good to all the said purposes, either inward or outward, but a great deal weaker.

It is a most admirable remedy for such whose lives are annoyed either by heat or cold. The liver is the former of blood, and blood the nourisher of the body, and Agrimony a strengthener of the liver.

WATER AGRIMONY.

IT is called in some countries water hemp, bastard hemp, and bastard agrimony; eupatorium and hepatorium, because it strengthens the liver.

Description.—The root continues a long time, having many long slender strings : the stalk grows up about two feet high, sometimes higher; they are of a dark purple colour : the branches are many, growing at distances the one from the other, the one from the one side of the stalk, the other from the opposite point : the leaves are winged, and much indented at the edges : the flowers grow at the

top of the branches, of a brown yellow colour, spotted
with black spots, having a substance within the midst of
them like that of a daisy ; if you rub them between your
fingers they smell like rosin or cedar when it is burnt : the
seeds are long, and easily stick to any woollen thing they
touch.

Place.—They delight not in heat, and therefore they are
not so frequently found in the southern parts of England as
in the northern, where they grow frequently. You may
look for them in cold grounds by the sides of ponds and
ditches, as also by running waters ; sometimes you may
find them grow in the midst of the waters.

Time.—They all flower in July or August, and the seed
is ripe presently after.

Government and Virtues.—It is a plant of Jupiter, as well
as the other Agrimony, only this belongs to the celestial sign Cancer. It healeth and drieth, cutteth and
cleanseth thick and tough humours of the breast, and for
this I hold it inferior to few herbs that grow ; it helps the
cachexia or evil disposition of the body, the dropsy, and
yellow jaundice ; it opens the obstructions of the liver,
mollifies the hardness of the spleen, being applied outwardly : it breaks imposthumes, taken inwardly : it is an
excellent remedy for the third day ague : it provokes urine
and the terms : it kills worms, and cleanseth the body of
sharp humours, which are the cause of itch and scabs ; the
herb being burnt, the smoke thereof drives away flies,
wasps, &c. : It strengthens the lungs exceedingly. Country
people give it to their cattle when they are troubled with
cough, or are broken winded.

ALEHOOF, OR GROUND-IVY.

SEVERAL counties give it different names, so that there is
scarcely an herb growing of that size, that has got so
many. It is called cat's-foot, ground-ivy, gill-go-by-ground,
and gill-creep-by-ground, turn-hoof, hay-maids, and ale-
hoof.

Description.—This well known herb lieth, spreadeth, and
creepeth upon the ground, shooteth forth roots at the corners of tender jointed stalks, set with two round leaves at

every joint, somewhat hairy, crumbled, and unevenly dented about the edges with round dents ; at the joints, likewise, with the leaves towards the end of the branches, come forth hollow long flowers, of a blueish purple colour, with small white spots upon the lips that hang down. The root is small, with strings.

Place.—It is commonly found under edges and on the sides of ditches, under houses, or in shadowed lanes and other waste lands in almost every part of the land.

Time.—They flower somewhat early, and abide a great while ; the leaves continue green until winter, and sometimes abide, except the winter be very sharp and cold.

Government and Virtues.—It is under Venus, and therefore cures the diseases she causes by sympathy, and those of Mars by antipathy ; you may easily find it all the year, except the year be extremely frosty ; it is quick, sharp, and bitter in taste, and is thereby found to be hot and dry ; a singular herb for all inward wounds, ulcerated lungs, or other parts, either by itself, or boiled with other like herbs ; and being drank, in a short time it easeth all griping pains, windy and choleric humours in the stomach, spleen or belly ; helps the yellow jaundice by opening the stoppings of the gall and liver, and melancholy, by opening the stoppings of the spleen ; expelleth venom or poison, and also the plague : it provokes urine and women's courses. The decoction of it in wine drank for some time together, procureth ease in sciatica, or hip gout ; as also the gout in the hands, knees or feet ; if you put to the decoction some honey and a little burnt alum, it is excellent to gargle any sore mouth or throat, and to wash the sores and ulcers in man or woman ; it speedily heals green wounds, being bruised and bound thereto. The juice of it boiled with a little honey and verdigrease, wonderfully cleanses fistulas, ulcers, and stayeth the spreading or eating of cancers and ulcers ; it helpeth the itch, scabs, weals, and other breakings out in any part of the body. The juice of Celandine, field Daises, and Ground-Ivy clarified and a little fine sugar dissolved therein, and dropped into the eyes, is a sovereign remedy for all pains, redness and watering of them ; as also for the pin and web, skins and films growing over the sight. The juice dropped into the ear cures the noise and singing of them, and restores the hearing which is decayed. It is good to tun up with new drink, for it will clarify it in a night, that it will be the fitter to be drank the next morning; or if any drink be thick with removing or any other accident, it will do the like in a few hours.

ALEXANDER.

IT is also called alisander, horse parsley, and wild parsley, and the black pot-herb; the seed of it is that which is usually sold in apothecaries' shops for Macedonian parsley-seed.

Description.—It is usually sown in all the gardens in Europe, and so well known, that it needs no further description.

Time.—It flowereth in June and July: the seed is ripe in August.

Government and Virtues.—It is under Jupiter, and therefore friendly to nature, for it warmeth a cold stomach, and openeth a stoppage to the liver and spleen; it is good to move women's courses, to expel the after-birth, to break wind, to provoke urine, and helpeth the strangury; and these things the seeds will do likewise. If either of them be boiled in wine, or bruised and taken in wine, is also effectual in the biting of serpents. And you know what Alexander pottage is good for, that you may no longer eat it out of ignorance, but out of knowledge.

THE BLACK ALDER TREE.

Description.—This tree seldom groweth to any great size, but for the most part abideth like a hedge-bush, or a tree spreading its branches, the woods of the body being white, and a dark red cole or heart; the outward bark is of a blackish colour, with many whitish spots therein; but the inner bark next the wood is yellow, which being chewed, will turn the spittle near into a saffron colour. The leaves are somewhat like those of an ordinary alder-tree, or the female cornet, or Dog-berry tree, called in Sussex dog-wood, but blacker, and not so long: the flowers are white, coming forth with the leaves at the joints, which turn into small round berries first green, afterwards red, but blackish when they are thoroughly ripe, divided as it were into two parts, wherein is contained two small round and flat seeds. The root runneth not deep into the ground, but spreads rather under the upper crust of the earth.

Place.—This tree or shrub may be found plentifully in St. John's wood, by Hornsey, and the woods on Hampstead-heath; as also in a wood called Old Park, in Barcomb, Essex, near the brook's side.

Time.—It flowereth in May, and the berries are ripe in September.

Government and Virtues.—It is a tree of Venus, and under the celestial sign Cancer. The inner yellow bark hereof purgeth downwards both choler and phlegm, and the watery humours of such that have the dropsy, and strengthens the inward parts again by binding. If the bark hereof be boiled with agrimony, wormwood, dodder, hops, and some fennel with smallage, endive, and succory roots, and a reasonable draught taken every morning for some time, it is very effectual against the jaundice, dropsy, and the evil disposition of the body, especially if some suitable purging medicines have been taken before, to void the grosser excrements; it purgeth and strengtheneth the liver and spleen, cleansing them from such evil humours and hardness as they are afflicted with. It is to be understood that these things are performed by the dry bark; for the fresh green bark taken inwardly provokes strong vomitings, pains in the stomach, and gripings in the belly; yet if the decoction may stand and settle two or three days, until the yellow colour be changed black, it will not work so strongly as before, but will strengthen the stomach, and procure an appetite for meat. The outward bark contrariwise doth bind the body, and is helpful for all lasks and fluxes thereof, but this also must be dried first, whereby it will work the better. The inner bark thereof boiled in vinegar is an approved remedy to kill lice, to cure the itch, and take away scabs, by drying them up in a short time. It is singularly good to wash the teeth, and to take away the pains, to fasten those that are loose, to cleanse them,

B

and keep them sound. The leaves are good fodder for kine, to make them give more milk.

In spring-time use the herbs before-mentioned, and take a handful of each of them, adding a handful of elder buds, and having bruised them all, boil them in a gallon of ordinary beer when it is new; and having boiled them half an hour, add to this three gallons more, and let them work together, and drink every morning half a pint, or thereabouts ; it is an excellent purge for the spring, to consume the phlegmatic quality the winter has left behind it, and withal to keep your body in health, and consume those evil humours which the heat of summer will readily stir up. Esteem it as a jewel.

THE COMMON ALDER TREE.

Description.—Groweth to a reasonable height, and spreads much if it like the place. It is so generally well known by country people, that I conceive it needless to tell that which is no news.

Place and Time.—It delighteth to grow in moist woods and watery places ; flowereth in April and May, and yielding ripe seed in September.

Government and Use.—It is a tree under the dominions of Venus, and of some watery sign or other, I suppose Pisces, and therefore the decoction, or distilled water of the leaves, is excellent against burnings and inflammations, either with wounds or without, to bathe the place grieved with, and especially for inflammation of the breast.

If you cannot get the leaves, which in winter is impossible, make use of the bark in the same manner.

The leaves and bark of the Alder tree are cooling, drying, and binding. The fresh leaves laid upon swellings dissolve them, and stay the inflammations. The leaves put under the bare feet galled with travelling, are a great refreshing to them. The said leaves gathered while the morning dew is on them, and brought into a chamber troubled with fleas, will gather them thereunto, which being suddenly cast out, will rid the chamber of these troublesome bedfellows.

ANGELICA.

To write a description of that which is so well known to be growing almost in every garden, I suppose is altogether needless; yet for its virtues it is of admirable use.

In time of heathenism, when men had found out any excellent herb, they dedicated it to their god, as the bay-tree to Apollo, the oak to Jupiter, the vine to Bacchus, the poplar to Hercules. These the papist following as the patriarchs, they dedicate to their saints; as our lady's Thistle to the Blessed Virgin, St. John's Wort to St. John, and another Wort to St. Peter, &c. Our physicians must imitate like apes, though they cannot come off so cleverly, for they blasphemously call Pansies, or Heart's Ease, *an herb for the Trinity*, because it is of three colours; and a certain ointment *an ointment of the Apostles*, because it consists of twelve ingredients. The papists called this an herb of the Holy Ghost; others more moderate called it Angelca, because of its angelical virtues, and that name it retains still, and all nations follow it so near as their dialect will permit.

Government and Virtues.—It is an herb of the Sun in Leo; let it be gathered when he is there, the Moon applying to his good aspect; let it be gathered either in his hour, or in the hour of Jupiter; let Sol be angular: observe the like in gathering the herbs of other planets, and you may happen to do wonders. In all epidemical diseases caused by Saturn, that is as good a preservative as grows. It resists poison by defending and comforting the heart, blood, and spirits; it doth the like against the plague and all spirits; it doth the like against the plague and all epidemical diseases, if the root be taken in powder to the weight of half a drachm at a time, with some treacle in Carduus water, and the party thereupon laid to sweat in his bed: if treacle be not to be had, take it alone in Carduus water or Angelica water. The stalks or roots candied and eaten fasting, are good preservatives in time of infection; and at other times to warm and comfort a cold stomach: the root also steeped in vinegar, and a little of that vinegar taken sometimes fasting, and the root

smelled unto is good for the same purpose : a water distilled from the root simply, as steeped in wine and distilled in a glass, is much more effectual than the water of
the leaves ; and this water, drank two or three spoonsful
at a time, easeth all pains and torments coming of cold
and wind, so that the body be not bound ; and taken with
some of the root in powder at the beginning, helpeth the
pleurisy, as also all other diseases of the lungs and breast,
as coughs, phthisic, and shortness of breath ; and a syrup
of the stalks doth the like. It relieves the pains of the
colic, the strangury and stoppage of the urine, procureth
women's courses, and expelleth the after birth ; openeth
the stoppage of the liver and the spleen, and briefly easeth
and discusseth all windiness and inward swellings. The
decoction drank before the fit of an ague, that they may
sweat, if possible, before the fit comes, will, in two or three
times taking, drive it away ; it helps digestion, and is a
remedy for a surfeit. The juice, or the water being dropped into the eyes or ears helps dimness of sight and deafness : the juice put into the hollow of the teeth easeth
their pain. The root in powder, made up into plaster
with a little pitch, and laid on the biting of mad dogs or
any other venomous creature, doth wonderfully help.
The juice or the water dropped, or tents wet therein, and
applied to old filthy ulcers, or the powder of the root, in
want of either, doth cleanse and cause them to heal quickly, by covering the naked bones with flesh ; the distilled
water applied to places pained with the gout, or sciatica,
doth give a great deal of ease.

The wild angelica is not so effectual as the garden ; although it may be safely used to all the purposes aforesaid.

AMARANTHUS.

BESIDES its common name, by which it is best known
by the florists of our days, it is called flower gentle, flower
velure, floramor, and velvet flower.

Description.—It being a garden flower, and well known
to every one that keeps it, I might forbear the description ; yet, notwithstanding, because some desire it, I shall
give it. It runneth up with a stalk a cubit high, streaked,

and somewhat reddish towards the root, but very smooth, divided towards the top with small branches, among which stand long broad leaves of a reddish green colour, slippery ; the flowers are not properly flowers, but tuffs, very beautiful to behold, but of no smell, of reddish colour ; if you bruise them, they yield juice of the same colour ; being gathered, they keep their beauty a long time : the seed is of a shining black colour.

Time.—They continue in flower from August till the time the frost nips them.

Government and Virtues.—It is under the dominion of Saturn, and is an excellent qualifier of the unruly actions and passions of Venus, though Mars should also join with her. The flowers dried and beaten into powder, stop the terms in women, and so do almost all other red things. And by the icon or image of every herb, the ancients at first found out their virtues. Modern writers laugh at them for it ; but I wonder how the virtues of herbs came at first to be known, if not by their signatures ; the moderns have them from the writings of the ancients ; the ancients had no writings to have them from. — The flowers stop all fluxes of blood, whether in man or woman, bleeding either at the nose or wound. There is also a sort of amaranthus that bears a white flower, which restrains the whites, and the running of the reins in men, and is a most gallant anti-venereal, and a singular remedy for the French pox.

ANEMONE.

CALLED also wind flower, because they say the flowers never open but when the wind bloweth. Pliny is my author ; if it be not so blame him. The seed is downy, and flies away with the wind.

Place and Time. —They are sown usually in the gardens of the curious, and flower in the spring-time. As for description, I shall pass it, being well known to all those that sow them.

Government and Virtues.—It is under the dominion of Mars, being supposed to be a kind of crow-foot. The leaves provoke the terms mightily, being boiled and the decoction drank. The body being bathed with the decoction of them, cures the leprosy : the leaves being stamped, and the juice snuffed up the nose, purgeth the head mightily ; so doth the root being chewed in the mouth, for it procureth much spitting, and bringeth away many watery and phlegmatic humours, and is therefore good for lethargy. And when all is done, let physicians prate what they please, all the pills in the dispensary purge not the head like to hot things held in the mouth. Being made into an ointment, and the eye-lids anointed with it, it helps inflammations of the eyes ; whereby it is palpable, that every stronger draweth its weaker like. The same ointment is excellent good to cleanse malignant and corroding ulcers.

GARDEN ARRACH.

CALLED also orach, and arage.

Description.—It is so commonly known to every housewife, it were labour lost to describe it.

Time.—It flowereth and seedeth from June to the end of August.

Government and Virtues.—It is under the government of the Moon : in quality cold and moist like unto her. It softeneth and looseneth the body of man, being eaten, and fortifieth the expulsive faculty in him. The herb, whether it be bruised and applied to the throat, or boiled, and in like manner applied, it matters not much, it is good for swellings in the throat ; the best way is to boil it, having drunk the decoction inwardly, and apply the herb outwardly. The decoction of it besides is an excellent remedy for the yellow jaundice.

ARRACH, WILD AND STINKING.

CALLED also vulvaria, from that part of the body upon which the operation is most ; also dog's arrach, goat's arrach, and stinking mother wort.

Description.—This hath small and almost round leaves, yet a little pointed, and almost without dent or cut, of a dusky mealy colour, growing on the slender stalks and branches that spread on the ground, with small flowers in clusters set with the leaves, and small seeds succeeding like the rest, perishing yearly, and rising again with its own sowing. It smells like rotten fish, or something worse.

Place.—It grows usually upon dunghills.

Time.— They flower in June and July, and their seed is ripe quickly after.

Government and Virtues.—Stinking Arrach is used as a remedy to help women pained, and almost strangled with the mother, by smelling it ; but inwardly taken there is no better remedy for that disease. It is an herb under the dominion of Venus, and under the sign Scorpio ; it is common almost upon every dunghill. The works of God are given freely to man, his medicines are common and cheap, and easy to be found. I commend it for a universal medicine of the womb, and such a medicine as will easily, safely, and speedily cure any diseases thereof, as fits of the mother, dislocation or falling out thereof : it cools the womb when overheated. And let me tell you that heat of the womb is one of the greatest causes of hard labour in child-birth. It makes barren women fruitful : it cleanseth the womb if it be foul, and strengthens it exceedingly : it provokes the terms if they be stopped, and stops them if they flow immoderately ; you can desire no good to your womb but this herb will effect it ; therefore if you love children, if you love health, if you love ease, keep a syrup always by you made of the juice of this herb, and sugar, or honey, if it be to cleanse the womb ; and let such as be rich keep it for their poor neighbours.

ARCHANGEL.

To put a gloss upon their practice, the physicians call an herb (which country people vulgarly know by the name of the dead nettle) archangel : whether they favour more of supersition or folly, I leave to the judicious reader. There is more curiosity than courtesy to my countrymen used by others in the explanation as well of the names, as description of this so well known herb ; which, that I may not also be guilty of, take this short description, first of the red archangel.

Description.—This hath divers square stalks, somewhat hairy, at the joints whereöf grow two sad green leaves dented about the edges, opposite to one another to the lowermost, upon long foot stalks, but without any toward the tops, which are somewhat round yet pointed, and a little crumpled and hairy; round about the upper joints, where the leaves grow thick, are sundry gaping flowers of a pale reddish colour; after which come the seeds three or four in a husk; the root is smaller and thready, perishing every year; the whole plant hath a strong scent, but not stinking.

White archangel hath divers square stalks, none standing straight upward, but bending downward, wherein stand two leaves at a joint, larger and more pointed than the other, dented about the edges, and greener also, more like unto nettle leaves, but not stinking, yet hairy. At the joints with the leaves stand larger and more open gaping white flowers, husks round about the stalks, but not with such a bush of leaves as flowers set in the top, as is on the other, wherein stand small roundish black seed: the root is white, with many strings at it, not growing downward, but lying under the upper crust of the earth, and abideth many years increasing: this has not so strong a scent as the former.

Yellow Archangel is like the white in the stalks and leaves; but that the stalks are more straight and upright, and the joints with leaves are farther asunder, having larger leaves than the former, and the flowers a little longer and more gaping, of a fair yellow colour in most, in some paler: the roots are like white, only they creep not so much under the ground.

Place.—They grow almost everywhere; the yellow most usually in the wet grounds of woods, and sometimes in the drier, in divers counties of this nation.

Time.—They flower from the beginning of spring all the summer long.

Virtues and Use.—The Archangels are somewhat hot and drier than the stinging nettles, and used with better success for the stopping and hardness of the spleen, than by using the decoction of the herb in wine, and afterwards applying the herb hot into the region of the spleen as plaster, or the decoction with sponges. Flowers of the white Archangel are preserved or conserved to be used to stay the whites, and the flowers of the red to stay the reds in women. It makes the heart merry, drives away melancholy, quickens the spirits, is good against the quartan agues, stauncheth bleeding at the mouth and nose if it be stamped and applied to the nape of the neck ; the herb also bruised, and with some salt and vinegar and hog's grease laid upon an hard tumour or swelling, or that vulgarily called the king's evil, do help to dissolve or discuss them : and being in like manner applied, doth much allay the pains, and give ease to the gout, sciatica, and other pains of the joints and sinews. It is also very effectual to heal green wounds and old ulcers ; also to stay their fretting, gnawing, and spreading ; it draweth forth splinters, and such like things gotten into the flesh, and is very good against bruises and burnings. But the yellow Archangel is most commended for old, filthy, corrupt sores and ulcers, yea, although they be hollow ; and to dissolve tumours. The chief use of them is for women, it being an herb of Venus, and may be found in my Guide for Women.

ARSSMART.

THE hot Arssmart is called also Water-pepper, or Culrage. The mild Arssmart is called dead Arssmart Percicaria, or Peachwort, because the leaves are so like the leaves of a peach-tree : it is also called Plumbago.

Description of the Mild.—This hath broad leaves at the great red joints of the stalks, with semi-circular blackish marks on them usually either bluish or whitish, with such like seed following. The root is long, with many strings thereat, perishing yearly ; this hath no sharp taste (as another sort hath, which is quick and biting) but rather sour like Sorrel, or else a little drying, or without taste.

Place.—It groweth in watery places, ditches, and the like, which for the most part are dry in summer.

Time.—It flowereth in June, and the seed is ripe in August.

Government and Virtues.—As the virtue of both these is

various, so is also their government ; for that which is hot and biting is under the dominion of Mars, but Saturn challengeth the other, as appears by that leaden coloured spot he hath placed upon the leaf.

It is of a cooling and drying quality, and very effectual for putrid ulcers in man or beast, to kill worms and cleanse putrified places. The juice thereof dropped in, or otherwise applied, consumeth all cold swellings, and dissolveth the congealed blood of bruises by strokes, falls, &c. A piece of the root, or some of the seeds bruised and held to an aching tooth, taketh away the pain : the leaves bruised and laid to the joint that hath a felon thereon, taketh it away ; the juice destroyeth worms in the ears, being dropped into them : if the hot Arssmart be strewed in a chamber, it will soon kill all the fleas ; and the herb or juice of the cold Arssmart put to a horse or other cattle's fores, will drive away the fly in the hottest day of summer : a good handful of the hot biting Arssmart put under a horse's saddle, will make him travel the better, although he were half tired before. The mild Arssmart is good against all imposthumes and inflammations at the beginning, and to heal all green wounds.

All authors chop the virtues of both sorts of Arssmart together, as men chop herbs to the pot, when both of them are of clean contrary qualities. The hot Arssmart groweth not so high nor so tall as the mild doth, but hath many leaves of the colour of peach leaves, very seldom or never spotted ; in other particulars it is like the former, but may easily be known from it if you will be pleased to break a leaf of it across your tongue for the hot will make your tongue to smart, so will not the cold. If you see them together you may easily distinguish them, because the mild hath far broader leaves : and our College Physicians, out of their learned care of the public good, *anglice*, their own gain, mistake the one for the other in their *New Masterpiece*, whereby they discover,—1. Their ignorance ; 2. Their carelessness ; and he that hath but half an eye may see their pride without a pair of spectacles. I have done what I could to distinguish them in the virtues, and when you find not the contrary named, use the cold.

ASARABACCA.

Description.—Asarabacca hath many heads rising from the roots, from whence come many smooth leaves, every one upon his own foot stalks which are rounder and bigger than violet leaves, thicker also, and of a dark green shining colour on the upper side, and of a pale yellow green underneath, little or nothing dented about the edges, from among which rise small, round, hollow, brown green husks, upon short stalks, about an inch long, divided at the brims into five divisions, very like the cups or heads of the Henbane seed, but that they are smaller ; and these be all the flowers it carrieth, which are somewhat sweet being smelled unto, and wherein, when they are ripe, are contained small corned rough seeds, very like the kernel or stones of grapes or raisins. The roots are small and whitish, spreading divers ways in the ground, increasing into divers heads : but not running or creeping under the ground as some other creeping herbs do. They are somewhat sweet in smell, resembling nardus, but more when they are dry than green ; and of a sharp but not unpleasant taste.

Place.—It groweth frequently in gardens.

Time.—They keep their leaves green all winter ; but shoot forth new in the spring, and with them come forth those heads or flowers which give ripe seed about Midsummer, or somewhat after.

Government and Virtues.—'Tis a plant under the dominion of Mars, and therefore inimical to nature. This herb being drank, not only provoketh vomiting, but purgeth downward, and by urine also, purgeth both choler and phlegm. If you add some spikenard, with the whey of goat's milk, or honeyed water, it is made more strong ; but it purgeth phlegm more manifestly than choler, and therefore doth much help pains in the hips and other parts : being boiled in whey they wonderfully help the obstructions of the liver and spleen, and therefore profitable for the dropsy and jaundice : being steeped in wine and drank, it helps those continual agues that come by the plenty of stubborn humours : an oil made thereof by setting in the sun, with some laudanum added to it, provoketh sweating, (the ridge of the back anointed therewith) and thereby driveth away the shaking fits of the ague. It will not abide any long boiling, for it loseth its chief strength thereby : nor much beating, for the finer powder doth provoke vomits and urine, and the coarser purgeth downwards.

The common use hereof is to take the juice of five or seven leaves in a little drink to cause vomiting ; the roots have also the same virtue, though they do not operate so forcibly ; they are very effectual against the biting of serpents, and therefore are put in as an ingredient both into Mithridate and Venice treacle. The leaves and roots being boiled in lye, and the head often washed therewith while it was warm, comforteth the head and brain that is ill affected by taking cold, and helpeth the memory.

The roots purge more gently, and may prove beneficial to such as have cancers, or old putrifying ulcers, or fistulas upon their bodies, to take a drachm of them in powder in a quarter of a pint of white wine in the morning. The truth is, I fancy purging and vomiting medicines as little as any man breathing doth, for they weaken nature, nor shall ever advise them to be used unless upon urgent necessity. If a physician be nature's servant, it is his duty to strengthen his mistress as much as he can, and weaken her as little as may be.

ASPARAGUS, SPARAGUS or SPERAGE.

Description.—It riseth up at first with divers white and green scaly heads, very brittle or easy to break while they are young, which afterwards rise up in very long and slender green stalks, of the size of an ordinary riding wand, at the bottom of most, or bigger or lesser, as the roots are of growth ; on which are set divers branches of green leaves, shorter and smaller than fennel, to the top ; at the joints whereof come forth small yellowish flowers, which run into round berries, green at first, and of an excellent red colour when they are ripe, showing like bead or coral, wherein are contained exceeding hard black seeds : the roots are dispersed from a spongeous head into many long, thick, and round strings, wherein is sucked much nourishment out of the ground, and increaseth plentifully thereby.

PRICKLY ASPARAGUS or SPERAGE.

Description.— It groweth usually in gardens, and some of it grows wild in Appleton meadows, in Gloucestershire, where the poor people do gather the buds of young shoots, and sell them cheaper than our garden asparagus is sold in London.

Time.—They do for the most part flower and bear their berries late in the year, or not at all, although they are housed in winter.

Government and Virtues.—They are both under the dominion of Jupiter. The young buds or branches boiled in ordinary broth, make the belly soluble and open ; and boiled in white wine, provoke urine being stopped, and is good against the stranguary, or difficulty in making water ; it expelleth the gravel and stone out of the kidneys, and helpeth pains in the reins : and boiled in white wine or vinegar, it is prevalent for them that have their arteries loosened, or are troubled with hip-gout or sciatica. The decoction of the roots boiled in wine, and taken, is good to clear the sight, and being held in the mouth easeth the tooth-ache ; and being taken fasting several mornings together, stirreth up bodily lust in man or woman, whatever some have written to the contrary. The garden asparagus nourisheth more than the wild, yet hath it the same effects in all the afore-mentioned diseases. The decoction of the roots in white wine, and the back and belly bathed therewith, or kneeling or lying down in the same, or sitting therein as a bath, hath been found effectual against pains of the reins and bladder, pains of the mother and colic, and generally against all pains that happen to the lower parts of the body, and no less effectual against stiff and benumbed sinews, or those that are shrunk by cramps and convulsions, and helpeth the sciatica.

ASH TREE.

This is so well known, that time will be misspent in writing a description of it : and therefore I shall only insist upon the virtues of it.

Government and Virtues.— It is governed by the Sun ; and

the young tender tops, with the leaves taken inwardly, and some of them outwardly applied, are very good against the biting of an adder, viper, or any other venomous beast; and the water distilled therefrom being taken, a small quantity every morning fasting, is a singular medicine for those that are subject to the dropsy, or to abate the greatness of those that are too gross or fat. The decoction of the leaves in white wine helpeth to break the stone and expel it, and cure the jaundice. The ashes of the bark of the ash made into lye, and those heads bathed therewith which are leprous, scabby, or scald, they are thereby cured. The kernels within the husks commonly called ashen keys prevail against stitches and pains in the side, proceeding of wind and voiding away the stone, by provoking urine.

I can justly except against none of this, save only the first viz.—That ash-tree tops are good against biting of serpents and vipers. I suppose this had its rise from Gerard or Pliny, both which hold, that there is such an antipathy between an adder and ash-tree, that if an adder be encompassed round with ash tree leaves, she will sooner run through fire than through the leaves; the contrary to which is the truth, as both my eyes are witness. The rest are virtues something likely, only if it be in winter when you cannot get the leaves, you may safely use the bark instead of them. The keys you may easily keep all the year, gathering them when they are ripe.

AVENS, called also COLEWORT, and HERB BONNET.

Description.—The ordinary avens have many long, rough, dark green winged leaves rising from the root, every one made of many leaves set on each side of the middle rib, the largest three whereof grow at the end, and are snipped or dented round about the edges; the other being small pieces, sometimes two and sometime four, standing on each side of the middle rib underneath them : among which do rise up divers rough or hairy stalks, about two feet high, branching forth with leaves at every joint, not so long as those below, but almost as much cut in on the edges, some into three, some into more. On the tops of the branches stand small, pale yellow flowers, consisting of five leaves, like the flowers of cinque-foil, but large, in the middle whereof stand-eth a small green herb, which when the flower is fallen, groweth to be sound, being made of many long greenish purple seeds like grains, which will stick upon your clothes. The root consists of many brownish strings or fibres, smelling somewhat like unto cloves, especially those which grow in the higher, hotter, and drier grounds, and in clear air.

Place.—They grow wild in many places under hedges' sides, and by the path-ways in fields ; yet they rather delight to grow in shadowy than in sunny places.

Time.—They flower in May and June for the most part, and their seed is ripe in July at the farthest.

Government and Virtues.—It is governed by Jupiter. and it must be a wholesome, healthful herb. It is good for the diseases of the chest or breast, for pains and stitches in the side, and to expel crude and raw humours from the belly and stomach, by the sweet savour and warming quality. It dissolves the inward congealed blood happening by falls or bruises, and the spitting of blood, if the roots, either green or dry, be boiled in wine and drank : as also all manner of inward wounds, or outward, if washed or bathed therewith. The decoction also being drank, comforts the heart, and strengthens the stomach and a cold brain, and therefore is good in the spring-time to open obstructions of the liver, and helpeth the wind colic : it is good in fluxes, and in ruptures : it taketh away spots or marks in the face being washed therewith. The juice of the fresh root, or powder of the dried root, have the same effect as the decoction. The root in the spring-time, steeped in wine, gives it a delicate savour and taste, and being drank fasting every morning, comforteth the heart, and is a good preservative against the plague. It promoteth digestion, warmeth a cold stomach, and openeth obstructions of the liver and spleen.

It is very safe; you need have no dose prescribed ; and is very fit to be kept in every body's house.

BALM.

This herb is so well known to grow almost in every garden, that I shall not give any description of it.

Government and Virtues.—It is an herb of Jupiter; and under Cancer, and strengthens nature much. Let a syrup made with the juice of it and sugar (as directed at the end of the book) be kept in every gentlewoman's house to relieve the weak stomachs and sick bodies of their poor and sickly neighbours; as also the herb kept dry in the house, that so with other convenient simples, you may make it into an electuary with honey, according as the disease is, you shall be taught at the end of my book. The Arabian physicians have extolled the virtues thereof to the skies; although the Greeks thought it not worth mentioning. Seraphio saith, it causeth the mind and heart to become merry, and reviveth the heart in faintings and swoonings, especially of such who are overtaken in sleep, and driveth away all troublesome cares and thoughts out of the mind, arising from melancholy and black choler: which Avicen also confirmeth. It promotes digestion, and opens obstructions of the brain, and hath so much purging quality in it, (saith Avicen) as to expel those melancholy vapours from the spirits and blood which are in the heart and arteries, although it cannot do so in other parts of the body. Dioscorides saith, that the leaves steeped in wine, and the wine drank, and the leaves externally applied, is a remedy against the sting of a scorpion, and the biting of mad dogs; and commendeth the decoction for women to bathe or sit in to procure their courses; it is good to wash aching teeth therewith, and profitable to those that have the bloody-flux. The leaves also, with a little nitre taken in drink, are good against the surfeit of mushrooms, and help the griping pains of the belly; and being made into an electuary, it is good for difficult breathing: used with salt, it takes away the wens, kernels, or hard swellings in the flesh or throat: it cleanseth foul sores, and easeth pains of the gout. It is good for the liver and spleen. A tansy or caudle made with eggs, and juice thereof, while it is young, with sugar and rosewater, is good for a woman in child-bed, when the afterbirth is not thoroughly voided, and for their faintings in their travail. The herb bruised and boiled in a little white wine and oil, and laid warm on a bile, will ripen and break it.

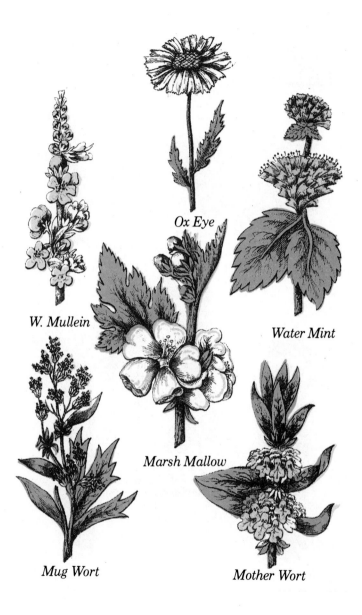

W. Mullein

Ox Eye

Water Mint

Marsh Mallow

Mug Wort

Mother Wort

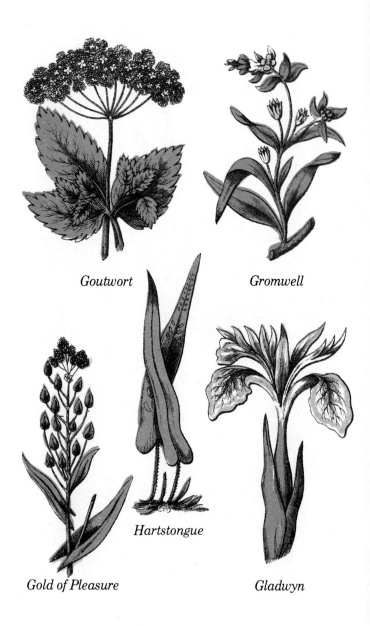

Goutwort

Gromwell

Hartstongue

Gold of Pleasure

Gladwyn

BARBERRY.

THE shrub is so well known by every boy and girl that has but attained to the age of seven years, that it needs no description.

Government and Virtues.—Mars owns the shrub, and presents it to the use of my countrymen to purge their bodies of choler. The inner rind of the Barberry tree boiled in white wine, and a quarter of a pint drank every morning, is an excellent remedy to cleanse the body of choleric humours, and free it from such diseases as choler causeth, such as scabs, itch, tetters, ringworms, yellow jaundice, biles, &c. It is excellent for hot agues, burnings, scaldings, heat of the blood, heat of the liver, bloody flux, for the berries are as good as the bark, and more pleasing; they get a man a good stomach to his victuals, by strengthening the attractive faculty which is under Mars. The hair washed with the lye made of ashes of the tree and water, will turn it yellow, viz. of Mars' own colour. The fruit and rind of the shrub, the flowers of broom and of heath, or furze, cleanse the body of choler by sympathy, as the flowers, leaves, and bark of the Peach tree do by antipathy; because these are under Mars, that under Venus.

BARLEY.

THE continual usefulness hereof hath made all in general so acquainted herewith, that it is altogether needless to describe it, several kinds hereof plentifully growing, being yearly sown in this land. The virtues thereof take as followeth.

Government and Virtues.— It is a notable plant of Saturn; if you view diligently its effects by sympathy and antipathy, you may easily perceive a reason of them; as also why barley-bread is so unwholesome for melancholy people. Barley, in all the parts and composition thereof, except malt, is more cooling than wheat, and a little cleansing; and all the preparations thereof, as barley-water and other things made thereof, give great nourishment to persons troubled with fevers, agues, and heats in the stomach. A poultice made of barley-meal or flour boiled in vinegar and

C

honey, and a few dried figs put in them, dissolveth all hard imposthumes, and assuageth inflammation, being thereto applied : and being boiled with melilot and camomile flowers, and some linseed, fenugreek and rue in powder, and applied warm, it easeth pains in the side and stomach, and windiness of the spleen. The meal of barley and fleaworts boiled in water, and made a poultice with honey and oil of lilies, and applied warm, cureth swellings under the ears, throat, neck, and such like ; and a plaster made thereof with tar, wax, and oil, helpeth the king's evil in the throat ; boiled with sharp vinegar into a poultice, and laid on hot, helpeth the leprosy ; being boiled in red wine with pomegranate rind, and Myrtles, stayeth the lask or other flux of the belly ; boiled with vinegar and quince, it easeth the pains of the gout : barley flour, white salt, honey, and vinegar mingled together, taketh away the itch speedily and certainly. The water distilled from the green barley, in the end of May, is very good for those that have defluctions of humours fallen into their eyes, and easeth the pain being dropped into them : or white bread steeped therein, and bound on the eyes, doth the same.

GARDEN BAZIL, OR SWEET BAZIL.

Description.—The greater or ordinary Bazil riseth up usually with one upright stalk diversely branching forth on all sides, with two leaves at every joint, which are somewhat broad and round, yet pointed, of a pale green colour, but fresh ; a little snipped about the edges, and of a strong healthy scent. The flowers are small and white, and standing at the tops of the branches, with two small leaves at the joints, in some places green, in others brown, after which come black seed. The root perisheth at the approach of winter and therefore must be sown every year.

Place.—It groweth in gardens.

Time.—It must be sown late, and flowers in the heart of summer, it being a very tender plant.

Government and Virtues.—This is the herb which all authors are together by the ears about, and rail at one another, like lawyers. Galen and Dioscorides hold it not fitting to be taken inwardly, and Chrysipus rails at it with downright Billinsgate rhetoric : Pliny and the Arabian physicians defend it.

For my own part, I presently found that speech true ;
Non nostrum inter nos tantas componere lites.

And away to Dr. Reason went I, who told me it was an herb of Mars, and under the Scorpion, and therefore called basilicon, and it is no marvel if it carry a kind of virulent quality with it. Being applied to the place bitten by venomous beasts, or stung by a wasp or hornet, it speedily draws the poison to it.—*Every like draws its like.* Mizaldus affirms, that being laid to rot in horse-dung, it will breed venomous beasts. Something is the matter ; this herb and Rue will never grow together, no, nor near one another ; and we know Rue is as great an enemy to poison as any that grows.

To conclude. It expelleth both birth and after birth ; and as it helps the deficiency of Venus in one kind, so it spoils all her actions in another.

THE BAY TREE.

THIS is so well known that it needs no description

Government and Virtues.—It is a tree of the Sun, and under the celestial sign Leo, and resisteth witchcraft potently, and all the evils old Saturn can do the body of man, and they are not a few ; for it is the speech of one, I think of Mizaldus, that neither witch nor devil, thunder nor lightning, will hurt a man where a Bay tree is. Galen said, that the leaves or bark dry and heal very much, and the berries more than the leaves ; the bark of the root is less sharp and hot, but more bitter, and hath some astriction, whereby it is effectual to break the stone, and good to open obstructions of the liver, spleen, and other inward parts which bring the jaundice, dropsy, &c. The berries are very effectual against all poisons of venomous creatures, and the sting of wasps and bees, as also against infectious diseases, and therefore put into treacle for that purpose. They likewise procure women's courses ; and seven of them given to a woman in sore travail of child-birth, cause a speedy delivery, and expel the after-birth, and therefore not to be taken by such as have not gone out of their time, lest they procure abortion, or cause labour too soon. They wonderfully help all cold and rheumatic distillations from the brain to the eyes, lungs, or other parts; and being made into an electuary with honey, do help in consumptions, old coughs, shortness of breath, and thin rheums, as also the megrum. They expel wind, and provoke urine; help the mother, and kill worms. The leaves also work the like effects. A bath of the decoction of the leaves and berries, is good for women to sit in that are troubled with the mother, or the diseases thereof, or the stoppings of their courses, or for the diseases of the bladder, pains in the bowels by wind and stopping of urine. A decoction of equal parts of Bay berries, Cuminseed, Hyssop, Origanum, and Euphorbium, with some honey, and the head bathed therewith, doth wonderfully help distillations and rheums, and settleth the palate of the mouth into its place. The oil made of the berries is very comfortable in all cold griefs of the joints, nerves, arteries, stomach, belly, or womb; and helpeth palsies, convulsions, cramp, aches, trembling, and numbness in any part, weariness also, and pains of sore travailing. All griefs and pains proceeding from wind, either in the head, stomach, back, belly, or womb, by anointing the parts affected therewith; and pains of the ears are also cured by dropping in some of the oil, or by receiving into the ears the fume of the decoction of the berries through a funnel. The oil takes away the marks of the skin and flesh caused by bruises, falls, &c., and dissolveth the congealed blood in them. It cures the itch, scabs, and weals in the skin.

BEANS.

Both the garden and field beans are well known.

Government and Virtues.—They are plants of Venus, and the distilled water of the flower of garden beans is good to clean the face from spots and wrinkles; and the meal or flower of them, or the small beans, doth the same. The water distilled from the green husks, is held to be very effectual against the stone, and to provoke urine. Bean flour is used in poultices to assuage inflammations rising upon wounds, and the swelling of women's breasts, caused by curdling of their milk, and represseth their milk. Flour of Beans and Fenugreek mixed with honey, and applied to felons, biles, bruises, or blue marks by blows, or the imposthumes in the kernels of the ears, helpeth them all, and with rose leaves, Frankincense, and the white of an egg, being applied to the eyes, helpeth them that are swollen or do water, or have received any blow upon them, if used in wine. If a bean be parted in two, the skin being taken away, and laid on the place where the leech hath been set that bleedeth too much, stayeth the bleeding. Bean flour boiled to a poultice with wine and vinegar, and some oil put thereto, easeth both pains and swelling of the testicles. The husks boiled in water to the consumption of a third part thereof, stayeth a lask, and the ashes of the husks, made up with hog's grease, helpeth the old pains, contusions, and wound of the sinews, the sciatica and gout. The field Beans have all the aforementioned virtues as the garden Beans. Beans eaten are extremely windy meat; but if after the Dutch fashion, when they are half boiled you husk them and then stew them, they are wholesome food.

FRENCH BEANS.

Description.—This French or Kidney Bean ariseth at first but with one stalk, which afterwards divides itself into many arms or branches, but all so weak that if they be not sustained with sticks or poles, they will be fruitless upon the ground. At several places of these branches grow foot stalks, each with three broad, round and pointed green leaves at the end of them; towards the top come forth divers flowers made like unto pea blossom, of the same colour for the most part that the fruit will be of—that is to say, white, yellow, red, blackish, or of a deep purple, but white is the most usual; after which come long and slender flat pods, some crooked, some straight, with a string running down the back thereof, wherein is flattish round fruit made like a kidney: the root long, spreadeth with many strings annexed to it, and perisheth every year.

There is another sort of French beans commonly growing with us in this land, which is called the Scarlet flowering bean, or Scarlet Runners.

This ariseth with sundry branches as the other, but runs higher to the length of hop poles, about which they grow twining, but turning contrary to the sun, having foot stalks with three leaves on each, as on the other, the flowers also are like the other, and of a most orient scarlet colour. The beans are larger than the ordinary kind, of a dead purple colour, turning black when ripe and dry. The root perisheth in winter.

Government and Virtues.—These belong to Venus, and being dried and beat to powder, are as great strengtheners of the kidneys as any are ; a drachm at a time taken in white wine, to prevent the stone, or to cleanse the kidneys, of gravel. The ordinary French beans are of an easy digestion ; they move the belly, provoke urine, enlarge the breast that is straightened with shortness of breath, engender sperm, and incite to venery. And the scarlet-coloured beans, in regard of the glorious beauty of their colour, being set near a quickset hedge, will bravely adorn the same by climbing up thereon, so that they may be discerned a great way, not without admiration of the beholders at a distance.

LADIES' BED-STRAW

BESIDES the common name above written, it is called Cheese Rennet, because it performs the same offices ; as also Gallion, Pettimugget, and Maid-hair ; and by some Wild Rosemary.

Description.—This riseth up with divers small, brown, and square upright stalks, a yard high or more ; sometimes branches forth into divers parts full of joints, and with divers very fine small leaves at every one of them, little or nothing rough at all ; at the tops of the branches grow many long tufts or branches of yellow flowers, very thick set together, from the several joints which consist of four leaves a piece, which smell somewhat strong, but not unpleasant. The seed is small and black, like poppy-seed, two for the most part joined together. The root is reddish, with many small threads fastened to it, which take strong hold of the ground, and creep a little ; and then the branches leaning a little down to the ground, take root at the joints thereof, whereby it is easily increased.

There is another sort of Ladies' Bed-straw growing frequently in England, which beareth white flowers, as the other doth yellow ; but the branches of this are so weak, that unless it be sustained by the edges, or other things near which it groweth, it will lie down to the ground. The leaves a little bigger than the former, and the flowers not so plentiful as these, and the root hereof is also thready and abiding.

Place.—They grow in meadows and pastures, both wet and dry, and by the hedges.

Time.—They flower in May for the most part, and the seed is ripe in July and August.

Government and Virtues.—They are both herbs of Venus, and therefore strengthening the parts, both internal and external, which she rules. The decoction of the former of those being drank, is good to fret and break the stone, provoke urine, stayeth the inward bleeding, and healeth inward wounds : the herb or flower bruised and put into the nostrils, stayeth their bleeding likewise : the flowers and herb being made into an oil being set in the sun, and changed after it hath stood ten or twelve days ; or into an ointment, being boiled in salad oil, with some wax melted therein after it is strained; either the oil made thereof, or the ointment, cure burnings with fire, or scaldings with water. The same also, or the decoction of the herb and flower, is good to bathe the feet of travellers and lacquies, whose long running causeth weariness and stiffness in their sinews and joints. If the decoction be used warm and the joints afterwards anointed with ointment, it helpeth the dry scab and the itch in children ; and the herb with the white flower is also very good for the sinews, arteries, and joints, to comfort and strengthen them after travel, cold, and pains.

BEETS.

OF Beets there are two sorts which are best known generally, and whereof I shall principally treat at this time, viz. the white and red Beets, and their virtues.

Description.—The common white beet hath many great leaves next the ground, somewhat large, and of a whitish green colour. The stalk is great, strong, and ribbed, bearing a great store of leaves upon it, almost to the very top of it : the flowers grow in very long tufts, small at the end, and turning down their heads, which are small, pale greenish yellow buds, giving cornered prickly seeds. The root is great, long and hard, and when it hath given seed, is of no use at all,

The common red beet differeth not from the white, but only it is less, and the leaves and roots are somewhat red. The leaves are differently red, some only with red stalks or veins ; some of a fresh red, and others of a dark red ; the root thereof is red, spongy, and not eaten.

Government and Virtues.—The government of these two sorts of beet are far different : the red beet being under Saturn, and the white under Jupiter : therefore take the virtues of them apart, each by itself. The white beet doth much loosen the belly, and is of a cleansing, digesting quality, and provoketh urine : the juice of it openeth obstructions both of the liver and spleen, and is good for the headache and swimmings therein, and all affections of the brain : and is effectual also against all venomous creatures ; and applied upon the temples it stayeth inflammations in the eyes : it helpeth burnings, being used without oil, and with a little alum put to it is good for St. Anthony's fire. It is good for all weals, pushes, blisters, and blains in the skin : the herb boiled and laid upon chilblains or kibes, cures them : the decoction in water and vinegar, healeth the itch if bathed therewith, and cleanseth the head of dandriff, scurf, and dry scabs, and relieves running sores, ulcers, and cankers in the head, legs, or other parts, and is much commended against baldness and shedding the hair.

The red beet root is good to stay the bloody flux, women's courses, and the whites, and to help the yellow jaundice : the juice of the root put into the nostrils purgeth the head, helpeth the noise in the ears, and the toothache : the juice snuffed up the nose cures a stinking breath, if the cause lies in the nose, as many times it doth, if any bruise had been there ; as also want of smell coming that way.

WATER BETONY.

CALLED also brown wort : and in Yorkshire, bishop's leaves.

Description. —First, of the water betony, which riseth up with square, hard, greenish stalks, sometimes brown, set with broad dark green leaves dented about the edges with notches, somewhat resembling the leaves of the wood betony, but much larger too, for the most part set at a joint. The flowers are many, set at the tops of the stalks and branches, being round bellyed and opened at the brims, and divided into two parts the uppermost like a hood, and the lowermost like a hip hanging down, of a dark red colour, which passing, there comes in their places small round heads with small points at the ends, wherein lie small and brownish seeds. The root is a thick bush of strings and shreds growing from the head.

Place. —It groweth by the ditch side, brooks, and other water courses generally through this land, and is seldom found far from the water side.

Time. —It flowereth about July, and the seed is ripe in August.

Government and Virtues. —Water Betony is an herb of Jupiter in Cancer, and is appropriated more to wounds and hurts in breasts than wood betony, which follows ; it is an excellent remedy for sick hogs—it is of a cleansing quality. The leaves bruised and applied are effectual for old and filthy ulcers ; and especially if the juice of the leaves be boiled with a little honey and dipped therein, and the sores dressed therewith ; as also for bruises or hurts, whether inward or outward. The distilled water of the leaves is used for the same purpose, as also to bathe the face and hands spotted or blemished, or discoloured by sun burning.

I confess I do not much fancy distilled waters, I mean such waters as are distilled cold ; some virtues of the herb they may happily have. but this I am confident of, that being distilled in a pewter still, as the vulgar and apish fashion is, both chemical oil and salt are left behind, unless you burn them, and then all is spoiled, water and all, which was good for as little as can be by such a distillation in my translation of the London Dispensatory.

WOOD BETONY.

Description.—Common, or Wood Betony, hath many leaves rising from the root, which are somewhat broad and round at the end, roundly dented about the edges, standing upon long foot stalks, from among which rise up small, square, slender, but upright hairy stalks, with some leaves thereon to a piece at the joints, smaller than the lower, whereon are set several spiked heads of flowers like lavender, but thicker and shorter for the most part, and of a reddish or purple colour, spotted with white spots both in the upper and lower part, the seeds being contained in the husks that hold the flowers, are blackish, somewhat long and uneven. The roots are many white thready strings ; the stalk perisheth, but the roots with some leaves thereon, abide all the winter. The whole plant is somewhat small.

Place.—It groweth frequently in woods, and delighteth in shady places.

Time.—It flowereth in July, after which the seed is quickly ripe, yet in its prime in May.

Government and Virtues.—The herb is appropriated to the planet Jupiter, and the sign Aries. Antonius Musa, physician to the Emperor Augustus Cæsar, wrote a peculiar book of the virtues of this herb ; and among other virtues saith of it, that it preserveth the liver and body of man from the danger of epidemical diseases ; it helpeth those that loathe or cannot digest their meat, those that have weak stomachs, or sour belchings, or continual rising in their stomach, using it familiarly either green or dry : either the herb or root, or the flowers in broth, drink, or meat, or made into conserve, syrup, water, electuary, or powder, as every one may best frame themselves unto, or as the time or season requires ; taken any of the aforesaid ways, it cures the jaundice, falling sickness, the palsy, convulsions, shrinking of the sinews, the gout, and those that are inclined to dropsy, those that have continual pains in their heads, although it turn to phrensy. The powder mixed with pure honey is no less available for all sorts of coughs colds, wheezing, or shortness of breath, distillations of thin rheums upon the lungs, which cause consumptions. The decoction made with mead and a little penny-royal, is good for those that are troubled with putrid agues, whether quotidian, tertian, ar quartan, and to draw down and evacuate the blood and humours, that by falling into the eyes, do hinder the sight : the decoction thereof made in wine, and taken, killeth the worms in the belly, openeth obstructions both of the spleen and liver, cureth stitches and pains in the back or sides, the torments and griping pains of the bowels, and the windy colic : and mixed with honey purgeth the belly, helpeth to bring down women's courses, and is of special use for those that are troubled with the falling down of the mother, and pains thereof, and causeth an easy and speedy delivery of women in child-birth. It helpeth also to break and expel stone, either in the bladder or kidneys : the decoction with wine gargled in the mouth easeth the tooth-ache. It is a cure for the bite of mad dogs, being used inwardly and applied outwardly to the place. A drachm of the powder of Betony, taken with a little honey in some vinegar, will refresh those that are wearied by travel. It stayeth bleeding at the mouth and nose, and helpeth those that spit blood, or void it instead of urine, and those that have a rupture, and is good for such as are bruised by any fall or otherwise. The green herb bruised, or the juice applied to any inward hurt, or outward green wound in the head or body, will quickly heal and close it up : as also any veins or sinews that are cut ; and will draw forth a broken bone or splinter, thorn or other things got into the flesh. It is no less profitable for old filthy ulcers ; yea, though they be fistulous and hollow. But some do advise to put a little salt to this purpose, being applied with a little hog's lard, it helpeth a plague or sore and other biles and pushes. The fume of the decoction while it is warm received by a funnel into the ears, easeth the pains of them, destroys worms, and it cureth running sores, the juice dropped into them doth the same. The root of Betony is displeasing both to the taste and stomach, whereas the leaves and flowers, by their sweet and spicy taste, are comfortable both for meat and medicine.

These are some of the many virtues Antonius Musa, an expert physician, for it was not the practice of Augustus Cæsar to keep fools about him, appropriates to Betony : it is a very precious herb, that is certain, and most fitting to be kept in a man's house, both in syrup, conserve, oil, ointment, and plaster. The flowers are usually conserved.

THE BEECH-TREE.

In treating of this tree, you must understand that I mean the green mast-beech, which is by the way of distinction from that other small rough sort, called in Sussex the smaller beech, but in Essex horn bean.

I suppose it is needless to describe it, being already too well known to my countrymen.

Place.—It groweth in woods among oaks and other trees, and in parks, forests, and chases to feed deer, and in other places to fatten swine.

Time.—It bloometh in the end of April or the beginning of May for the most part, and the fruit is ripe in September.

Government and Virtues.—It is a plant of Saturn, and therefore performs his qualities and proportion in these operations. The leaves of the beech tree are cooling and binding, and therefore good to be applied to hot swellings to discuss them : the nuts much nourish such beasts as feed thereon. The water found in the hollow places of decaying beeches will cure both man and beast of any scurf, scab, or running tetters, if they be washed therewith : you may boil the leaves into a poultice, or make an ointment of them when time of year serves.

BILBERRIES, CALLED BY SOME WHORTS AND WHORTLE-BERRIES.

Description.—Of these there are two sorts which are common in England, viz.—the black and red berries. And first of the black.

The small bush creepeth along upon the ground, scarce rising half a yard high, with divers small dark green leaves set in the green branches, not always one against the other, and a little dented about the edges; at the foot of the leaves come forth small, hollow, pale, blueish coloured flowers, the brims ending in five points, with a reddish thread in the middle, which pass into small round berries of the size and colour of the Juniper berries, but of a purple, sweetish, sharp taste; the juice of them give a purplish colour to the hands and lips that eat and handle them, especially if they break them. The root groweth aslope under ground, shooting forth in sundry places as it creepeth. This loseth its leaves in winter.

The red Bilberry, or Whortle-bush, riseth up like the former, having sundry hard leaves, like the Boxtree leaves, green and round pointed, standing on the several branches, at the top whereof only, and not from the sides as in the former, come forth divers round, reddish, sappy berries, of a sharp taste when they are ripe. The root runneth in the ground as in the former, but the leaves of this abide all the winter.

Place.—The first groweth in forests, on the heath, and such like barren places. The red grows in the north parts of this land, as Lancashire, Yorkshire, &c.

Time.—They flower in March and April, and the fruit of the black is ripe in July and August.

Government and Virtues.—They are under the dominion of Jupiter. It is a pity they are used no more in physic than they are. The black Bilberries are good in hot agues, and to cool the heat of the liver and stomach : they do somewhat bind the belly, and stay the vomitings and loathings : the juice of the berries made into a syrup, or the pulp made into a conserve with sugar, is good for the purposes aforesaid, as also for an old cough, or an ulcer in the lungs, or other diseases therein. The red Worts are more binding, and stop women's courses, spitting of blood, or any other flux of blood or humours, being used as well outwardly as inwardly.

BIFOIL, OR TWABLADE.

Description.—This small herb, from a root somewhat sweet, shooting downwards many long strings, riseth up a round green stalk, bare or naked next the ground for an inch, two or three to the middle thereof, as it is in age or growth : as also from the middle upward to the flowers, having only two broad plantain-like leaves, but whiter, set at the middle of the stalk, one against another, compasseth it round at the bottom of them.

Place.—It is a usual inhabitant in woods, copses, and in many other places in this land.

There is another sort groweth in wet grounds and marshes, which is somewhat different from the former. It is a smaller plant, and greener, having sometimes three leaves ; the spike of the flowers is less than the former, and the roots of this do run or creep in the ground.

They are much and often used by many to good purposes for wounds, both green and old, to consolidate or knit ruptures, as well it may, being a plant of Saturn.

BIRCH TREE.

Description.—This groweth a goodly tall straight tree, fraught with many boughs and slender branches bending downward ; the old being covered with a discoloured chopped bark, and the younger being browner by much. The leaves at the first breaking out are crumpled, and afterwards like Beech leaves, but smaller and greener, and dented about the edges. It beareth small short cat-skins, somewhat like those of the Hazel-nut tree, which abide on the branches a long time until growing ripe they fall upon the ground, and their seed with them.

Place.—It usually groweth in woods.

Government and Virtues.—It is a tree of Venus. The juice of the leaves, while they are young, or the distilled water of them, or the water that comes from the tree being bored with an auger, and distilled afterwards ; any of these being drank for some days together, is available to break the stone in the kidneys and bladder, and is good also to wash sore mouths.

BIRD'S FOOT.

THIS small herb groweth not above a span high, with many branches spread upon the ground, set with many wings of small leaves. The flowers grow upon the branches, many small ones of a pale yellow colour being set a head together, which afterwards turneth into small jointed cods, well resembling the claws of small birds, whence it took its name.

There is another sort of Bird's Foot in all things like the former, but a little larger; the flowers of a pale whitish red colour, and the cods distinct by joints like the other, but a little more crooked, and the roots do carry many small white knots or kernels among the strings.

Place.—These grow on heaths, and many upon untilled places of this land.

Time.—They flower and seed in the end of summer.

Government and Virtues.—They belong to Saturn, are of a drying, binding quality, and therefore very good to be used in wound drinks; as also to apply outwardly for the same purpose. But the latter Bird's Foot is found by experience to break the stone in the back or kidneys, and drives them forth, if the decoction thereof be taken; and it wonderfully cures ruptures, being taken inwardly, and outwardly applied to the place.

All salts have best operations upon the stone, as ointments and plasters have upon wounds; and therefore you may make a salt of this for the stone.

BISHOP'S WEED.

BESIDES the common name, Bishop's Weed, it is usually known by the Greek name *ammi* and *ammios*; some call it Æthiopian Cummin-seed, and others Cummin-royal, as also Herb-William, and Bull Wort.

Description.—Common Bishop's Weed riseth up with a round straight stalk, sometimes as high as a man, but usually three or four feet high, beset with divers small, long, and somewhat broad leaves, cut in some places and dented about the edges, growing one against the other, of a dark green colour, having sundry branches on them, and at the top small umbels of white flowers, which turn into small round seeds, little bigger than Parsley-seeds, of a quick hot scent and taste ; the root is white and stringy, perishing yearly, and usually rising again on its own sowing.

Place.—It groweth wild in many places in England and Wales, as between Greenhithe and Gravesend.

Government and Virtues.—It is hot and dry in the third degree, of a bitter taste, and somewhat sharp withal : it provokes lust to purpose ; I suppose Venus owns it. It digesteth humours, provoketh urine and women's courses, dissolveth wind, and being taken in wine it easeth pain and griping in the bowels, and is good against the biting of serpents : it is used to good effect in those medicines which are given to hinder the poisonous operation of cantharides upon the passage of the urine : being mixed with honey, and applied to black or blue marks coming of blows or bruises, it takes them away : and being drank or outwardly applied, it abateth an high colour, and makes it pale.

BISTORT, OR SNAKEWEED.

It is called Snakeweed, English Serpentary, Dragon Wort, Osterick, and Passions.

Description.—It has a thick short knobbed root, blackish without, and somewhat reddish within, a little crooked or turned together, of a hard astringent taste, with divers black threads hanging there, from whence spring up every year divers leaves standing upon long foot-stalks, being somewhat broad and long like a dock leaf, and a little pointed at the ends, but that it is of a blueish green colour on the upper side, and of an ash-colour grey and a little purplish underneath, with divers veins therein, from among which rise up some small and slender stalks, two feet high, and almost naked and without leaves, or with a very few and narrow, bearing a spiky bush of pale-coloured flowers ; which being past, there abideth small seed, like unto Sorrel seed, but greater.

There are other sorts of Bistort growing in this land, but smaller, both in height, root, and stalks, and especially in the leaves. The root is blackish without, and somewhat whitish within ; of an austere binding taste, as the former.

Place.—They grow in shadowy moist woods and at the foot of hills, but are chiefly nourished up in gardens. The narrow leafed Bistort groweth in the north, in Lancashire, Yorkshire, and Cumberland.

Time.—They flower about the end of May, and the seed is ripe about the beginning of July.

Government and Virtues.—It belongs to Saturn, and is in operation cold and dry : both the leaves and roots have a powerful faculty to resist all poison. The root in powder taken in drink expelleth the venom of the plague, the small-pox, measles, purples, or any other infectious disease, driving it out by sweating. The root in powder, the decoction thereof in wine being drank, stayeth all manner of inward bleeding, or spitting of blood, and any fluxes in the body of either man or woman, or vomiting. It is also very available against ruptures, or all bruises or falls, dissolving the congealed blood, and easeth the pains that happen thereupon ; it is beneficial in jaundice.

The water distilled from the leaves and roots, is a good remedy to wash any place bitten or stung by any venomous creature ; and is very good to wash running sores or ulcers. The decoction of the root in wine being drank, prevents abortion or miscarriage in child-bearing. The leaves kill worms in children, and relieves those who cannot keep their water ; if the juice of the Plantain be added thereto, and outwardly applied, it cures gonorrhœha, or running of the veins. A drachm of the powder of the root taken in water thereof, wherein some red hot iron or steel hath been quenched, assists it, the body being first prepared and purged from the offensive humours. The leaves, seed, or roots, are all very good in decoctions, drinks, or lotions, for inward or outward wounds or sores ; and the powder strewed upon any cut or wound in a vein, stayeth the immoderate bleeding thereof. The decoction of the root in water, whereunto some Pomegranate peel and flowers are added, injected into the matrix, stayeth the immoderate flux of the courses. The root thereof with Pellitory of Spain and burnt alum, of each a little quantity, beaten small and made into paste with some honey, and a little piece thereof put into a hollow tooth, or held between the

D

teeth if there be no hollowness in them, stayeth the œ-fluxion of rheum upon them, which causeth pains, and helps to cleanse the head, and void much offensive water. The distilled water is very effectual to wash sores or cankers in the nose or any other part, if the powder of the root be applied thereunto afterwards. It is good also to fasten the gums, and to take away the heat and inflammations that happen in the jaws, almonds of the throat and and mouth, if the decoction of the leaves, roots, or seeds be bruised, or the juice of them be applied; but the roots are most effectual to the purposes aforesaid.

ONE-LEAF.

Description.—This small plant never beareth more than one leaf, but only when it riseth up with its stalk, which thereon beareth another, and seldom more, and are of a blueish green colour, broad at the bottom, and pointed with ribs or veins, like Plantain; at the top of the stalk grow many small flowers, star fashion, smelling somewhat sweet: after which cometh small reddish berries when they are ripe. The root small, of the size of a rush, lying and creeping under the upper crust of the earth, shooting forth in divers places.

Place.—It grows in moist, shadowy, grassy places of woods in parts of this realm.

Time.—It flowereth about May, and the berries are ripe in June, and then quickly perisheth until the next year, and it springeth from the same again.

Government and Virtues.—It is under the Sun, and therefore cordial: half a drachm, or a drachm, at most, of the roots in powder taken in wine and vinegar, of each a like quantity, and the party presently laid to sweat, is held to be a sovereign remedy for the plague, and sores, by expelling the poison and defending the heart and spirits from danger. It is also accounted a singular good wound herb, and therefore used with other herbs in making such balms as are necessary for curing wounds, either green or old, and especially if the nerves be hurt.

THE BRAMBLE, OR BLACKBERRY BUSH.

IT is so well known that it needeth no description.

Government and Virtues.—It is a plant of Venus in Aries. See directions at the end of this book for the gathering herbs, plants, &c. The buds, leaves, and branches, while they are green, are good for ulcers and putrid sores of the mouth and throat, and for the quinsy, and to heal fresh wounds and sores; but the flowers and fruits unripe are very binding, and restrain the bloody flux, lasks, and spitting of blood. Either the decoction or powder of the root being taken is good for gravel and the stone in the reins and kidneys. The leaves and brambles, green or dry, are excellent good lotions for sores in the mouth or secret parts: the decoction of them and of the dried branches, bind the belly, and restrain the profusion of women's courses: the berries of the flowers are a powerful remedy against the poison of the most venomous serpents: as well drank as outwardly applied, helpeth the sores of the fundament, and the piles; the juice of the berries mixed with the juice of Mulberries do bind more effectually, and help all fretting and eating sores and ulcers. The distilled water of the branches, leaves, and flowers, or of the fruit, is very pleasant in taste, and very effectual in fevers and hot distempers of the body, head, eyes, and other parts, and for the purposes aforesaid. The leaves boiled in lye, and the head washed therewith, healeth the itch and running sores thereof, and maketh the hair black. The powder of the leaves strewed on cankers and running ulcers, tends to heal them. The juice of the leaves and of the berries combined may be preserved for the aforesaid uses.

BLITES.

Description.—Of these there are two sorts, white and red. The white hath leaves resembling Beets, but smaller, rounder, and of a whitish green colour, every one standing upon a small long foot-stalk; the stalk rises up two or three feet high with such like leaves thereon; the flowers grow at the top in long round tufts or clusters. wherein are contained small and round seeds : the root is very full of threads or strings.

The red blite is in all things like the white, but that its leaves and tufted heads are exceeding red at first, and after turn more purplish.

There are other kinds of blites which grow differing from the two former sorts but little, but only the wild are smaller in every part.

Place.—They grow in gardens, and wild in many places in this land.

Time.—They seed in August and September.

Government and Virtues. — They are cooling, drying, and binding, serving to restrain the fluxes of blood in either man or woman, especially the red ; which restrains the menses, and the white blite stayeth the whites.   It is an excellent secret ; you cannot well fail in the use : they are all under the dominion of Venus.

There is another sort of wild blites like the other wild kinds, but have long and spiky heads of greenish seeds, seeming by the thick setting together to be all seed.

This sort fishes are delighted with, and it is a good and usual bait, for fishes will bite fast enough at them.

BORAGE AND BUGLOSS.

THESE are so well known to those who have gardens that it is needless to describe them.

To these I may add a third sort, which is not so common nor yet so well known, and therefore I shall give you its name and description.

It is called *langue de bœuf :* but why then should they call one herb by the name bugloss and another by the name *langue de bœuf?*   It is some question to me, seeing one signifies ox-tongue in Greek, and the other signifies the same in French.

Description.—The leaves thereof are smaller than those of bugloss, but much rougher ; the stalks arising up about a foot and a half high, and is most commonly of a red colour ; the flowers stand in scaly rough heads, being composed of many small yellow flowers, not much unlike to those of dandelions, and the seed flieth away in down as that doth ; you may easily know the flowers by their taste, for they are very bitter.

Place.—It groweth wild in many places of this land, and may be plentifully found near London, as between Rotherhithe and Deptford by the ditch side. Its virtues are held to be the same with borage and bugloss, only this is somewhat hotter.

Time.— They flower in June and July, and the seed is ripe shortly after.

Government and Virtues.—They are all three herbs of Jupiter, and under Leo, all great cordials and great strengtheners of nature. The leaves and roots are to very good purpose used in putrid fevers to defend the heart, and to resist and to expel the poison or venom of other creatures ; the seed is of the like effects ; and the seed and leaves are good to increase milk in women's breasts ; the leaves, flowers, and seed, all or any of them, are good to expel melancholy : it clarifies the blood, and mitigates heat in fevers. The juice made into a syrup prevaileth much to all the purposes aforesaid, and is put with other cooling, opening, and cleansing herbs to open obstructions and cure the yellow jaundice ; and mixed with fumitory, to cool, cleanse, and temper the blood, it cures the itch, ringworms, and tetters, or other spreading scabs and sores. The flowers candied or made into a conserve, are helpful in the former cases, but are chiefly used as a cordial, and are good for those that are weak by long sickness, and to comfort the heart and spirits of those that are in a consumption, or troubled often with swoonings, or passions of the heart. The distilled water is no less effectual to all the purposes aforesaid, and abates redness and inflammations of the eyes being washed therewith : the dried herb is never used, but the green : yet the ashes thereof boiled in mead or honeyed water, is available in inflammations and ulcers in the mouth or throat, as a gargle, the roots of bugloss are effectual, being made into electuary, for the cough, and to condensate phlegm, and the rheumatic distillations upon the lungs.

BLUE-BOTTLE.

It is called Cyanus, Hurtsickle, because it turns the edges of the sickles that reap the corn, blue-blow, corn-blue-blow, corn-flower, and blue-bottle.

Description.—Its leaves spread upon the ground, being of a whitish green colour, somewhat on the edges like those of of Corn Scabious, amongst which ariseth up a stalk divided into divers branches beset with long leaves of a greenish colour, either but very little indented or not at all : the flowers are of a blue colour, from whence it took its name, consisting of an innumerable company of small flowers set in a scaly head, not much unlike those of Knap-weed ; the seed is smooth, bright, and shining, wrapped up in a woolly mantle ; the root perisheth every year.

Place.—They grow in corn-fields, amongst all sorts of corn, peas, beans, and tares excepted. If you transplant them into your garden, especially towards the full moon, they will grow more double, and many times change colour.

Time.—They flower from the beginning of May to the end of harvest.

Government and Virtues.—As they are naturally cold, dry, and binding, so they are under the dominion of Saturn. The powder or dried leaves of the Blue-Bottle, or Corn Flower, is given with good success to those that are bruised by a fall, or have broken a vein inwardly, and void much blood at the mouth : being taken in the water of plantaine, horse-tail, or the greater comfrey, it is a remedy against the poison of the scorpion, and resisteth all venoms and poison. The seed or leaves taken in wine, is good for the plague, all infectious diseases, and in pestilential fevers : the juice put into fresh or green wounds quickly closes the lips together, and it heals ulcers and sores in the mouth ; the juice dropped into the eyes takes away heat and inflammation ; the distilled water of this herb hath the same properties.

BRANK URSINE.

Besides the common name Brank Ursine, it is also called Bear's Breech, and Acanthus, though I think our English names to be more proper.

Description.—This thistle shooteth forth very many large, thick, sad green smooth leaves upon the ground, with a very thick and juicy middle rib ; the leaves are parted with sundry deep gashes on the edges ; the leaves remain a long time before any stalk appears, afterwards riseth up a moderate-sized stalk, three or four feet high, and nicely decked with flowers from the middle of the stalk upwards, for on the lower part of the stalk there is neither branches nor leaf : the flowers are hooded and gaping, being white in colour, and standing in brownish husks, with a long, small, undivided leaf under each leaf : they seldom seed in our country. Its roots are many, great, and thick, blackish without and whitish within, full of a clammy sap. A piece of them if you set in the garden, and defend it from the winter cold, will grow and flourish.

Place.—They are only cultivated in the gardens in England, where they will grow very well

Time.—It flowereth in June and July.

Government and Virtues.—This excellent plant is under the dominion of the moon. It should be kept in all gardens : the leaves boiled and used in clysters, wonderfully soften the belly, and make the passage slippery : the decoction drank is good for the bloody flux : the leaves being bruised, or rather boiled, and applied like a poultice help to unite broken bones, and strengthen joints that have been put out ; the decoction of either leaves or roots being drank, and the decoction of leaves applied to the place, is good for the king's evil that is broken and runneth ; for by the influence of the moon it reviveth the ends of the veins which are relaxed ; there is scarcely a better remedy to be applied to burns, for it extracts fire, and heals without a scar : it reduces rupture, and relieves cramp and gout : it is good in hectic fevers, and restores radical moisture to such as are in consumptions.

BRIONY, or WILD VINE.

It is called wild and wood vine, tamus or ladies seal. The white is called white vine by some, and the black, black vine.

Description.—The common White Briony groweth rampant in hedges, sending forth many long, rough, tender branches at the beginning, with many rough and broad leaves thereon, cut (for the most part) into five partitions, in form like a vine leaf, but smaller, rough, and of a whitish hoary green colour, spreading very far, and twining with his small claspers, (that come forth at the joints with the leaves) very far on whatsoever standeth next to it. At the several joints also, especially towards the top of branches, it has a long stalk, bearing many white flowers together on a long tuft, consisting of five small leaves a-piece laid open like a star, after which come the berries separated one from another, more than a cluster of grapes, green at first and very red when they are ripe, of no good scent, but of a most loathsome taste, provoking vomit. The root groweth to be large, with many long twines or branches going from it, of a pale whitish colour on the outside, and more white within, and of a sharp bitter, loathsome taste.

Place.— It groweth on banks or under hedges, through this land : the roots lie very deep.

*Time.—*It flowereth in July and August, some earlier, and some later than the other.

*Government and Virtues.—*They are furious martial plants. The root of briony purges with great violence, troubling the stomach and burning the liver, and therefore not rashly to be taken ; but being corrected, is very profitable for diseases of the head, as falling sickness, giddiness and swimmings, by drawing away much phlegm and rheumatic humours that oppress the head, and the joints and sinews ; and is therefore good for palsies, convulsions, cramps, and stitches in the side, and the dropsy, and in provoking urine : it cleanseth the reins and kidneys from gravel and stone, by opening the obstruction of the spleen, and consumeth the hardness and swelling thereof. The decoction of the root in wine drank once a week at going to bed, strengthens the womb and expelleth the dead child ; a drachm of the root in powder taken in white wine promotes the courses. An electuary made of the roots and honey, cleanses the chest of corrupt phlegm, and relieves an old cough, to those that are troubled with shortness of breath, and is very good for them that are bruised inward-ly, to help to expel congealed blood. The leaves, fruit, and root, cleanse old sores, are good against all fretting and running cankers, gangrenes, and tetters, and therefore the berries are by some country-people called tetter berries. The root cleanseth the skin wonderfully from all black and blue spots, freckles, morphew, leprosy, foul scars, or other deformity whatsoever : also all running scabs and manginess are healed by the powder of the dried root or the juice thereof, but especially by the fine white hardened juice. The distilled water of the root worketh the same effects, but more weakly : the root bruised and applied of itself to any place where the bones are broken, helpeth to draw them forth, as also splinters and thorns in the flesh ; and being applied with a little wine mixed therewith, it break-eth biles, and helpeth whitlows on the joints.

As for the former diseases where it must be taken in-wardly, it purgeth violently, and needs an abler hand to correct it than most country people have ; therefore it is a better way for them, to let the simple alone, and take the compound water of it mentioned in my Dispensatory.

BROOK LIME, or WATER PIMPERNAL.

Description.—This sendeth forth from a creeping root that shooteth forth strings at every joint as it runneth, divers and sundry green stalks, round and sappy, with some branches on them, somewhat broad, round, deep green and thick leaves set by couples thereon ; from the bottom whereof shoot forth long foot-stalks with sundry small blue flowers on them, that consist of five small round pointed leaves a-piece.

There is another sort nothing differing from the form er that but it is greater, and the flowers are of a paler green colour.

Place.—They grow in small standing waters, and usually near water-cresses.

Time.—And flower in June and July, giving seed the next month after.

Government and Virtues.—It is a hot and biting martial plant. Brook-lime and water cresses are generally used

together in diet drink with other things serving to purge
the blood and body from all ill humours that would destroy
health, and are helpful to the scurvy.   They provoke urine,
and help to break the stone and void it : they procure
women's courses, and expel the dead child.   Being fried
with butter and vinegar, and applied warm, it cures
tumours, swellings, and inflammations.   Such drinks
ought to be made of various herbs according to the malady.

BUTCHER'S BROOM.

It is called ruscus, and bruscus, kneeholm, kneeholy,
kneehulver, and pettigree.

Description.—The first shoots that sprout from the root
of butcher's broom are thick, whitish, and short, somewhat
like those of asparagus, but greater, they rising up to be a
foot and a half high, are spread into divers branches, green,
and somewhat cressed with the roundness, tough and flexi-
ble, whereon are set somewhat broad and almost round
hard leaves and prickly, pointed at the end, of a dark green
colour, two for the most part set at a place very close and
near together ; about the middle of the leaf, on the back
and lower side from the middle rib, breaketh forth a small
whitish green flower, consisting of four small round pointed
leaves standing upon little or no foot-stalk, and in the
place whereof cometh a small round berry, green at the
first and red when it is ripe, wherein are two or three
white, hard round seeds contained.   The root is thick,
white, and great at the head, and from thence sendeth
forth divers thick, white, long tough strings.

Place.—It groweth in copses, upon heaths and waste
grounds, and often under or near the Holly bushes.

Time.— It shooteth forth its young buds in the spring,
and the berries are ripe about September, the branches of
leaves abiding green all the winter.

Government and Virtues.—'Tis a plant of Mars, having a
cleansing and opening quality.   The decoction of the root
made with wine openeth obstructions, provoketh urine,
expelleth gravel and stone, the strangury and women's
courses, also the yellow jaundice and the headache : and
with some honey or sugar, cleanseth the breast of phlegm,

and the chest of its clammy humours. The decoction of the root drank, and a poultice made of the berries and leaves being applied are effectual in knitting and consolidating broken bones or parts out of joint. The common way of using it is to boil the root, and parsley, fennel, and smallage in white wine, and drink the decoction, adding the like quantity of grass root to them : the more of the root you boil the stronger will the decoction be ; it works no ill effects.

BROOM, AND BROOM-RAPE.

To describe it is needless, as it is used by all the good housewives almost throughout this land to sweep their houses with, and therefore well known to all sorts of people.

The Broom-rape springeth up on many places from the roots of the Broom, but more often in fields, as by hedgesides and on heaths : the stalk whereof is of the size of a finger or thumb, above two feet high, having a show of leaves on them, and many flowers at the top of a reddish yellow colour, as also the stalks and leaves are.

Place.—They grow in many places of this land commonly, and as commonly spoil all the land they grow in.

Time.—And flower in the summer months, and give their seed before winter.

Government and Virtues.—The juice or decoction of the young branches, or seed, or the powder of the seed taken in drink purgeth downwards, and draweth phlegmatic and watery humours from the joints, whereby it cures the dropsy, gout, sciatica, and pains of the hips and joints ; it also provoketh strong vomits, and relieves the pains of the sides, and swelling of the spleen ; cleanseth also the reins or kidneys, and the bladder of stone, provoketh urine abundantly, and hindereth the growing again of the stone in the body. The continual use of the powder of the leaves and seed cures the black jaundice : the distilled water of the flowers is profitable for the same purposes : it is good in surfeits, and altereth the fits of agues, if three or four ounces thereof with as much of the water of the lesser centuary, and a little sugar put therein, be taken a little before the fit cometh, and the party be laid down to sweat in his bed : the oil or water that is drawn from the end of the green sticks heated in the fire, relieves toothache : the juice of the young branches made into an ointment with hog's lard, and anointed, or the young branches bruised and heated in oil or hog's lard, and laid to the sides pained by wind, as in stitches or the spleen, easeth them in once or twice using it : the same boiled in oil is the surest medicine to kill lice in the head or body, if any : and is an especial remedy for joint aches and swollen knees, that come by the falling down of humours.

The Broom-rape also is not without its virtues.

The decoction thereof in wine is thought to be as effectual to void the stone in the kidneys and bladder, and to provoke urine as the broom itself ; the juice thereof is a singular cure for green wounds, filthy sores, and malignant ulcers; the insolate oil wherein there hath been three or four infusions of the top stalks, with flowers strained, cleanseth the skin from spots, marks, and freckles that riseth either by the heat of the sun or the malignity of the humours.

BUCK'S-HORN PLAINTAIN

Description. — This being sown of seed, riseth up at first with small, long, narrow, hairy, dark green leaves like grass, without any division or gash in them ; but those that follow are gashed in on both sides, the leaves into three or four gashes, and pointed at the ends, resembling the knags of a buck's horn, whereof it took its name, and being well ground round about the root upon the ground, in order one by another, thereby resembling the form of a star, from among which rise up divers hairy stalks about a hand's breadth high, bearing every one a long, small, spiky head, like those of the common Plantain, having such like bloomings and seed after them. The root is single, long, and small, with divers strings at it.

Place. — They grow in sandy grounds as in Tothill-fields, by Westminster, and divers other places of this land.

Time.—They flower and seed in May, June, and July, and their green leaves do in a manner abide fresh all the winter.

Government and Virtues.—It is under Saturn, and is of a drying and binding quality. Boiled in wine, and drank, and some of the leaves put to the hurt place, is a good remedy for the biting of the viper or adder. The same being also drank, relieves stone in the kidneys, cooling the heat of the parts afflicted, and strengthening them ; also weak stomachs that cannot retain their meat. It restrains bleeding at the mouth and nose, bloody urine, or the bloody flux, and stoppeth the lask or looseness of the belly and bowels. The leaves bruised and laid to their sides that have an ague, suddenly easeth the fit : and the leaves and roots being beaten with some bay salt, and applied to the wrists, have the same effects. The herb boiled in ale or wine, and given morning and night for some days, stops the distillation of hot and sharp rheums falling into the eyes from the head, and is good for sore eyes.

BUCK S HORN.

IT is called Harts-horn, Herba-stellaria, Sanguinaria, Herb-eve, Herb-ivy, Wort-cresses, and Swine-cresses.

Description.—They have many small and weak straggling branches trailing here and there upon the ground ; the leaves are many, small, and jagged, not much unlike to those of Buck's Horn Plantain, but much smaller and not so hairy : the flowers grow among the leaves in small, rough, whitish clusters : the seeds are much smaller and brownish, of a bitter taste.

Place.—They grow in dry, barren sandy grounds.

Time.—They flower and seed when the rest of the Plantains do.

Government and Virtues.—It is under the dominion of Saturn ; the virtues are held to be the same as Buck's-horn Plantain, and therefore by all authors it is joined with it : the leaves bruised and applied to the place, stops bleeding ; the herb bruised and applied to warts, will make them consume and waste away in a short time.

BUGLE.

BESIDES the name Bugle, it is called Middle Confound and Middle Comfrey, Brown Bugle, and by some Sickle-wort and Herb-carpenter ; though in Essex we call another herb by that name.

Description. — It has larger leaves than those of the Self-heal, but of the same shape, or rather longer, in some green on the upper side, and in others more brownish, dented about the edges, somewhat hairy, as the square stalk is also, which riseth up to be half a yard high some-times, with the leaves set by couples from the middle al-most, whereof upward stand the flowers, together with many smaller and browner leaves than the rest on the stalk below set at a distance, and the stalk bare betwixt them ; among which flowers are also small ones of a blue-ish and sometimes of an ash colour, fashioned like the flowers of Ground-Ivy, after which come small, round, blackish seeds : the root is composed of many strings, and spreadeth upon the ground.

The white flowered Bugle differeth not in form or great-ness from the former, saving that the leaves and stalk are always green, and never brown like the other, and the flowers thereof are white.

Place. — They grow in woods, copses, and fields generally throughout England, but the white flowered Bugle is not so plentiful as the former.

Time. — They flower from May until July, and in the meantime perfect their seed : the roots and leaves next thereunto upon the ground abiding all the winter.

Government and Virtues. — This herb is under Venus : if the virtues of it make you fall in love with it, (as they will if you be wise) keep a syrup of it to take inwardly, and an ointment and plaster of it to use outwardly, always by you.

The decoction of the leaves and flowers in wine, dissolv-eth the congealed blood in those that are bruised inwardly by a fall or otherwise, and is very effectual for any inward wounds, thrusts, or stabs in the body or bowels ; and is an especial help in all wound-drinks, and for those that are

liver-grown, as they call it.   It is wonderful in curing all
ulcers and sores, gangrenes, and fistulas, if the leaves
bruised and applied, or their juice be used to wash and
bathe the place, and the same made into a lotion and some
honey and alum, cureth the worst sores in the mouth and
gums ; and worketh no less effectually for such ulcers and
sores in the secret parts of men and women.   Being also
taken inwardly, or outwardly applied, it helpeth those that
have broken any bone, or have any member out of joint.
An ointment made with the leaves of bugle, scabious and
sanicle bruised and boiled in hog's lard until the herbs be
dry, and then strained into a pot for such occasions as shall
require ; it is so efficacious for all sorts of hurts in the body,
that none should be without it.

I have known this herb cure some diseases of Saturn.
Drunkards are troubled with strange fancies, strange
sights in the night time, and some with voices, as also with
the nightmare.   I take the reason of this to be (according
to Fernelius) a melancholy vapour made thin by excessive
drinking strong liquor, and so flies up and disturbs the
brain, and breeds imaginations, fearful and troublesome ;
these I have known cured by taking only two spoonfuls of
the syrup of this herb after supper.   But whether this
does it by sympathy or antipathy is some doubt in astrology.   I know there is a great antipathy between Saturn and
Venus in the matter of procreation ; yea, such a one, that
the barrenness of Saturn can be removed by none but Venus ; nor the lust of Venus be repelled by none but Saturn,
but I am not of opinion this is done this way, and my reason is, because these vapours, though in quality melancholy,
yet by their flying upward seem to be somewhat aerial ;
therefore I rather think it is done by sympathy, Saturn
being exalted in Libra in the house of Venus.

BURNET.

It is called sanguisorbia, pimpinella, &c.   The common
garden burnet is so well known that it needeth no description.

Description.—The great wild burnet hath winged leaves

rising from the roots like the garden burnet, but not so many ; yet each of these leaves is twice as large as the other, and nicked in the same manner about the edges, of a greyish colour on the under side ; the stalks are greater and rise higher, with many such like leaves thereon, and greater heads at the top of a brownish colour, and out of them come small dark purple flowers like the former, but larger ; the root is black and long like the other. It hath almost neither scent nor taste, like the garden kind.

Place.—The first grows in some gardens. The wild kind groweth in various counties ; in meadows, waysides, and in moist places.

Time.—They flower about the end of June and beginning of July, and their seed is ripe in August.

Government and Virtues.—It is under the Sun, and is a most precious herb, little inferior to betony : the continual use of it preserves the body in health and the spirit in vigour : for if the sun be the preserver of life under God, his herbs are the best in the world to do it. They are accounted to be both of one property, but the lesser is more effectual, because quicker and more aromatical. It is a friend to the heart, liver, and other principal parts of a man's body. Two or three of the stalks with leaves put into a cup of wine, especially claret, are known to quicken the spirits, refresh and clear the heart, and drive away melancholy. It is a special help to defend the heart from noisome vapours, and from infection of the pestilence, the juice thereof being taken in some drink, and the party laid to sweat thereupon. They have also an astringent quality ; whereby they are available in all manner of fluxes of blood or humours, to staunch bleedings inward or outward, lasks, scourgings, the bloody-flux, too abundant courses, the whites, and the choleric belchings and castings of the stomach, and is a capital wound herb for all sorts of wounds both of the head and body, either inward or outward ; for all old ulcers, running cankers, and most sores, to be used either by the juice or decoction of the herb, or by the powder of the herb or root, or the water of the distilled herb or ointment by itself, or with other things to be kept ; the seed is also no less effectual both to fluxes, and dry up

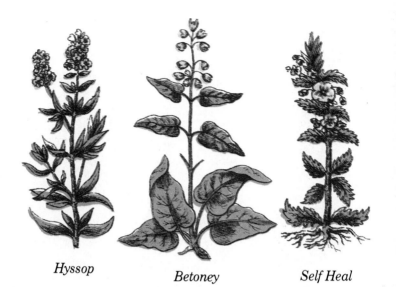

Hyssop   *Betoney*   *Self Heal*

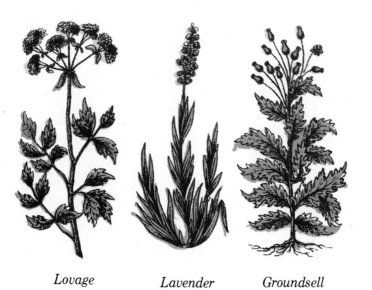

Lovage   *Lavender*   *Groundsell*

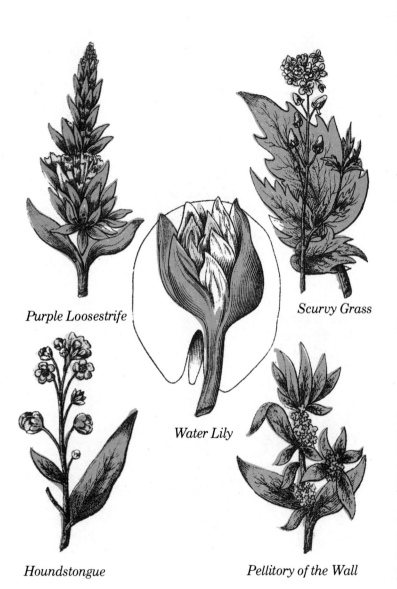

Purple Loosestrife

Scurvy Grass

Water Lily

Houndstongue

Pellitory of the Wall

moist sores, being taken in powder inwardly in wine or steeled water, that is, wherein hot gads of steel have been quenched : or the powder, or the seed mixed with the ointments.

BUTTER-BUR, OR PETASITIS.

Description.—This riseth up in February, with a thick stalk about a foot high, whereon are set a few small leaves, or rather pieces, and at the tops a long spike head ; flowers of a blush or deep red colour, according to the soil where it groweth, and before the stalk with the flowers have abiden a month above ground it will be withered and gone, and blown away with the wind, and the leaves will begin to spring, which being full grown are very large and broad, being somewhat thin and almost round, whose thick red foot stalks above a foot long, stand towards the middle of the leaves ; the lower part being divided into two round parts close almost one to another, and are of a pale green colour, and hairy underneath : the root is long, and spreadeth under ground, being in some places no larger than one's finger, in others much bigger, blackish on the outside, and whitish within, of a bitter and unpleasant taste.

Place and Time.—They grow in low and wet grounds by rivers and water-sides ; their flowers, as is said, rising and decaying in February and March before their leaves, which appear in April.

Government and Virtues.—It is under the dominion of the Sun, and therefore is a great strengthener of the heart and cheerer of the vital spirits : the roots thereof are by long experience found to be very available against pestilential fevers, by provoking sweat : if the powder thereof be taken in wine, it also resisteth the force of any other poison : the decoction of the root, in wine, is good for those who wheeze much, or are short-winded. It provoketh urine also, and women's courses, and killeth worms. The powder of the root will dry up the moisture of sores hard to be cured, and taketh away all spots and blemishes of the skin. It were well if gentlewomen would keep this root preserved to help their poor neighbours.

E

BURDOCK.

It is well known by little boys, who pull off the burs to throw at one another because they stick so.

Place.—They grow plentifully by ditches and water-sides and by the high-ways almost every where through this land.

Government and Virtues.—Venus challengeth this herb for her own : and by its leaf or seed you may draw the womb which way you please, either upward by applying it to the crown of the head in case it falls out ; or down-wards in fits of the mother, by applying it to the soles of the feet : or if you would stay it in its place, apply it to the navel, and that is one good way to stay the child in it.

Burdock leaves are cooling, moderately drying, and dis-cussing withal, whereby it is good for old ulcers and sores. A drachm of the roots taken with pine kernels, helpeth those who spit corrupt or bloody phlegm. The leaves ap-plied to the places troubled with the shrinking of the sinews or arteries, give much ease : the juice of the leaves, or the roots, given to drink with old wine, cure the bites of serpents ; the root beaten with a little salt and laid on the place, suddenly easeth the pain, and cures the bite of a mad dog : the juice of the leaves drank with honey, promotes urine and easeth pain of the bladder : the seed being drank in wine some days, relieves sciatica : the leaves bruised with the white of an egg and applied to any burn, taketh out the fire, gives sudden ease, and heals it up afterwards ; the decoction of the fomented on any fret-ting sore or canker, stayeth the corroding quality, if after-wards anointed with an ointment made of the same liquor, hog's lard, nitre, and vinegar boiled together. The root may be preserved with sugar, and taken fasting or at other times for the same purposes, and for consumptions, the stone, and diarrhœa. The seed is effectual to break the stone, and expel it by urine. It is often used with other seeds and herbs for that purpose.

CABBAGES and COLEWORTS.

THESE are well known, and need not to be described.

Place.—They are generally planted in gardens.

Time.—Their flower time is towards the middle or end of July, and the seed is ripe in August.

Government and Virtues.—The cabbages or coleworts boiled in broth, and eaten, open the body, but the second decoction doth bind the body. The juice promotes women's courses; being taken with honey it soon cures hoarseness or loss of the voice. The pulp, or middle ribs of coleworts boiled in almond milk, and made up into an electuary with honey, being taken often is very profitable for those that are short winded. Being boiled twice, and an old cock boiled in the broth and drank, it relieveth the pains, and the obstructions of the liver and spleen, and the stone in the kidneys. The juice boiled with honey, and dropped into the corners of the eyes, cleareth the sight by consuming any cloud or film beginning to dim it : it also consumeth the canker growing therein. They soon make a man sober; for, as they say, there is such an antipathy or enmity between the vine and the coleworts, that not one will die where the other groweth. The decoction of coleworts relieves pains and aches, and reduces the swellings of sores and gouty legs and knees, wherein many gross and watery humours are fallen, the place being bathed therewith warm. It cures old and filthy sores being bathed therewith, and healeth small scabs in the skin : the ashes of colewort stalks mixed with hog's lard, are very effectual to anoint the sides of those that have had long pains therein, or any other place pained with melancholy and windy humours. This was surely Chrysippus's god, and therefore he wrote a whole volume of their virtues, he appropriates them to every disease in every part of the body ; and honest old Cato, they say, used no other physic. But cabbages are extremely windy whether you take them as meat or as medicine ; yea, as windy meat as can be eaten, unless you eat bag-pipes or bellows, and they are but seldom eaten in our days. Colewort flowers are more tolerable, and the wholesomer food of the two : the Moon challengeth the dominion of the plant.

THE SEA COLEWORTS.

Description.—This hath divers somewhat long and broad, large and thick wrinkled leaves somewhat crumpled about the edges, and growing each upon a thick foot-stalk, very brittle, of a greyish green colour, from among which riseth up a strong thick stalk two feet high and better, with some leaves thereon to the top, where it branches forth much ; on every branch standeth a large bush of pale whitish flowers, consisting of four leaves a piece : the root is somewhat great, shooteth forth many branches under ground, keeping the leaves green all the winter.

Place.—They grow in many places upon the sea coasts, on the Essex shores, and Lid, in Kent, Colchester, in Essex, and other places in this land.

Time.—They flower and seed about the time that other kinds do.

Government and Virtues.—The Moon claims the dominion of these also. The decoction of the sea colewort by the sharp, nitrous, and bitter qualities therein, forms a good purge ; it cleanseth and digests more powerfully than the other kind : the seed bruised and drank, killeth worms : the leaves or the juice of them applied to sores or ulcers cleanseth and healeth them, and dissolveth swellings, and taketh away inflammations.

CALAMINT, OR MOUNTAIN-MINT.

Description.—This is a small herb, seldom rising above a foot high, with square, hairy, and woody stalks, and two small hoary leaves set at a joint, about the size of marjoram, or not much bigger, a little dented about the edges, and of a very fierce or quick scent, as the whole herb is ; the flowers stand at several spaces of the stalks from the middle almost upwards, which are small and gaping like to those of mints, and of a pale blueish colour ; after which follow small, round, blackish seed : the root is small and woody, with divers small strings spreading within the ground, and dieth not, but abideth many years.

Place.— It groweth on heaths and uplands, and dry grounds in many places of this land.

Time. —They flower in July, and their seed is ripe quickly after.

Government and Virtues.—It is under Mercury, and is very efficacious in all afflictions of the brain ; the decoction promotes women's courses, and provoketh urine ; it reduces rupture, and relieves convulsions and cramps, shortness of breath or choleric pains in the stomach or bowels : it cures the yellow jaundice, and stayeth vomiting being taken in wine : taken with salt and honey it killeth worms. It relieves those who have the leprosy, taken inwardly, drinking whey after it, or the green herb outwardly applied : it hindereth conception ; it takes away black and blue marks in the face, and maketh black scars become well coloured, if the green herb (not the dry) be boiled in wine and laid to the place, or the place washed therewith. The juice being dropped into the ears, killeth worms in them ; the leaves boiled in wine, provoke sweat, and open obstructions of the liver and spleen. It helpeth them that have a tertian ague (the body being first purged,) by taking away the cold fits ; the decoction hereof, with sugar, it is a remedy for the overflowing of the gall, and old cough, and shortness of breath, cold distemper of their bowels, and hardness of the spleen, for all which purposes both the powder, called diacaluminthes, and compound syrup of calamint (which are to be had at the apothecaries) are the most effectual.

CAMOMILE.

It is so well known every where, that it is needless to describe it.

A decoction made of camomile, taketh away all pains and stitches in the side : the flowers of camomile beaten and made up into balls with oil, cure all sorts of agues, if the part grieved be anointed with the oil, taken from the flowers, and afterward laid to sweat in bed, and he sweats well. It is most beneficial to the sides and region of the liver and spleen. Bathing with a decoction of camomile taketh away weariness, easeth pains to what parts soever they be applied. It comforteth the sinews when over-strained, mollifieth all swellings : it comforteth all parts that have need of warmth, digesteth whatsoever hath need thereof by a wonderful speedy property : it relieves the colic and stone, and all pains and torments of the belly, and gently provokes urine. The flowers boiled in posset-drink provoke sweat, and help to expel all colds, aches and pains, and promotes women's courses. Syrup made of the juice of camomile, with the flowers in white wine, is a remedy against jaundice and dropsy : the flowers boiled in ley, are good to wash the head and comfort both it and the brain : the oil made of the flowers of camomile is much used for all hard swellings, pains or aches, shrinking of the sinews, cramps or pains in the joints, or any other part of the body. As a clyster it expels the wind and pains in the belly ; as an ointment it relieves pains and stitches in the sides.

The Egyptians dedicated it to the Sun, because it cures agues. Bachinus, Bena, and Lobel, commend the syrup made of the juice of it with sugar, taken inwardly, to be excellent for the spleen. It certainly breaks the stone ; some take it in syrup or decoction, others inject the juice of it into the bladder with a syringe. My opinion is, that the salt of it taken half a drachm in the morning in a little white wine, is better than either : that it is excellent for the stone appears in this which I have seen tried, viz. — That a stone that hath been taken out of the body of a man, being wrapped in camomile, will in a little time dissolve.

WATER CALTROPS.

THEY are called also tribulus aquaticus, tribulus lacuso-ris, tribulus marinus, caltrop, saligos, water nuts, and water chestnuts.

Description. —As for the greater sort of water caltrop, it is not found here, or very rarely : two other sorts there are, which I shall here describe ; the first hath a long creeping and jointed root, sending forth tufts at each joint, from which joints arise long, flat, slender-knotted stalks, even to the top of the water, divided towards the top into many branches, each carrying two leaves on both sides, being about two inches long and a half inch broad, thin and almost transparent, they look as if they were torn; the flowers are long, thick, and whitish, set together almost like a bunch of grapes, which being gone, there succeeds for the most part sharp pointed grains altogether, containing a small white kernal in them.

The second differs not much from this, save that it delights in more clear water; its stalks are not flat, but round; its leaves are not so long but more pointed. As for the place we need not determine, for their name showeth they grow in water.

Government and Virtues.—They are under the dominion of the Moon, and being made into a poultice, are excellent for hot inflammations, swellings, cankers, sore mouths and throats, being washed in the decoction: it cleanseth and strengtheneth the neck and throat, and heals those swellings which, when people have, they say the almonds of their ears are fallen down; it is good for the rankness of the gums, a safe and present remedy for the king's evil; for the stone and gravel, especially the nuts dried.

CAMPION WILD.

Description.—The wild white campion hath many long and rather broad dark green leaves lying upon the ground, and divers ribs therein, somewhat like plantain but somewhat hairy; broader, and not so long; the hairy stalks rise up in the middle of them three or four feet high, and sometimes more, with divers great white joints at several places thereon, and two such like leaves thereat up to the top, sending forth branches at several joints also; all which bear on several footstalks white flowers at the tops of them, consisting of five broad-pointed leaves, every one cut in on the end unto the middle, making them seem to be two a-piece, smelling somewhat sweet, and each of them standing in a large green striped hairy husk, large and round below next to the stalk: the seed is small and greyish in

the hard heads that come up afterwards : the root is white
and long, spreading fangs in the ground.

The red wild campion groweth in the same manner as
the white, but the leaves are not so plainly ribbed, somewhat shorter, rounder, and more woolly in handling.   The
flowers are of the same form and size ; but in some of a
pale, in others of a bright red colour, cut in at the ends
more finely, which makes the leaves look more in number
than the other.   The seeds and the roots are alike, the
roots of both sorts abiding many years.

There are forty-five kinds of campion more ; those of
them which are of a physical use having the like virtues
with those above described.

Place.—They grow commonly through this land by fields
and hedge sides and ditches.

Time.—They flower in summer, some earlier than others,
and some abiding longer than others.

Government and Virtues.—They belong unto Saturn ; and
the decoction of the herb, either in white or red wine, being drank stops inward bleedings, and applied outwardly
it doth the like ; and being drank, it expelleth urine,
gravel, or stone in the kidneys.   Two drachms of the seed
drank in wine purgeth the body of choleric humours, and
helpeth those that are stung by scorpions or other venomous beasts.   It is of very great use in old sores, ulcers,
cankers, fistulas, and the like, to cleanse and heal them by
consuming the moist humours falling into them, and cor-
recting the putrefaction of humours offending them.

CARDUUS BENEDICTUS.

It is called carduus benedictus, or blessed thistle, or holy
thistle.   It is well known, and needs no description.

Time.—They flower in August, and seed soon after.

Government and Virtues.—It is an herb of Mars, and under the sign of Aries.   It relieves swimming and giddiness
of the head, or the disease called vertigo, because Aries is
in the house of Mars.   It is an excellent remedy for the
yellow jaundice and other infirmities of the gall, because
Mars governs choler.   It strengthens the attractive faculty

in man, and clarifies the blood, because the one is ruled by Mars. The habitual drinking of the decoction of it, cures red faces, tetters, and ringworms, because Mars causeth them. It cures sores, boils, and itch, the bitings of mad dogs, and venomous beasts ; all which infirmities are under Mars.

By antipathy to other planets it cureth the French pox. By antipathy to Venus, who governs it, it strengthens the memory, and cures deafness by antipathy to Saturn, who hath his fall in Aries, which rules the head. It cures quartan agues and diseases of melancholy, and adjusts choler, by sympathy to Saturn, Mars being exalted in Capricorn. It provokes urine, the stopping of which is usually caused by Mars or the Moon.

CARROTS.

GARDEN carrots are so well known that they need no description ; but because they are of less physical use than the wild kind (as indeed almost in all herbs the wild are the most effectual in physic, as being more powerful in operation than the garden kinds) I shall therefore briefly describe the wild carrot.

Description.—It groweth in a manner like the tame, but the leaves and stalks are somewhat whiter and rougher. The stalks bear large tufts of white flowers, with a deep purple spot in the middle, which are contracted together when the seed begins to ripen, that the middle part being hollow and low, and the outward stalk rising high, maketh the whole umbel look like a bird's nest : the root small, long, and hard, and unfit for meat, being somewhat sharp and strong.

Place.—The wild kind groweth in various parts of this land, plentifully by the field sides and untilled places.

Time.—They flower and seed in the end of summer.

Government and Virtues.—Wild carrots belong to Mercury, and expel wind and remove stitches in the side, promote the flow of urine and women's courses, and break and expel the stone : the seed has the same effect, and is good for dropsy, and those whose bowels are swollen with wind :

It cures colic, stone, and rising of the mother ; being taken in wine, or boiled in wine and taken, it helpeth conception. The leaves being applied with honey to running sores or ulcers cleanse them. I suppose the seeds of them perform this better than the roots : and though Galen recommended garden carrots highly to expel wind, yet they breed it first, and we may thank nature for expelling it, not they ; the seeds of them expel wind, and so mend what the root marreth.

CARRAWAY.

Description.—It beareth many stalks of fine cut leaves lying upon the ground, somewhat like the leaves of carrots, but not bushing so thick, of a little quick taste in them, from among which riseth up a square stalk, not so high as the carrot, at whose joints are set the like leaves, but smaller and fitter, and at the top small open tufts or um· bels of white flowers, which turn into small blackish seed, smaller than the aniseeds, and of a quicker and better taste. The root is whitish, small, and long, somewhat like unto parsnip, but with more wrinkled bark, and much less, of a little hot and quick taste, and stronger than the parsnip, and abideth after seed time.

Place.—It is usually sown with us in gardens.

Time.—They flower in June and July, and seed quickly after.

Government and Virtues.—This is also a Mercurial plant. Carraway seed hath a sharp quality, and expels wind and promotes urine, which also the herb doth. The root is better food than the parsnips ; it is pleasant and comfortable to the stomach, and promoteth digestion. The seed clears the head and warms the stomach and bowels, and expels the wind in them, and benefits the eye-sight. The powder of the seed put into a poultice taketh away black and blue spots of blows and bruises. The herb itself, or with some of the seeds bruised and fried, laid hot in a bag or double cloth to the lower parts of the belly, easeth the pains of the windy cholic.

The roots of carraways eaten as parsnips, strengthen the

stomach of old people exceedingly, and ought to be grown in every garden.

CELANDINE.

Description.—This hath several tender, round, whitish green stalks, with greater joints than ordinary in other herbs, as it were knees, very brittle and easy to break, from whence grow branches with large tender broad leaves divided into many parts, each of them cut in on the edges, set at the joint on both sides of the branches, of a dark blueish green colour on the upper side like columbines, and of a more pale blueish green underneath, full of yellow sap when any part is broken, of a bitter taste and strong scent. The root is somewhat large, shooting forth long roots and small strings, reddish on the outside, and yellow within, full of yellow sap therein.

Place.—They grow in many places by old walls, hedges, and way-sides, in untilled places *;* and being once planted in the garden, especially in some shady places, it will remain there.

Time.—They flower all the summer long, and the seed ripeneth in the meantime.

Government and Virtues.—This is an herb of the Sun, and under the celestial Lion, and is one of the best cures for sore eyes, for all that know anything in astrology know that the eyes are subject to the luminaries ; let it then be gathered when the Sun is in Leo, and the Moon in Aries, applying to this time ; let Leo arise, then you may make it into an oil or ointment, to anoint your sore eyes with : I can prove it both by my own experience and the experience of very many, that most desperate sore eyes have been cured by this medicine ; and is not this far better than endangering the eyes by the art of the needle ? For if this doth not absolutely take away the film, it will so facilitate the work, that it may be done without danger : the herb or root, boiled in white wine and drank, a few aniseeds being boiled therewith, openeth obstructions of the liver and gall, cures the yellow jaundice ; and often using it cures the dropsy and the itch, and old sores in the legs or other parts of the body ; the juice thereof taken fasting, is of great use against the pestilence : the distilled water with a little sugar and a little good treacle mixed therewith (the person taking it being laid down to sweat a little) hath the same effect ; the juice dropped into the eyes cleanseth them from films and cloudiness that darken the sight, but it is best to allay the sharpness of the juice with a little breast-milk. It is good in old filthy ulcers, to stay their malignity of fretting and running, and to cause them to heal speedily : the juice often applied to tetters, ring-worms, or other spreading cankers, will quickly heal them : and rubbed often upon warts will take them away : the herb with the root bruised and bathed with the oil of camomile, and applied to the naval, taketh away the griping pains in the bowels, and all the pains of the mother ; and applied to women's breasts, restrains the immoderate flow of the courses : the juice or decoction of the herb gargled between the teeth that ache, eases the pain, and the powder of the root laid upon any aching, hollow, or loose tooth, will cause it to fall out : the juice mixed with flour of brimstone is good against the itch, and taketh away all discolourings of the skin ; and if it cause itchings, or inflammations, by bathing the place with a little vinegar it is allayed.

Another ill-favoured trick bave physicians with the eye, and that is worse than the needle ; which is to take away films by corroding medicines ; this I protest against, 1. Because the tunicles of the eyes are very thin, and therefore soon eaten asunder.—2. The film that they would eat away is seldom of an equal thickness in every place, and then the tunicle may be eaten asunder in one place before the film may be consumed in another, and so extinguish the sight.

It is called chelidonium, from the Greek word *chelidon*, which signifies a swallow, because they say that if you put out the eyes of young swallows when they are in the nest, the old ones will recover them again with this herb : this I am confident, for I have tried it, that if we mar the very apple of their eyes with a needle, she will recover them again ; but whether with this herb or not I know not.

Also I have read, and it seems to be somewhat probable.

that the herb, being gathered as I showed before, and the elements drawn apart from it by the art of the alchymist, and after they are drawn apart rectified, the earthly quality still in rectifying them added to the *terra damnata* (as alchymists call it,) or *terra sacratissima* (as some philosophers call it.) the elements so rectified are sufficient for the cure of all diseases, the humours offending being known, and the contrary elements given. It is an experiment worth trying, and can do no harm.

THE LESSER CELANDINE, USUALLY KNOWN BY THE NAMES OF PILEWORT AND FOGWORT.

I WONDER what ailed the ancients to give this the name of celandine, which resembleth it neither in nature or form ; it acquired the name of pilewort from its virtues, and it being no great matter where I set it down, so as I do set it down, I humoured Dr. Tradition so much as to set him down here.

Description.—This celandine or pilewort spreads many round pale green leaves, set on weak and trailing branches, which lie on the ground, and are flat, smooth, and shining. and in some places marked with black spots, each standing on a long foot-stalk, among which rise small yellow flowers consisting of nine or ten small narrow leaves upon slender foot-stalks, very like crow's foot, whereunto the seed is not unlike, being many small kernels, like a grain of corn, sometimes twice as long as others, of a whitish colour, with some fibres at the end of them.

Place.—It groweth in moist corners of fields and places near watersides, yet will abide in drier ground if it be but a little shady.

Time.—It flowereth about March or April, and is quite gone by May.

Government and Virtues.—It is under the dominion of Mars, and mark another verification of the learning of the ancients, viz., that the virtue of an herb may be known by its signature, as plainly appears in this ; for if you dig up the root of it, you will see the perfect image of the disease which they commonly call the piles. It is certain by good experience that the decoction of the leaves and roots doth wonderfully relieve or cure piles also kernels near the ears and throat, called the king's evil, or any other hard wens or tumours.

Pilewort made into an oil, ointment or plaster cures the piles, and the king's evil; the herb borne about one's body next the skin helps in such diseases, though it never touch the place grieved ; let poor people make much of it for those uses ; with this I cured my own daughter of the king's evil, broke this sore, drow out a quarter of a pint of corruption, cured without any scar at all.

THE ORDINARY SMALL CENTAURY.

Description.—This groweth up most usually but with one round and somewhat crusted stalk, about a foot high or better, branching forth from the top into many sprigs, and some also from the joints of the stalks below : the flowers thus stand at the tops in one umbel or tuft, are of a pale red, tending to carnation colour, consisting of five, sometimes six small leaves very like those of St. John's wort, opening themselves in the day time and closing at night, after which come seeds in little short husks, in form like wheat corn ; the leaves are small and somewhat round : the root small and hard, perishing every year ; the whole plant has a bitter taste.

There is another sort in all things like the former, save only it beareth white flowers.

Place.—They grow ordinarily in fields, pastures, and woods, but that with the white flowers not so frequently as the other.

Time.—They flower in July or thereabouts, and seed within a month after.

Government and Virtues.—They are under the dominion of the Sun, as their flowers open and shut as the sun showeth or hideth his face : this herb boiled and drank, purgeth coleric and gross humours, and helpeth the sciatica : it openeth obstructions of the liver, gall, and spleen, helpeth the jaundice, and easeth pains in the sides and hardness of the spleen, used outwardly, and is given with very good effect in agues. It is good for the dropsy, or the green sickness; it killeth worms, the decoction of the tops of the stalks, with the leaves and flowers is good against the colic, and to bring down women's courses, helpeth to void the dead birth, and easeth pains of the mother, and is very effectual in pains of the joints, as the gout, cramp, or convulsions. A drachm of the powder taken in wine, cures the bite of an adder: the juice of the herb with a little honey put to it, is good to clear the eyes from dimness, mist, and clouds that hinder the sight. It is good both for green and fresh wounds, as also for old ulcers and sores, to close up the one and cleanse the other, and perfectly to cure them both, although they are hollow or fistulous; the green herb especialy being bruised and laid thereto: the decoction thereof dropped into the ears, cleanseth them from worms, cleanseth the foul ulcers and spreading scabs of the head, and taketh away all freckles, spots and marks in the skin, being washed with it; the herb is so safe you cannot fail in the using of it, only giving it inwardly for inward diseases: 'tis very wholesome, but not very toothsome.

There is, besides these, another small centaury, which beareth a yellow flower; in all other respects it is like the former, save that the leaves are larger, and of a darker green, and the stalk passeth through the midst of them. They are all of them, under the government of the Sun; yet this observe, in diseases of the blood, use the red centaury; if of choler, use the yellow; but for phlegm or water, you will find the white best.

THE CHERRY-TREE.

This is well known.

Place.—It is grown in every orchard.

Government and Virtues.—It is a tree of Venus. Cherries, as they are of different tastes, so they are of different qualities: the sweet pass through the stomach and the belly more speedily, but are of little nourishment: the tart or sour are more pleasing to a hot stomach, procure an appetite, and help to cut tough phlegm and gross humours: but when they are dried, they are more binding to the belly than when they are fresh, being cooling in hot diseases and welcome to the stomach, and provoke urine : the gum of the cherry-tree dissolved in wine, is good for a cold, cough, and hoarseness of the throat ; mending the colour in the face, sharpeneth the eye-sight, and helpeth to break and expel the stone : the black cherries bruised with the stones and dissolved, the water thereof cures the stone, and expels gravel and wind.

WINTER CHERRIES.

Description.— The winter cherry hath a running or creeping root in the ground, of the size of one's little finger, shooting forth at several joints in several places, whereby it quickly spreads over a great compass of ground ; the stalk riseth not above a yard high, whereon are set many broad and long green leaves, somewhat like night shade, but larger : at the joints whereof come forth whitish flowers made of five leaves a-piece, which afterwards turn into green berries inclosed with thin skins, which change to be reddish when they grow ripe, the berries likewise being reddish and as large as a cherry, wherein are many flat and yellowish seeds lying within the pulp, which being gathered and strung up, are kept all the year to be used upon occasion.

Place.—They grow not naturally in this land, but are cherished in gardens for their virtues.

Time.—They flower not until the middle or latter end of July ; and the fruit is ripe in August or the beginning of September.

Government and Virtues.—This is a plant of Venus, and of great use in physic ; the leaves being cooling, may be used in inflammations, but they are not as opening as the berries and fruit are ; which promotes the urine profusely when it is stopped or grown hot, and painful in the passage ; it is good to expel the stone and gravel out of the reins, kidneys, and bladder, helping to dissolve the stone, and voiding it by grit or gravel sent forth in the urine : it cleanses inward imposthumes or ulcers in the reins or bladder, or those that void a bloody or foul urine : the distilled water of the fruit, or the leaves with them, or the berries green or dry, distilled with a little milk and drank morning and evening with a little sugar is effectual to all the purposes before specified, and especially against the heat and sharpness of the urine. I shall mention one way to cause the berries, to be effectual for the urine and the stone :—take three or four good handsful of the berries, either green, or fresh, or dried, and having bruised them, put them into so many gallons of beer or ale when it is new and tunned : this drink taken daily hath been found to do much good to many, both to ease the pains and expel urine and the stone, and to cause the stone not to engender : the decoction of the berries in wine and water is the most usual way, but the powder of them taken in drink is more effectual.

CHERVIL.

It is called cerefolium, mirrhis, and mirrha, chervil, sweet chervil, and sweet cicely.

Description. — The garden chervil at first resembles parsley, but after it is better grown the leaves are more cut in and jagged, resembling hemlock, being a little hairy, and of a whitish green colour, sometimes turning reddish in the summer, with the stalks also : it riseth a little above half a foot high, bearing white flowers in spiked tufts, which turn into long and round seeds pointed at the ends, and blackish when they are ripe ; of a sweet taste but no smell, though the herb itself smelleth reasonably well : the root is small and long, and perisheth every year, and must be sown in spring for seed, and after July for autumn salad.

The wild chervil groweth two or three feet high, with yellow stalks and joints, set with broader and more hairy leaves divided into sundry parts, nicked about the edges, and of a dark green colour, which likewise grow reddish with the stalks; at the tops whereof stand small white tufts of flowers, afterward smaller and longer seed : the root is white, hard, and endureth long. This hath little or no scent.

F

Place.— The first is sown in gardens for a salad herb; the second groweth wild in many of the meadows of this land, and by the hedge-sides and on heaths.

Time.—They flower and seed early, and thereupon are sown again in the end of the summer.

Government and Virtues.—The garden chervil being eaten, doth moderately warm the stomach, and is a certain remedy (saith Tragus) to dissolve congealed or clotted blood in the body, or that which is clotted by bruises, falls, &c. : the juice or distilled water thereof being drunk, and the bruised leaves laid to the place, being taken either in meat or drink, it promotes the flow of urine, or expels the stone in the kidneys, and it promotes the monthly coures, and is good for the pleurisy and pricking of the sides.

The wild chervil bruised and applied dissolveth swellings in any part, or the marks of congealed blood by bruises or blows in a little space.

SWEET CHERVIL, OR SWEET CICELY.

Description.— This groweth very like the great hemlock, having large spread leaves cut into divers parts, but of a fresher green colour than hemlock, tasting as sweet as the aniseed. The stalks rise up a yard high, or better, being cressed or hollow, having leaves at the joints, but lesser ; and at the tops of the branched stalks, umbels or tufts of white flowers ; after which come large and long crested black shining seed, pointed at both ends, tasting quick, yet sweet and pleasant. The root is great and white, growing deep in the ground, and spreading sundry long branches therein, in taste and smell stronger than the leaves or seeds, and continuing many years.

Place.—This groweth in gardens.

Government and Virtues.—It is under Jupiter. This plant, besides its pleasantness in salads, hath its physical virtue. The roots boiled and eaten with oil and vinegar, or without oil, warms old and cold stomachs oppressed with wind and phlegm, or those that have the phthisic or consumption of the lungs ; the same drank with wine is a preservation from the plague : it provoketh women's courses and expelleth the after-birth ; procureth an appetite to meat, and expelleth wind : the juice is good to heal the ulcers of the head and face : the candied roots hereof are held as effectual as angelica to preserve from infection in the time of a plague, and to warm and comfort a cold weak stomach. It is so harmless you cannot use it amiss.

CHESTNUT TREE.

THE tree is under the dominion of Jupiter, and therefore the fruit must promote good blood, and yield good nourishment to the body ; yet if eaten over much, they make the blood thick, cause headache, and bind the body ; the inner skin that covereth the nut is of so binding a quality, that a scruple of it being taken by a man, or ten grains by a child, soon stops any flux whatsoever : the whole nut being dried and beat into powder, and a drachm taken at a time, is good to stop the terms in women. If you dry chestnuts, (only the kernels I mean) both the barks being taken away, beat them into powder, and make the powder up into an electuary with honey, it is a first-rate remedy for cough and spitting of blood

EARTH CHESTNUTS.

THEY are called earth nuts, earth chestnuts, ground nuts, ciper nuts, and in Sussex pig nuts. A description of them were needless, for every child knows them.

Government and Virtues.—They are something hot and dry in quality, under the dominion of Venus, they provoke lust exceedingly ; the seed is excellent good to provoke urine : and so also is the root, but it doth not perform it so forcibly as the seed doth. The root being dried and beaten into a powder, and the powder made into an electuary, is a first-rate remedy for spitting and voiding blood, or voiding it by urine.

CHICKWEED.

IT is so well known to most people, that I shall not give a description of it.

Place.—They are usually found in moist and watery places, by wood sides and elsewhere.

Time.—They flower about June, and their seed is ripe in July.

Government and Virtues.—It is a fine soft pleasing herb under the dominion of the Moon. It is as effectual as purslain in all its applications except for meat. The herb bruised or the juice applied with cloths or sponges dipped therein to the region of the liver, and as they dry to have it fresh applied, wonderfully abates inflammation of it ; it is effectual for all imposthumes and swellings, for all redness in the face, wheals, itch, scabs : the juice either simply used or boiled with hog's lard and applied, relieves cramp, convulsions, and palsy. The juice, or distilled water, is of much use for all heat and redness in the eyes, to drop some thereof into them ; and is of good effect to ease pains from the heat and sharpness of the blood in piles, and generally all pains in the body that arise from heat. It is used also in hot and virulent ulcers and sores, in the privy parts of men and women, or on the legs or elsewhere. The leaves boiled with marsh-mallows, and made into a poultice with fenugreek and linseed, applied to swellings and imposthumes, ripen and break them, or assuage the swellings and ease the pains. It helpeth the sinews when they are shrunk by cramp or otherwise, and to extend and make them pliable again by this medicine. Boil a handful of chickweed and a handful of red rose leaves dried in a quart of muscadine until a fourth part be consumed, then put to them a pint of neat-foot oil ; let them boil a good while, stirring them well, which being strained, anoint the grieved part therewith warm against the fire, rubbing it well with one hand ; and bind also some of the herb to the place, and it will cure in three times dressing. It is good for cage birds, and makes a good dish like spinach, if carefully cooked.

CHICK-PEASE, OR CICERS.

Description.—The garden sorts, whether red, black, or white, bring forth stalks a yard long, whereon do grow many small and round leaves dented about the edges, set on both sides of a middle rib; at the joints come forth one or two flowers upon sharp foot-stalk, pease fashion, either white or whitish, or purplish red, lighter or deeper, according as the pease that follow will be, that are contained in small, thick and short pods, with one or two pease, more usually pointed at the lower end, and almost round at the head, yet a little cornered or sharp. The root is small, and perisheth yearly.

Place and Time.—They are sown in gardens or fields as pease, being sown later than pease, and gathered at the same time with them, or presently after.

Government and Virtues.—They are both under the dominion of Venus. They are less windy than beans, but nourish more; they provoke urine, and they have a cleansing faculty, whereby they break the stone; to drink the cream of them being boiled in water is the best way. It purges downwards, provokes women's courses, and urine, and increases both milk and seed. One ounce of cicers, two ounces of French barley, and a small handful of marshmallow roots, clean washed and cut, being boiled in the broth of a chicken, and four ounces taken in the morning, and fasting two hours after, is a good medicine for pains in the side. The white cicers are used more for meat than medicine, yet have the same effects, and are thought more powerful to increase milk and seed. The wild cicers are much more powerful than the garden kind, and effectually open obstructions, break the stone, and have all the properties of opening, digesting, and dissolving.

CINQUEFOIL, or FIVE-LEAVED GRASS, called in some Counties FIVE-FINGERED GRASS.

Description.—It spreads and creeps far upon the ground with long slender strings like strawberries, which take root again and shoot forth many leaves made of five parts, and sometimes seven, dented about the edges and rather hard. The stalks are slender, leaning downwards, and bear many small yellow flowers thereon, with some yellow threads in the middle standing about a smooth green head, which, when it is ripe, is a little rough, and containeth small brownish seeds. The root is of a blackish brown colour, the size of one's little finger, but growing long with some threads thereat; and by the small strings it quickly spreadeth over the ground.

Place.—It groweth by wood sides, hedge sides, the pathway in fields, and in the borders and corners of them, almost through this land.

Time.—It flowereth in summer, some sooner, some later.

Government and Virtues.—This is an herb of Jupiter, and therefore strengthens the part of the body it rules; let Jupiter be angular and strong when gathered; and if you give but a scruple (which is but twenty grains) of it at a time, in white wine, you shall seldom miss the cure of an ague, be it what ague soever, in three fits, as I have often proved to the admiration both of myself and others: let no man despise it because it is plain and easy, the ways of God are all such. It is an especial herb used in all inflammations and fevers, whether infectious or pestilential, or among other herbs to cool and temper the blood and humours in the body; as also for all lotions, gargles, and infections; for sore mouths, ulcers, cancers, fistulas, and other foul, or running sores. The juice drank, about four ounces at a time for certain days together, cureth the quinsey and yellow jaundice; and taken for thirty days, cureth the falling sickness. The roots boiled in milk and drank, is a most effectual remedy for all fluxes, whether the white or red, as also the bloody flux. The roots boiled in vinegar, and the decoction held in the mouth, easeth tooth-ache. The juice or decoction taken with a little honey removes hoarseness, and is very good for cough. The disilled water of both roots and leaves produceth the same effects as aforesaid; and if the hands be often washed therein, and suffered at every time to dry in of itself without wiping, it will in a short time relieve the palsy or shaking in them. The root boiled in vinegar cures knots, kernels, hard swellings, and lumps growing in any part of the flesh, being applied; as also inflammations and St. Anthony's fire; all imposthumes and painful sores with heat and putrefaction; the shingles also. and running and foul scabs, sores, and the itch. The same also boiled in wine, and applied to any joint full of pain, ache, or the gout in the hands or feet, or the hip gout, called the sciatica, and the decoction thereof drank the while, doth cure them, and easeth much pain in the bowels. The roots are also effectual to reduce ruptures, being used with other things available to that purpose, taken either inwardly or outwardly, or both ; as also bruises or hurts by blows, falls, or the like, and to stay the bleeding of wounds in any part, inward or outward.

Dioscorides says that one leaf cures a quotidian, three a tertian, and four a quartan ague ; I never stood so much upon the number of leaves, or whether I give it in powder or decoction : if Jupiter were strong, and the Moon applied to him, and his good aspect at the gathering, I never knew it miss the desired effect.

CIVES.

Called also rush leeks, chives, civet, and sweth.

Government and Virtues.—I confess I had not added these had it not been for a country gentleman, who, by a letter certified to me that amongst other herbs I had left these out ; they are indeed a kind of leeks, hot and dry in the fourth degree as they are, and so under the dominion of Mars ; if they be eaten raw, (I do not mean raw opposite to roasted or boiled, but raw opposite to chymical preparation) they send up very hurtful vapours to the brain, causing troublesome sleep, and spoiling the eye-sight ; yet of them, prepared by the art of the alchymist, may be made an excellent remedy for the stoppage of urine.

CLARY, OR MORE PROPERLY, CLEAR-EYE.

Description.—Our ordinary garden clary hath four square stalks, with broad, rough, wrinkled, whitish, or hoary green leaves, somewhat evenly cut in on the edges, and of a strong sweet scent, growing some near the ground, and some by couples upon stalks. The flowers grow at certain distances, with two small leaves at the joints under them, somewhat like unto flowers of sage, but smaller, and of a whitish blue colour. The seed is brownish and somewhat flat, or not so round as the wild. The roots are blackish, and spread not far, and perish after seed time. It is usually sown, for it seldom rises of its own sowing.

Place.—This groweth in gardens.

Time.—It flowereth in June and July, some a little later than others, and their seed is ripe in August, or thereabouts.

Government and Virtues.—It is under the dominion of the Moon. The seed put into the eyes clears them from motes and such like things gotten within the lids to offend them, as also clears them from white and red spots on them. The mucilage of the seed made with water, and applied to tumours or swellings removes them; as also draweth forth splinters, thorns, or other things gotten into the flesh. The leaves used with vinegar, either by itself with a little honey, cures boils, felons, and the hot inflammations that are gathered by their pains, if applied before it be grown too great. The powder of the dried root put into the nose, provoketh sneezing and thereby purgeth the head and brain of much rheum. The seeds or leaves taken in wine, provoketh to venery. It is of much use both for those who have weak backs, and it strengthens the reins. The fresh leaves dipped in a batter of flour, eggs, and a little milk, and fried in butter, is not unpleasant, but very profitable for those who have weak backs. The juice of the herb in ale or beer, and drank, promotes the courses.

WILD CLARY.

This useful plant is well known.

Description.—It is like the other clary but less with many stalks about a foot and a half high. The stalks are square, and a little hairy; the flowers of a bluish colour.

Place.—It grows commonly in barren places.

Time.—They flower from the beginning of June till the latter end of August.

Government and Virtues.—It is something hotter and drier than the garden clary is, yet nevertheless under the dominion of the Moon as well as that. The seeds of it being beaten to powder, and drank with wine, is an admirable help to provoke lust. A decoction of the leaves being drank, warms the stomach, and it is a wonder if it should not, the stomach being under Cancer, the house of the Moon : also it helps digestion, scatters congealed blood in any part of the body. The distilled water hereof cleanseth the eyes of redness, waterishness and heat : it is a gallant remedy for dimness of sight, to take one of the seeds of it and put it into the eyes, and there let it remain till it drops out of itself, the pain will be nothing to speak on ; it will cleanse the eyes of all filthy and putrid matter ; and repeating it will take off a film which covereth the sight.

CLEAVERS

It is also called aparine, goose-share, goose-grass and cleavers.

Description.—The common cleavers have several rough square stalks, and rising two or three yards high, and if it meet with any tall bushes or trees whereon it may climb, without claspers, or it creeps on the ground, full of joints, and at every one of them shooteth forth a branch besides the leaves, which are usually six, set in a round compass like a star ; from between the leaves or the joints towards the tops of the branches come forth very small white flowers, at every end upon small thready foot-stalks, which, after they fall, two small round and rough seeds appear united, which, when they are ripe, grow hard and whitish. Both stalks, leaves, and seeds are so rough, that they will stick to any thing that touches them. The root is small and thready, spreading much to the ground, but dieth every year.

Place.—It groweth by hedges and ditch-sides, and is so troublesome an inhabitant in gardens, that it is ready to choke whatever grows near it.

Time.—It flowereth in June or July, and the seed is ripe and falleth again in the end of July or August, from whence it springeth up again, and not from the old roots.

Government and Virtues.—It is under the dominion of

the Moon.   Taken in broth, it keeps them lean and lank that are apt to grow fat.   The distilled water drank twice a day cures the yellow jaundice; and the decoction of the herb is found to do the same, and stayeth lasks and bloody fluxes.   The juice of the leaves, a little bruised and applied to any bleeding wound, stayeth the bleeding.   The juice also is very good to close up the lips of green wounds, and the powder of the dried herb strewed thereupon doth the same, and heals old ulcers.   Being boiled in hog's lard, it reduces hard swellings or kernels in the throat, being anointed therewith.   The juice dropped into the ears removes pain.

It is a good remedy in the spring, eaten (being first chopped small and boiled well) in water gruel, to cleanse the blood and strengthen the liver, thereby to keep the body in health, and fitting it for that change of season that is coming.

CLOWN'S WOUNDWORT.

Description.—It groweth up sometimes to two or three feet high, but usually about two feet, with square, green, rough stalks, but slender, joined far asunder, and two very long, rather narrow dark green leaves bluntly dented about the edges thereof, ending in a long point.   The flowers stand towards the tops, compassing the stalks, at the joints with the leaves, and end in a spiked top, having long and much gaping hoods of a purplish red colour, with whitish spots, standing in rather round husks, wherein afterwards stand blackish round seeds.   The root is composed of many long strings with some tuberous long knobs growing among them, of a pale yellowish or whitish colour; yet some times of the year those knobby roots in many places are not seen in this plant.   It has a strong scent.

Place.—It groweth by path sides in the fields, and in or near ditches.

Time.—It flowereth in June or July, and the seed is ripe soon after.

Government and Virtues.—It is under the dominion of Saturn.   It is very effectual in all fresh wounds, and therefore has not this name for nought. It is very available in staunching blood, and to dry up the fluxes of humours in old fretting ulcers, cankers, &c. that hinder the healing of them.

A syrup made of the juice of it is inferior to no remedy for inward wounds, ruptures of veins, bloody flux, vessels broken, spitting, voiding, or vomiting blood. Ruptures are speedily and effectually cured by taking now and then a little of the syrup, and applying an ointment or plaster of this herb to the place. Also if any vein or muscle be swelled, apply a plaster of this herb to it, adding a little comfrey to it. The herb, reader, deserves commendation, though it has gotten such a clownish name ; and whoever tries it, as I have done, will commend it ; only take notice that it is of a dry earthy quality.

COCK'S HEAD, RED FITCHING, or MEDECK FETCH.

Description.—This hath divers weak but rough stalks half a yard long leaning downwards, but set with winged leaves longer and more pointed than those of lintels, and whitish underneath ; from the tops of these stalks arise up other slender stalks, naked without leaves to the tops, where there grow many small flowers in manner of a spike, of a pale reddish colour, tinged with blue ; after which rise up in their places, round, rough, and somewhat flat heads. The root is tough and woody, yet liveth and shooteth anew every year.

Place.—It groweth under hedges, and sometimes in the open fields.

Time.—They flower all the months of July and August, and the seed ripeneth in the meanwhile.

Government and Virtues.—It is under the dominion of Venus, it hath power to rarify and digest, and therefore the green leaves bruised, and made into a plaster, disperse knots, or kernels in the flesh ; and if when dry it be taken in wine, it cures the strangury ; and being anointed with oil it promotes sweat. It is a singular food for cattle, to cause them to give much milk ; and why may it not do the like, being boiled in ordinary drink for nurses ?

COLUMBINES.

THESE are well known growing almost in every garden.

Time.—They flower in May to the end of June, perfecting their seed in the meantime.

Government and Virtues.—It is an herb of Venus. The leaves of columbines are successfully used in lotions for sore mouths and throats. Tragus saith, that a drachm of the seed taken in wine with a little saffron, removes obstructions of the liver, and is good for the yellow jaundice, if the party after taking it, lying to sweat well in bed. The seed taken in wine, causeth a speedy child-birth ; if one draught suffice not, let her drink a second, and it will be effectual. The Spaniads used to eat a piece of the root thereof in a morning fasting, many days together, to help them when troubled with stone.

COLT'S FOOT.

CALLED also coughwort, foal's foot, horse's hoof, and bull's foot.

Description.—This shooteth up a tender stalk, with small yellowish flowers somewhat earlier, which fall away quickly, and after they are past come up nearly round leaves, sometimes dented about the edges, much less, thicker, and greener than those of butter-bur, with a little down or frieze over the green leaf on the upper side, which may be rubbed away, and whitish or mealy underneath. The root is small and white, spreading much underground, so that where it taketh it will hardly be driven away again if any little piece be abiding therein ; and from thence spring fresh leaves.

Place.—It groweth in wet ground as well as in drier places.

Time.—And flowereth in the end of February; the leaves begin to appear in March.

Government and Virtues.—The plant is under Venus:

the fresh leaves, or juice, or a syrup thereof, is good for a hot, dry cough, or wheezing, and shortness of breath. The dry leaves are best for those who have thin rheums and distillations upon their lungs, causing a cough; for which also the dried leaves taken as tobacco, or the root, is very good. The distilled water hereof simply, or with elderflowers and night-shade, is a good remedy for hot agues, to drink two ounces at a time, and apply cloths wet therein to the head and stomach, which also does much good being applied to any hot swellings or inflammations. It helpeth St. Anthony's fire, and burnings, and is good to take away wheals and pushes that arise through heat; as also the burning heat of the piles, or privy parts, cloths wet therein being thereunto applied.

COMFREY.

Description.—The common great comfrey hath very large hairy green leaves lying on the ground, so hairy or prickly, that if they touch any tender part of the hands, face or body, it will cause it to itch : the stalk that riseth from among them being two or three feet high, hollow and cornered, is very hairy also, having many such like leaves as grow below, but less and less up to the top ; at the joints of the stalks it is divided into many branches with some leaves thereon, and at the end stand many flowers in order one above another, which are somewhat long and hollow like the finger of a glove, of a pale whitish colour, after which come small black seeds. The roots are large and long, spreading great thick branches underground, black on the outside and whitish within, short and easy to break, and full of glutinous or clammy juice of little or no taste at all.

There is another sort like this, only less, and beareth flowers of a pale purple colour.

Place.--They grow by ditches and water-sides and in fields that are moist, for therein they chiefly delight to grow : the first generally through all the land, and the other but in some places. Sometimes it grows in dry places.

Time.—They flower in June or July, and give their seed in August

Government and Virtues.—It is under Saturn, and under the sign Capricorn; cold, dry, and earthy in quality. What was spoken of clown s wound-wort may be said of this. The great comfrey restrains spitting of blood, and bloody urine. The root boiled in water or wine, and the decoction drank, heals inward hurts, bruises, wounds, and ulcers of the lungs, and causes the phlegm that oppresses him to be easily spit forth. It cureth the defluctions of rheum from the head upon the lungs, the fluxes of blood or humours by the belly, women's immoderate courses, and the reds and whites and the running of the reins. A syrup made thereof is very effectual in inward hurts, and the distilled water for the same purpose also, and for outward wounds or sores in the fleshy or sinewy part of the body, and to abate the fits of agues, and to allay the sharpness of humours. A decoction of the leaves is good for those purposes, but not so effectual as the roots. The roots being outwardly applied, cure fresh wounds or cuts immediately, being bruised and laid thereto : and is special good for ruptures and broken bones ; so powerful to consolidate and knit together, that if they be boiled with dissevered pieces of flesh in a pot, it will join them together again. It is good for women's sore breasts ; also to repress profuse bleeding of the hæmorrhoids, or piles, to cool the inflammation of the parts thereabouts, and to ease pain. The roots of comfrey taken fresh, beaten small, and spread upon leather, and laid upon any place troubled with the gout, presently gives ease; and applied in the same manner it eases pained joints, and tends to heal running ulcers, gangrenes, mortifications, for which it hath by often experience being found helpful.

CORALWORT.

It is also called by some toothwort, tooth violet, dog-teeth violet, and dentaria.

Description.—Of the many sorts of this herb, two of them may be found growing in this nation ; the first of which shooteth forth one or two winged leaves upon long brownish foot-stalks, which are doubled down at their first coming out of the ground; when they are fully opened, they consist of seven leaves, most commonly of a sad green colour, dented about the edges, set on both sides the middle rib one against another, as the leaves of the ash-tree; the stalk beareth no leaves on the lower half of it : the upper half beareth sometimes three or four, each consisting of five leaves, sometimes of three; on the top stand four or five flowers upon short foot-stalks, with long husks; the flowers are very like the flowers of stock gilliflowers, of a pale purplish colour, consisting of four leaves each, after which come small pods which contain the seed; the root is very small, white, and shining; it doth not grow downwards, but creeping along under the upper crust of the ground, and consisteth of divers small round knobs set together; towards the top of the stalk there grows some single leaves, by each of which cometh a small cloven bulb, which when it is ripe, if it be set in the ground, will grow to be a root.

As for the other coralwort which groweth in this nation, it is more scarce than this, being a very small plant much like crowfoot.

Place.—The first groweth in Sussex, also in woods and copses.

Time.—They flower from the latter end of April to the middle of May, and before the middle of July they are gone, and not to be found.

Government and Virtues.—It is under the dominion of the Moon. It cleanseth the bladder and provoketh urine, expels gravel and the stone; it easeth pains in the sides and bowels, is very good for inward wounds, especially such as are made in the breast or lungs, by taking a drachm of the powder of the root every morning in wine; the same is excellent for ruptures, as also to stop fluxes : an ointment made of it is good for wounds and ulcers, for it soon dries up the watery humours which hinder the cure.

COSTMARY, OR ALCOST, OR BALSAM HERB.

THIS inhabitant in almost every garden is well known.
Time.—It flowereth in June and July.

Government and Virtues.—It is under the dominion of Jupiter. The ordinary costmary, as well as maudlin, provoketh urine abundantly, and softens the hardness of the mother ; it gently purgeth choler and phlegm, extenuating that which is gross, and cutting that which is tough and glutinous, cleanseth that which is foul, and prevents putrefaction ; it openeth obstructions and relieves their bad effects, and it is beneficial in all sorts of dry agues. It is astringent to the stomach, and strengtheneth the liver and other viscera : and taken in whey, worketh more effectually. Taken fasting in the morning, it relieves chronic pains in the head, and to stay, dry up, and consume all thin rheums or distillations from the head into the stomach, and helpeth much to digest raw humours gathered therein. It is very profitable for those that are fallen into a continual evil disposition of the body, called cachexy, especially in the beginning of the disease. It is good for weak and cold livers. The seed is given to children for worms, and so is the infusion of flowers in white wine, about two ounces at a time : it maketh an excellent salve to heal old ulcers, being bo led with oil of olive, and adder's tongue with it ; and after it is strained, put a little wax, rosin, and turpentine to make it as thick as required.

CUDWEED, OR COTTONWEED.

BESIDES cudweed and cottonweed, it is called chaffweed, dwarf cotton, and petty cotton.

Description.—The common cudweed riseth up with one stalk sometimes, and sometimes with two or three, thick set on all sides, with small, long, and narrow whitish and woody leaves, from the middle of the stalk almost up to the top; with every leaf stands a small flower of a dun or brownish yellow colour, or not so yellow as others : in which herbs, after the flowers are fallen come small seed wrapped up with the down therein, and is carried away with the wind : the root is small and thready.

There are other sorts hereof, which are rather less than the former, not much different, save only that the stalks and leaves are shorter, so the flowers are paler and more open.

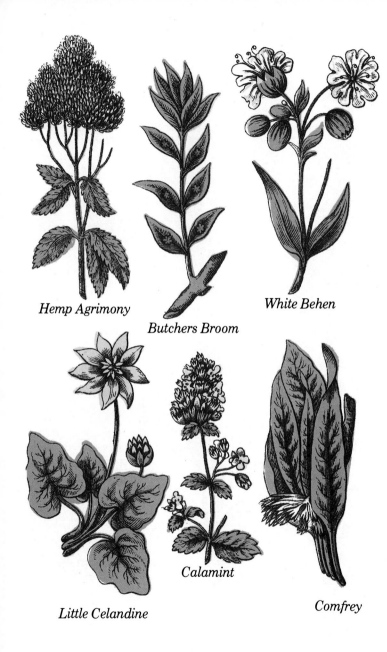

Hemp Agrimony

Butchers Broom

White Behen

Little Celandine

Calamint

Comfrey

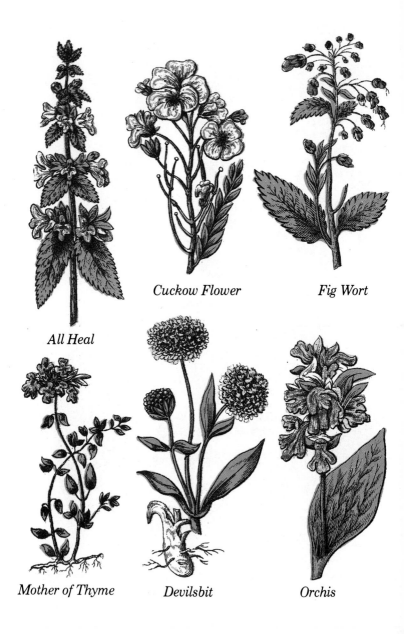

Cuckow Flower

Fig Wort

All Heal

Mother of Thyme

Devilsbit

Orchis

Place.—They grow in dry, barren, sandy, and gravelly grounds in many places of this land.

Time.—They flower about July, some earlier, some later, and their seed is ripe in August.

Government and Virtues.—Venus governs it. It is astringent, binding, or drying, and therefore profitable for all defluxions of rheum from the head, and to stay fluxes of blood, the decoction being made with red wine and drank, or the powder taken therein. It restrains the bloody flux, and easeth the pains, stayeth the immoderate courses of women, and is also good for inward or outward wounds, hurts, or bruises, and in children cures worms ; and being drank or injected for the disease called tenusmus, or inclination to stool without doing anything. The green leaves bruised and laid to any green wound, stayeth the bleeding, and soon healeth it. The juice of the herb is, as Pliny saith, a sovereign remedy against the mumps and quinsey ; and that whosoever shall so take it, shall never be troubled with that disease again.

COWSLIPS, OR PEAGLES.

BOTH the wild and garden are well known.

Time.—They flower in April and May.

Government and Virtues.—Venus lays claim to this herb as her own, and it is under the sign Aries, and our city dames know well enough the ointment or distilled water of it adds to beauty, or at least restores it when it is lost. The flowers are held to be more effectual than the leaves, and the roots of little use. An ointment being made with them, taketh away spots and wrinkles of the skin, sunburnings and freckles, and promotes beauty, they remedy all infirmities of the head coming of heat and wind, as vertigo, false apparitions, phrensies, falling sickness, palsies, convulsions, cramps, pains in the nerves ; the roots ease pains in the back and bladder, and open the passages of the urine. The leaves are good in wounds, and the flowers take away trembling. If the flowers be not well dried and kept in a warm place, they will soon putrify and look green. If you let them see the sun now and then, it will do neither the sun nor them harm.

G

Because they strengthen the brain and nerves, and remedy palsies, the Greeks gave them the name *paralysis*. The flowers preserved or conserved, and the quantity of a nutmeg taken every morning, is a sufficient dose for inward diseases, but for wounds, spots, wrinkles, and sunburnings, an ointment is made of the leaves and hog's lard.

CRAB'S CLAWS.

CALLED also water seagreen, knight's pond water, water houseleek, pond weed, and fresh-water soldier.

Description.—It hath sundry long narrow leaves, with sharp prickles on the edges of them, also very sharp-pointed; the stalks which bear flowers seldom grow so high as the leaves, bearing a forked head like a crab's claw, out of which comes a white flower, consisting of three leaves, with yellowish hairy threads in the middle: it taketh root in the mud in the bottom of the water.

Place.—It groweth plentifully in the fens in Lincolnshire.

Time.—It flowereth in June, and usually from thence till August.

Government and Virtues.—It is a plant under the dominion of Venus, and therefore a great strengthener of the reins: it is excellent good in that inflammation which is commonly called St. Anthony's fire: it reduces inflammations and swellings in wounds, and an ointment made of it is good to heal them: there is scarce a better remedy than this for injuries in their kidneys, and the flow of blood instead of urine: a drachm of the powder of the herb taken every morning, is a very good remedy to stop the terms.

BLACK CRESSES.

Description.—It hath long leaves deeply cut and jagged on both sides, not much unlike wild mustard; the stalk small, very limber, though tough: you may twist them round as you may a willow before they break. The stones are very small and yellow, after which come small pods which contain the seed.

Place.—It is a common herb growing usually by the wayside, and sometimes upon mud and old stone walls, but it delights most to grow among stones and rubbish.

Time.—It flowers in June and July, and the seed is ripe in August and September.

Government and Virtues.—It is a plant of a hot and biting nature, under the dominion of Mars. The seed of black cresses strengthens the brain exceedingly, being, in performing that office, little inferior to mustard seed, if at all ; they are excellent to stay those rheums which may fall down from the head upon the lungs ; beat the seed into powder, and make it into an electuary with honey ; so you have an excellent remedy for cough, yellow jaundice, and sciatica. The herb boiled into a poultice is an excellent remedy for inflammations, both in women's breasts and in men's testicles.

SCIATICA CRESSES.

Description.—These are of two kinds ; the first riseth up with a round stalk about two feet high, spread into divers branches, whose lower leaves are somewhat larger than the upper, yet all of them cut or torn on the edges, somewhat like garden cresses, but smaller ; the flowers are small and white, growing at the tops of branches, where afterwards grow husks with small brownish seeds therein, very strong and sharp in taste, more than the cresses of the garden : the root is long, white, and woody.

The other hath the lower leaves whole, somewhat long and broad, not torn at all, but only somewhat deeply dented about the edges towards the ends ; but those that grow up higher are less. The flowers and seeds are like the former, and so is the root likewise, and both root and seeds as sharp as it.

Place.—They grow by the way-sides in untilled places, and by the sides of old walls.

Time.—They flower in the end of June, and their seed is ripe in July.

Government and Virtues.—It is a Saturnine plant. The leaves, but especially the root, taken fresh in summer time, beaten or made into a poultice or salve with hog's lard, and applied to the places pained with the sciatica, to continue thereon four hours if it be on a man, and two hours on a woman ; the place afterwards bathed with wine and oil mixed, and then wrapped with wool or skins after they have sweat a little, will not only cure the same disease in hips, or other of the joints, as gout in the hands or feet, but all other old griefs of the head, (as inveterate rheums) and other parts of the body that are hard to be cured ; and if of the former griefs any parts remain, the same medicine after twenty days is to be applied again. The same is also effectual in the diseases of the spleen ; and applied to the skin it taketh away the blemishes thereof, whether they be scars, leprosy, scabs, or scurf, which, although it ulcerated the part, yet that is to be cured afterwards with a salve made of oil and wax. Esteem this as another secret.

WATER CRESSES.

Description.—Our ordinary water cresses spread forth with many weak, hollow, sappy stalks, shooting out fibres at the joints, and upwards long winged leaves made of sundry broad sappy almost round leaves, of a brownish colour. The flowers are many and white, standing on long foot-stalks, after which come small yellow seed, contained in small long pods like horns. The whole plant abideth green in the winter, and tasteth hot and sharp.

Place.—They grow for the most part in small standing waters, and in small rivulets of running water.

Time.—They flower and seed in the beginning of the summer.

Government and Virtues.—It is under the dominion of the Moon. They are more powerful against the scurvy and to cleanse the blood and humours, than brook-lime is, and serve in all the other uses in which brook-lime is available, as to break the stone, and provoke urine and women's courses. The decoction thereof cleanseth ulcers by washing them therewith. The leaves bruised, or the juice, is good to be applied to the face or other parts troubled with freckles, pimples, spots, or the like, at night, and washed away in the morning. The juice mixed with vinegar, and the fore-part of the head bathed therewith, is very good for those that are dull and drowsy, or have the lethargy.

Water-cress pottage is a good remedy to cleanse the blood in the spring, and helps headaches, and consumes the gross humours winter hath left behind : those that would live in health should use it freely. If any fancy not pottage, they may eat the herb as a salad.

CROSSWORT.

Description. — Common crosswort groweth up with square hairy brown stalks, a little above a foot high, having four small broad and pointed, hairy, yet smooth thin leaves growing at every joint, each against other crossway, which has caused the name. Towards the tóps of the stalks at the joints, with the leaves in three or four rows downwards, stand small, pale, yellow flowers, after which come small blackish round seeds, four for the most part set in every husk.

The root is very small, and full of fibres, or threads, taking good hold of the ground, and spreading with the branches a great deal of ground, which perish not in winter, although the leaves die every year, and spring again anew.

Place.—It groweth in moist grounds, and in meadows.

Time.—It flowers from May all the summer long, in one place or another, as they are more open to the sun : the seed ripeneth soon after.

Government and Virtues.—It is under the dominion of Saturn. This is a good wound herb, and is used inwardly not only to stay bleeding of wounds, but to consolidate them, as it doth outwardly any green wound, which it quickly closes and healeth. The decoction of the herb in wine expectorates phlegm from the chest, and is good for obstructions .in the breast, stomach, or bowels, and improves a bad appetite. It is also good to wash any wound or sore with, to cleanse and heal it. The herb bruised and boiled, applied outwardly for certain days, renewing it often ; and in the meantime the decoction of the herb in wine, taken inwardly every day, it cures rupture, if it be not too inveterate , but very speedily, if it be fresh and lately taken.

CROWFOOT.

MANY are the names this biting herb hath obtained, it is called frog's-foot from the Greek name *barrakion;* crowfoot, goldknobs, gold cups, king's knobs, baffiners, troilflowers, polts, locket goulions, and butter flowers.

Abundance are the sorts of this herb, that to describe them all would tire the patience of Socrates himself ; but because I have not yet attained to the spirits of Socrates, I shall but describe the most usual.

Description.—The most common crowfoot hath many thin green leaves cut into divers parts, in taste biting and sharp, biting and blistering the tongue ; it bears many flowers of a bright resplendent yellow eolour ; I do not remember that I ever saw any thing yellower—virgins in ancient times used to make powder of them to furrow bride-beds—after which flowers come small heads, some spiked and rugged like a pine apple.

Place.—They grow very common every where ; unless you turn your head into a hedge you cannot but see them as you walk.

Time.—They flower in May and June, even until September.

Government aud Virtues.—This fiery and hot-spirited herb of Mars is no way fit to be given inwardly, but an ointment of the leaves or flowers will draw a blister, and may be so fitly applied to the nape of the neck to draw back rheum from the eyes. The herb being bruised and mixed with a little mustard, draws a blister as perfectly as cantharides, and with far less danger to the vessels of urine, which cantharides naturally delight to wrong. I knew the herb once applied to a pestilential rising that was fallen down, and it saved life even beyond hope : it were good to keep an ointment and plaster of it, if it were but for that.

CUCKOW-PINT.

IT is called janus, calve's foot, ramp, starchwort, cuckowpintle, priest's pintle, and wake robin.

Description. —This shooteth forth three, four, or five leaves at the most from one root, every one whereof is rather large and long, broad at the bottom next the stalk, and forked but ending in a point, without a cut on the edge, of a full green colour, each standing upon a thick round stalk, of a hand-breadth long, among which, after two or three months that they begin to wither, riseth up a bare, round, whitish green stalk, spotted and streaked with purple, somewhat higher than the leaves; at the top whereof standeth a long hollow husk close at the bottom, but open from the middle upwards, ending in a point; in the middle whereof stand the small, long pestle or clapper, smaller at the bottom than at the top, of a dark purple colour, as the husk is on the inside, though green without, which after some time, the husk and clapper decay, and the foot of it groweth to be a small long bunch of berries, green at first, and of a yellowish red colour when ripe, the size of a hazel-nut kernel, which abideth thereon almost until winter; the root is round and rather long, lying along, the leaves shooting forth at the largest end, which, when it beareth its berries, are rather wrinkled and loose, another growing under it which is solid and firm, with many small threads hanging thereat. The plant is of a sharp bitter taste, prickling the tongue as nettles do the hands. The root thereof was anciently used instead of starch to starch linen with.

There is another sort of cuckow-pint with less leaves than the former, and sometimes harder, having blackish spots upon them, which abide longer green in summer than the former, and both leaves and roots are more sharp and fierce than it; in all things else it is like the former.

Place.—These two sorts grow frequently almost under every hedge side in many places of this land.

Time.—They shoot forth leaves in the spring, and continue but until the middle of summer or a little later; their husks appearing before they fall away, and their fruit showing in April.

Government and Virtues.—It is under the dominion of Mars. Tragus reporteth that a drachm weight, or more if need be, of the spotted wake robin either fresh and green or dried, beaten and taken, is a sure remedy for poison and the plague. The juice of the herb taken to the quantity of a spoonful hath the same effect; but if a little vinegar and the root be added, it allayeth its sharp biting taste upon the tongue. The green leaves as a poultice, extracts the poison from bad sores. A drachm of the powder of the dried root taken with twice as much sugar in the form of an electuary, or the green root, it relieves those that are pursy and short-winded, and those that have a cough; it breaketh, and raiseth phlegm from the stomach, chest, and lungs: the milk in which the root hath been boiled is effectual also for the same purpose. The said powder taken in wine or other drink, or the juice of the berries, or the powder of them, or the wine wherein they have been boiled, provoketh urine, and bringeth down women's courses, and purgeth them effectually after child-bearing. Taken with sheep's milk it healeth the inward ulcers of the bowels: the distilled water thereof is effectual for the same purposes. A spoonful taken often healeth the itch: and an ounce or more taken at a time for some days benefits rupture. The leaves either green or dry, or the juice of them, doth cleanse filthy ulcers, and sores in the nose, called polypus. The water wherein the root hath been boiled, dropped into the eyes, cleanseth them from any film or skin, cloud or mists, which begin to hinder the sight, and cures the watering and redness of them, or when they become black and blue. The root mixed with bean flower and applied to the throat or jaws that are inflamed, relieveth them. The juice of the berries boiled in oil of roses, or beaten into powder mixed with the oil, and dropped into the ears, easeth pains in them. The berries or the roots beaten with hot ox-dung, and applied, easeth the pains of the gout. The leaves and roots boiled in wine with a little oil and applied to the piles, or the falling down of the fundament, easeth them, and so doth sitting over the hot fumes thereof. The fresh roots bruised and distilled with milk, yield a sovereign water to cleanse the skin from scurf, freckles, spots, or blemishes.

CUCUMBERS.

Government and Virtues.—They are under the dominion of the Moon, though they are so much cried out against for their coldness, and if they were but one degree colder they would be poison. The best of Galenists hold it to be cold and moist in the second degree, and then not so hot as either lettuces or purslain : they are good for a hot stomach and hot liver ; the unrestrained use of them will fill the body full of raw humours, and so indeed the unmeasureable use of any thing else doth harm. The face being washed in their juice cleanseth the skin, and is excellent good for hot rheums in the eyes : the seed promotes urine, and cleanseth the passages thereof when they are stopped ; there is not a better remedy for ulcers in the bladder than cucumbers are. The usual course is to use the seed in emulsions, as they make almond milk ; or take the cucumbers and bruise them well and distil the water from them, and let such as are troubled with ulcers in the bladder drink no other drink. The face being washed with the same water cureth the reddest face that is ; it is also good for sun-burnings, freckles, and morphew.

DAISIES.

Government and Virtues.—The herb is under the sign Cancer, and under the dominion of Venus, and therefore good for wounds in the breast, and very fitting to be kept both in oils, ointments, plasters, and syrup. The greater wild daisy is a wound herb of good respect, often used in those drinks and salves that are for wounds, either inward or outward. The juice or distilled water of these, or the small daisy, reduces the heat of choler, and refreshes the liver and other inward parts. A decoction made of them and drunk, cures wounds of the breast : also cureth ulcers and pustules in the mouth or tongue, or in the secret parts. The leaves bruised and applied to the testicles or any other part that is swollen and hot, reduces the heat. A decoction made thereof, with wall-wort and agrimony, and places fomented or bathed therewith warm, giveth great ease in palsy, sciatica, or the gout. The same also cures knots or kernels in any part of the body, and bruises and hurts that come of falls and blows ; they are used successfully for ruptures and inward burnings. An ointment made thereof heals all wounds that have inflammations about them, or by reason of running, are kept long from healing. The juice of them dropped into the running eyes of any, cures them. As a poultice for sores they are good.

DANDELIONS, VULGARLY CALLED PISS-A-BEDS.

Description.—It has many long and deep gashed leaves lying on the ground; the ends of each gash or jag, on both sides looking downwards towards the roots; the middle rib being white, which being broken yieldeth abundance of bitter milk, but the root much more; from among the leaves, which always abide green, arise many slender, weak, naked foot-stalks, every one of them bearing at the top one large yellow flower, consisting of many rows of yellow leaves, broad at the points, and nicked in with deep spots of yellow in the middle, which growing ripe, the green husk wherein the flowers stood turns itself down to the stalk, and the head of down becomes as round as a ball, with long reddish seed underneath, bearing a part of the down on the head of every one, which together is blown away with the wind, or may be at once blown away with one's mouth. The root grows very deep, which being broken off within the ground, will yet shoot forth again, and will hardly be destroyed where it hath once taken deep root in the ground.

Place.—It groweth frequently in all meadows and pasture grounds.

Time.—It flowereth in one place or another almost all the year long.

Government and Virtues.—It is under the dominion of Jupiter. It is of an opening and cleansing quality, and therefore very effectual for the obstructions of the liver, gall, and spleen, and the diseases that arise from them, as the jaundice and hypochondriac; it openeth the passages of the urine both in young and old; powerfully cleanseth imposthumes and inward ulcers in the urinary passages, and by its drying and temperate quality doth afterwards heal them; for which purpose the decoction of the roots or leaves in white wine, or the leaves chopped as pot herbs with a few alisanders, and boiled in their broth, are very effectual. And whoever is drawing towards a consumption, or an evil disposition of the whole body called ca-chexy, by the use hereof for some time together shall find a wonderful help. It helpeth also to procure rest and sleep to bodies distempered by the heat of ague fits, or otherwise; the distilled water is effectual to drink in pestilential fevers, and to wash the sores.

Great are the virtues of this common herb, and that is the reason the French and Dutch so often eat them in the spring.

DARNEL.

It is called jum and wray; in Sussex they call it crop, it being a pestilent enemy among the corn.

Description.—This hath, all the winter long, sundry long, flat, and rough leaves, which, when the stalk riseth, which is slender and jointed, are narrower but rough still; on the top groweth a long spike composed of many heads set one above another, containing two or three husks with sharp but short beards or awns at the ends; the seed is easily shook out of the ear, the husk itself being somewhat rough.

Place.—The country husbandmen know this too well to grow among their corn, or in the borders or pathways of other fields that are fallow.

Government and Virtues.—It is a malicious part of sullen Saturn. As it is not without some vices, so hath it also many virtues. The meal of darnel is very good to stay gangrenes and other such like fretting and eating cankers and putrid sores; it also cleanseth the skin of all scurvy, morphews, ring-worms, if it be used with salt and reddish roots. And being used with quick brimstone and vinegar, it dissolveth hard knots and kernels, being boiled in wine with pigeon's dung and linseed. A decoction thereof made with water and honey, and the places bathed therewith cures the sciatica. Darnel meal applied in a poultice draweth forth splinters and broken bones in the flesh. The red darnel boiled in port wine and taken, stayeth the lask and all other fluxes and women's bloody issues, and restraineth urine that passeth away too suddenly.

DILL.

Description.—The common dill groweth up with seldom more than one stalk, neither so high nor so great usually as fennel, being round and fewer joints thereon, whose leaves are sadder and somewhat long, and so like fennel that it deceiveth many, but harder in handling, and somewhat thicker, and of a stronger unpleasant scent; the tops of the stalks have four branches, and smaller umbels of yellow flowers, which turn into small seed, somewhat flatter and thinner than fennel seed. The root is somewhat small and woody, perisheth every year after it hath borne seed, and is also unprofitable, being never put to any use.

Place.—It is most usually sown in gardens and grounds for the purpose, and is also found wild in many places.

Government and Virtues.—Mercury hath the dominion of this plant, and therefore it strengthens the brain. The dill boiled and drunk, is good to ease swellings and pains; it also stayeth the belly and stomach from casting. The decoction is good for pains in the womb. It stayeth the hiccup, being boiled in wine, and but smelled unto, being tied in a cloth. The seed is of more use than the leaves, and more effectual to digest raw and viscous humours, and is used in medicines that serve to expel wind, and the pains proceeding therefrom. The seed being roasted or fried, and used in oils or plasters, dissolves imposthumes in the fundament, and drieth up all moist humours especially in the fundament : an oil made of dill is effectual to warm or dissolve humours or imposthumes, to ease pains, and to procure rest. The decoction of dill, be it herb or seed, (only if you boil the seed you must bruise it) in white wine, being drunk, it is a gallant expeller of wind, and provoker of the terms.

DEVIL'S BIT.

Description.—This riseth up with a round green smooth stalk about two feet high, set with divers long and somewhat narrow, smooth, dark green leaves, somewhat nipped about the edges for the most part, being else all whole and not divided, or but very seldom, even at the tops of the branches, which are yet smaller than those below, with one rib only in the middle. At the end of each branch standeth a round head of many flowers set together in the same manner, or more neatly than scabious, and of a more blueish purple colour, which being past, there followeth seed that falleth away. The root somewhat thick, but short and blackish, with many strings, abiding after seed time many years. This root was longer, until the devil (as the friars say) bit away the rest of it for spite, envying its usefulness to mankind.

There are two sorts hereof, in nothing unlike the former, save that the one beareth white, and the other blush-coloured flowers.

Place.—The first groweth as well in dry meadows and fields as moist, in many places of this land : but the other two are more rare and hard to be met with, yet they are both found growing wild about Appledore, near Rye, in Kent.

Time.—They flower not usually until August.

Government and Virtues.—The plant is venereal, pleasing and harmless. The herb or the root being boiled in wine and drunk, is very powerful against the plague, and all pestilential diseases or fevers, and poisons : it helpeth also all that are inwardly bruised by any casualty, or outwardly by falls or blows, dissolving the clotted blood ; and the herb or root beaten and outwardly applied, taketh away black and blue marks in the skin. The decoction of the herb, with honey of roses put therein, is very effectual to help the inveterate tumours and swellings of the almonds and throat, by often gargling the mouth therewith. It procures women's courses, and easeth all pains of the mother, and expels wind from the bowels. The powder of the root taken in drink, expels worms. The juice or distilled water of the herb, is very effectual for green wounds or old sores, and cleanseth the body inwardly, and the seed outwardly, from sores, scurf, itch, pimples, freckles, morphew, or other deformities thereof, especially if a little vitriol be dissolved therein.

DOCK.

It needs no description.

Government and Virtues.—All docks are under Jupiter, of which the red dock, which is commonly called blood wort, cleanseth the blood and strengthens the liver; but the yellow dock root is best to be taken when either the blood or liver is affected by choler. All of them have a kind of cooling (but not all alike) drying quality, the sorrel being most cold, and the blood worts most drying. Of the burdock I have spoken already by itself. The seed of most of the other kinds, whether in gardens or fields, restrains lasks and fluxes of all sorts, the loathing of the stomach through choler, and is helpful for those that spit blood. The roots boiled in vinegar cureth the itch, scabs, and breaking out of the skin, if it be bathed therewith. The distilled water of the herb and roots have the same virtue, and cleanseth the skin from freckles, morphews, and all other spots and discolourings therein.

Blood wort is very strengthening to the liver, and procures good blood, being as wholesome a pot herb as any growing in a garden; yet such is the nicety of our times, forsooth! that women will not put it into a pot because it makes the pottage black; pride and ignorance preferring nicety before health.

DODDER of THYME, EPITHYMUM, AND OTHER DODDERS.

Description.—This first, from seed, giveth roots in the ground, which shoot forth threads or strings, grosser or finer as the property of the plant wherein it groweth and the climate doth suffer, creeping and spreading on that plant whereon it fasteneth, be it high or low. The strings have no leaves at all upon them, but wind and interlace themselves so thick upon a small plant, that it taketh away all comfort of the sun from it; and is ready to choke or strangle it. After these strings are risen up to that height, that they may draw nourishment from that plant, they seem to be broken off from the ground, either by the strength of their rising or withered by the heat of the sun.

Upon these strings are found clusters of small heads or husks, out of which shoot forth whitish flowers, which afterwards give small pale white-coloured seed, somewhat flat, and twice as big as a poppy-seed. It generally participates of the nature of the plants it climbeth upon ; but the dodder of thyme is accounted the best.

Government and Virtues.—All dodders are under Saturn. We confess thyme is the hottest herb it usually grows upon, and therefore that which grows upon thyme is hotter than that which grows upon colder herbs; for it draws nourishment from what it grows upon, as well as from the earth where its root is, and thus you see old Saturn is wise enough to have two strings to his bow. This is accounted the most effectual for melancholy diseases, and to purge black or burnt choler, which is the cause of many diseases of the head and brain, as also for the trembling of the heart, faintings, and swoonings. It is helpful in all diseases and griefs of the spleen, and melancholy that arises from the windiness of the hypochondria. It purgeth also the reins or kidneys by urine ; it openeth obstructions of the gall, whereby it profiteth them that have the jaundice ; as also the leaves, the spleen ; purging the veins of choleric and phlegmatic humours, and cures children in agues, a little worm seed being added.

The other dodders participate of the nature of those plants whereon they grow : as that which hath been found growing upon nettles in the west country, hath by experience been found very effectual to procure plenty of urine, where it hath been stopped or hindered.

Sympathy and antipathy are two hinges upon which the whole model of physic turns ; and that physician who minds them not, is like a door off from the hooks, more like to do a man mischief than to secure him. Then all the diseases Saturn causes this helps by sympathy, and strengthens all the parts of the body he rules ; such as be caused by Sol it helps by antipathy.

DOG'S GRASS, OR COUCH GRASS

Description.—Some call it *Quick.* It is well known that this grass creepeth far about underground, with long white jointed roots, and small fibres almost at every joint, very sweet in taste, as the rest of the herb is, and interlacing one another, from whence shoot forth many fair grassy leaves, small at the ends, and cutting or sharp on the edges. The stalks are jointed like corn, with the like leaves on them, and a large spiked head, with a long husk in them, and hard rough seeds in them. If you know it not by this description, watch the dogs when they are sick, and they will quickly lead you to it.

Place.—It groweth commonly in ploughed grounds, to the no small trouble of the husbandman, as also of the gardener, in gardens to weed it out if they can ; for it is a constant customer to the place it gets footing in.

Government and Virtues.—'Tis under the dominion of Jupiter, and is the most medicinal of all the quick grasses. Being boiled and drunk it openeth obstructions of the liver and gall, and the stoppings of urine, and easeth the griping pains of the belly, and inflammations ; wasteth the matter of the stone in the bladder, and the ulcers thereof also. The roots bruised and applied do consolidate wounds. The seeds doth powerfully expel urine, and stayeth the lask and vomiting. The distilled water alone, or with a little worm-seed, killeth worms in children.

The way to use it, is to bruise the roots, and having boiled them in white wine, drink the decoction ; it is opening, but not purging, very safe ; 'tis a remedy against all diseases coming of stopping, and such are half those that are incident to the body of man ; and although a gardener be of another opinion, yet a physician holds half an acre of them to be worth five acres of carrots twice told over.

DOVE'S FOOT, or CRANE'S BILL.

Description.—This hath some small, round, pale green leaves cut in about the edges, much like mallows, standing upon long, reddish, hairy stalks, lying in a round compass upon the ground, among which rise up two, or three, or more reddish jointed, slender, weak, hairy stalks with such like leaves thereon, but smaller, and more cut in up to the tops, where grow many very small, bright, red flowers of five leaves a-piece ; after which follow small heads with small short beaks pointed, as other sorts of this herb do.

Place.—It groweth in pasture grounds, and by the path-sides in many places and will also be in gardens.

Time.—It flowereth in June, July, and August, some earlier and some later.

Government and Virtues.—It is a very gentle, though martial plant. It is found by experience to be good for colic, and to expel stone and gravel. The decoction there-of in wine, is a good cure for those that have inward wounds, hurts, or bruises, both to stay the bleeding, to dissolve and expel the congealed blood, and to heal the parts, as also to cleanse and heal outward sores, ulcers, and fistulas ; and for green wounds many do only bruise the herb and apply it to the place, and it healeth them quickly. The same decoction in wine fomented to any place pained with gout, or to joint-ache, or pains of the sinews, giveth much ease. The powder or decoction of the herb taken for some time together, is found by experi-ence to be very good for ruptures.

DUCK'S MEAT.

THIS is so well known to swim on the tops of standing waters, as ponds, and ditches.

Government and Virtues.—Cancer claims the herb, and the Moon will be lady of it : a word is enough to a wise man. It is effectual to help inflammations and St. Anthony's fire, as also gout, either applied by itself or in a poultice with barley meal. The distilled water is highly esteemed by some against all inward inflammations and pestilential fevers ; as also to help the redness of the eyes and swellings of the testicles, and of the breasts before they be grown too much. The fresh herb applied to the forehead, easeth the pains of the headache coming of heat.

DOWN, or COTTON-THISTLE.

Description.—This hath large leaves lying on the ground, somewhat cut in, and as it were crumpled on the edges, of a green colour on the upper side, but covered with long hairy wool or cotton down, set with most sharp and cruel pricks, from the middle of whose heads of flowers thrust forth many purplish crimson threads, and sometimes, although very seldom, white ones. The seed that followeth in the heads, lying in a great deal of white down, is somewhat large, long, and round like the seed of ladies' thistle, but somewhat paler. The root is great and thick, spreading much, yet it usually dieth after seed time.

Place.—It groweth in ditches, banks, and in corn fields and highways, and other places.

Time.—It flowereth and beareth seed about the end of summer, when other thistles flower and seed.

Government and Virtues.—Mars owns the plant, and manifests to the world, that though it may hurt your finger, it will help your body; for I fancy it much for the ensuing virtues. Pliny and Dioscorides write that the leaves and roots taken in drink relieve those that have a crick in their neck, whereby they cannot turn their neck but their whole body must turn also. Galen saith, that the roots and leaves are healing, and are good for such persons as have their bodies drawn together by some spasm or convulsions, as it is with children that have the rickets.

DRAGONS.

THEY are well known as a garden plant; at the lower end of the stalks, and see how like a snake they look.

Government and Virtues.—The plant is under the dominion of Mars, and therefore it would be a wonder if it should want some obnoxious quality or other: in all herbs in an alembic, in what vehicle you please, or else to press out the juice and distil that in a glass still in sand. It scoureth and cleanseth the internal parts also, being externally applied, from freckles, morphew, and sun-burnings; your best way to use it externally is to mix it with vinegar: an ointment of it is held to be good in wounds and ulcers; it consumes cankers, and polypus: also the distilled water being dropped into the eyes taketh away spots, or the pin and webs, and mends dimness of sight; it is good against pestilence and poison. Pliny and Dioscorides affirm, that no serpent will meddle with him that carries the herb about him.

THE ELDER-TREE.

It is needless to describe this, since every boy that plays with a pop-gun will not·mistake another tree instead of the elder. I shall chiefly describe the dwarf elder, called also dead-wort and wall-wort.

THE DWARF ELDER.

Description.—This is but an herb, every year dying with his stalks to the ground, and rising fresh every spring, and is like unto the elder both in form and quality, rising up with a square rough hairy stalk four feet high, or more sometimes. The winged leaves are sometimes narrower than the elder, but else like them. The flowers are white with a dash of purple, standing upon umbels, very like the elder also, but more sweet in scent : after which come small blackish berries full of juice while they are fresh, wherein is small hard seed. The root doth creep under the upper crust of the ground, springing in various places, being of the size of one's finger or thumb sometimes.

Place.—The elder tree groweth in hedges, being planted there to strengthen the fences and partitions of ground, and to hold the banks by ditches and water courses. The dwarf elder groweth wild in many places of England, where being once gotten into the ground, it is not easily got rid of.

Time.—Most of the elder trees flower in June, and their fruit is ripe for the most part in August. But the dwarf elder or wall-wort flowereth somewhat later, and its fruit is not ripe until September.

Government and Virtues.—Both elder and dwarf trees are under the dominion of Venus. The first shoots of the common elder boiled like asparagus, and the young leaves and stalks boiled in fat broth, doth mightily carry forth phlegm and choler. The middle or inward bark boiled in water and given in drink worketh much more violently; and the berries either green or dry, expel the same humour, and are often given with good success in dropsy ; the bark of the root boiled in wine, or the juice thereof drunk, worketh the same effects but more powerfully than either the leaves or fruit. The juice of the root taken, causes vomitings, and purgeth the watery humours of the dropsy. It molifieth the hardness of the mother if women sit thereon, and openeth their veins and bring down their courses. The berries boiled in wine worketh the same effect; and the hair of the head washed therewith is made black. The juice of the green leaves applied to the hot inflammations of the eyes, assuageth them: the juice of the leaves snuffed up into the nostrils, purgeth the brain: the juice of the berries boiled with honey and dropped into the ears, relieveth the pains of them: the decoction of the berries in wine being drunk, provoketh urine: the distilled water of the flowers is of much use to free the skin from sun-burning, freckles, morphew, or the like; and taketh away the headache, coming of a cold cause, the head being bathed therewith. The leaves or flowers distilled in the month of May, and the legs often washed with the said distilled water, it taketh away the ulcers and sores of them. The eyes washed therewith, it cures the redness and blood shot; and the hands washed morning and evening therewith, is good for the palsy and shaking of them.

The dwarf elder is more powerful than the common elder in opening and purging choler, phlegm, and water; in curing the gout, piles, and women's diseases; it coloureth the hair black, cures inflammation of the eyes, pains in the ears, the biting of serpents and mad dogs, burnings and scaldings, colic and stone, the difficulty of voiding urine; it cures old sores and fistulous ulcers. Either leaves or bark of elder stripped upwards as you gather it, causeth vomiting. Dr. Butler, in a manuscript of his, commends dwarf elder to the skies for dropsies, being boiled in white wine and drank.

THE ELM TREE.

This tree is so well known, that it is needless to describe it.

Government and Virtues.—It is a cold Saturnine plant. The leaves bruised, heal green wounds, being bound thereon with its own bark. The leaves or bark used with vinegar, cureth scurf and leprosy very effectually. The decoction of the leaves, bark, or roots, being bathed, heals broken bones. The water that is found in the bladders on the leaves, while it is fresh, is very effectual to cleanse the skin and make it fair ; and if cloths be often wet therein and applied to the ruptures of children, it healeth them if they be well bound up with a truss. The said water put into a glass and set into the ground, or in a dung-heap for twenty-five days, the mouth thereof being close stopped, and the bottom set upon a lay of ordinary salt, that the fæces may settle and the water become clear, is a singular and sovereign balm for green wounds, being used with soft lint. The decoction of the bark of the root fomented, molifieth hard tumours, and the shrinking of the sinews. The roots of the elm boiled for a long time in water, and the fat arising on the top thereof being clean skimmed off, and the place anointed therewith that is grown bald, and the hair fallen away, will quickly restore them. The bark ground with brine and pickle until it come to the form of a poultice, and laid on the place pained with the gout, giveth great ease. The decoction of the bark in water, is excellent to bathe such places as have been burnt with fire.

ENDIVE.

Description.—Common garden endive beareth a longer and larger leaf than succory, and abideth but one year, quickly running up to stalk and seed, and then perisheth ; it hath blue flowers, and the seed of the ordinary endive is so like succory seed, that it is hard to distinguish them.

Government and Virtues.—It is a fine cooling, cleansing, plant. The decoction of the leaves, or the juice of the distilled water of endive, cooleth the excessive heat of the liver and stomach, and in the hot fits of agues, and all other inflammations in any part of the body : it cooleth the heat and sharpness of urine, and excoriations in the urinary parts. The seeds are of the same property, or rather more powerful, and besides are available for faintings, swoonings, and passions of the heart. Outwardly applied, they serve to temper the sharp humours of fretting ulcers, hot tumours, swellings and pestilential sores : and remove redness and inflammation of the eyes, and dimness of sight ; they are also used to allay pains of the gout ; a syrup of it is a fine cooling medicine for fevers.

ELECAMPANE.

Description.—It shooteth forth many large leaves, long and broad, lying near the ground, small at both ends, somewhat soft in handling, of a whitish green on the upper side and grey underneath, each set upon a short footstalk, from among which rise up divers great strong hairy stalks three or four feet high, with some leaves thereupon com·passing them about at the lower end, and are branched towards the tops, bearing great and large flowers like those of the corn marigold, both the borders of leaves and the middle thrum being yellow, which turn into down, with long small, brownish seeds among it, and is carried away with the wind. The root is large and thick, branching forth various ways, blackish on the outside and whitish within, of a very bitter taste, and strong but good scent, especially when they are dried, no part else of the plant having any smell.

Place.—It groweth in moist grounds and in shadowy places oftener than in the dry and open borders of fields and lanes, and in waste places.

Time.—It flowereth in the end of June and July, and the seed is ripe in August. The roots are gathered for use as well in the spring before the leaves come forth, as in autumn or winter.

Government and Virtues.—It is a plant under the dominion of Mercury. The fresh roots of elecampane preserved with sugar, or made into a conserve or a syrup, are very effectual to warm a cold windy stomach, and stitches in the sides caused by the spleen ; and to relieve cough, shortness of breath, and wheezing in the lungs. The dried root made into powder, and mixed with sugar and taken, serveth the same purpose ; and is also profitable for stoppage of urine, stopping of women's courses, pains of the mother, and of the stone in the reins, kidneys, or bladder ; it cures putrid and pestilential fevers, and even the plague. The roots and herbs beaten and put into new ale or beer, and daily drunk, cleareth, strengtheneth, and quickeneth the sight of the eyes. The decoction of the roots in wine, or the juice taken therein, destroys worms in the stomach and maw, and rectum ; and gargled in the mouth or the root chewed, fasteneth loose teeth and keeps them from putrefaction ; and being drunk, is good for spitting of blood ; it removes cramps or convulsions, gout, sciatica, pains in the joints, applied outwardly or inwardly, and is also good for those that are ruptured, or have any inward bruise. The root boiled well in vinegar, beaten afterwards, and made into an ointment with hog's suet or oil of trotters, is a most excellent remedy for scabs or itch in young or old ; the places also bathed or washed with the decoction doth the same ; it heals putrid sores or cankers. In the roots of this herb lieth the chief effect for the remedies aforesaid. The distilled water of the leaves and roots together, is very good to cleanse the skin of the face, or other parts, from any morphew, spots, or blemishes, and make it clear.

ERINGO, OR SEA HOLLY.

Description.—The first leaves of our ordinary sea holly are nothing so hard or prickly as when they grow old, being almost round and deep dented about the edges, hard and sharp-pointed, and a little crumpled, of a bluish green colour, every one upon a long foot-stalk ; but those that grow up higher with the stalk do as it were compass it about. The stalk itself is round and strong, yet somewhat crested with joints, and leaves set thereat, but more divided, sharp, and prickly, and branches rising from thence which have also other small branches, each of them having several bluish round prickly heads, with many small, jagged, prickly leaves under them standing like a star, and sometimes found greenish or whitish. The root groweth long, even to eight or ten feet in length, set with rings and circles towards the upper part, cut smooth and without joints down lower, brownish on the outside, and very white within, with a pith in the middle ; of a pleasant taste, but much more being candied with sugar.

Place.—It is found about the sea coast in almost every county of this land which bordereth on the sea.

Time.—It flowereth in the end of summer, and giveth ripe seed within a month after.

Government and Virtues.—The plant is venereal, and strengthens the spirits procreative; it is hot and moist, and under the celestial balance. The decoction of the root hereof in wine, is very effectual to open obstructions of the spleen and liver, and helpeth yellow jaundice, dropsy, pains of the loins and colic; provoketh urine, expelleth the stone, and procureth women's courses. The continued use of the decoction for fifteen days, taken fasting, and next to bedward, cures the strangury, the stopping of urine, stone, and all defects in the reins and kidneys; and if the said drink be continued longer, it is said that it cureth the stone. The roots bruised and applied outwardly, removes the kernels of the throat, called the king's evil; or taken inwardly, and applied to the place bitten or stung by any serpent, healeth it speedily. If the roots be bruised and boiled in hog's lard, or salted lard, and applied to broken bones, thorns, &c. in the flesh, they do not only draw them forth, but heal the place, gathering new flesh where it was consumed. The juice of the leaves dropped into the ear, helpeth imposthumes therein. The distilled water of the whole herb when the leaves and stalks are young, is profitably drunk for all the purposes aforesaid; and cures melancholy of the heart, and is available in quartan and quotidian agues, as also for them that have their necks drawn awry.

EYEBRIGHT.

Description.—Common eyebright is a small low herb, rising up usually but with one blackish green stalk a span high, or not much more, spread from the bottom into sundry branches, whereon are small and almost round, yet pointed, dark green leaves, finely snipped about the edges, two always set together, and very thick. At the joints with the leaves, from the middle upward, come forth small white flowers steeped with purple and yellow spots or stripes, after which follow small round heads with very small seeds therein. The root is long, small, and thready at the ends.

Place.—It groweth in meadows and grassy places of this land.

Government and Virtues.—It is under the sign of the Lion, and Sol claims dominion over it. If the herb was but as much used as it is neglected, it would half spoil the spectacle maker's trade ; and a man would think that reason should teach people to prefer the preservation of their natural before artificial spectacles, which that they may be instructed how to do, take the virtues of eyebright as followeth :— The juice or distilled water of the eyebright taken inwardly in white wine or broth, or dropped into the eyes for several days together, helpeth all infirmities of the eye that cause dimness of sight, Some make conserve of the flowers to the same effect. Being used any of the ways, it strengthens the weak brain or memory. This tunned with strong beer that it may work together, and drunk, or the powder of the dried herb, mixed with sugar, a little mace and fennel seed and drunk, or eaten in broth ; or the said powder made into an electuary with sugar, and taken, hath the same powerful effect to help and restore the sight decayed through age; and Arnoldus de Villa Nova saith, it hath restored sight to them that have been blind a long time.

FERN.

Description.—Of this there are two kinds principally to be treated of, viz. the male and female. The female groweth higher than the male but the leaves thereof are lesser, and more divided or dented, and of as strong a smell as the male. The virtues of them are alike.

Place.—They grow both in heaths and shady places near the hedge-sides in all counties of this land.

Time.—They flower and give their seed at Midsummer. The female fern is that plant which is in Sussex called brakes, the seed of which some authors hold to be so rare.

Government and Virtues.—It is under the dominion of Mercury, both male, and female. The roots of both sorts of fern being bruised and boiled in mead or honeyed water and drunk, killeth both the broad and long worms in the body, and abateth the swelling and hardness of the spleen. The green leaves eaten, purge the belly of choleric and waterish humours in the stomach. The roots bruised and boiled in oil or hog's lard, make a very profitable ointment to heal wounds. The powder used in foul ulcers, drieth up their malignant moisture, and causeth their speedier healing. Fern being burned, the smoke driveth away serpents, gnats, and other noisome creatures, which in fenny countries, in the night time, molest people lying in bed with their faces uncovered. It causeth barrenness.

OSMOND ROYAL, OR WATER FERN.

Description.—This shooteth forth in spring-time (for in the winter the leaves perish) many rough hard stalks half round and yellowish, or flat on the other side, two feet high, having divers branches of winged yellowish green leaves on all side, set one against another, longer, narrower, and not nicked at the edges as the former. From the top of some of these stalks grow a long bush of small and more yellow, green, scaly aglets, set in the same manner on the stalk as the leaves are, which are accounted the flowers and seed. The root is rough, thick, and scabby, with a white pith in the middle, which is called the heart.

Place.—It groweth on moors, bogs, and watery places.

Time.—It is green all the summer, and the root only abiding in the winter.

Government and Virtues.—Saturn owns the plant. It has all the virtues mentioned in the former fern, is much more effectual than both for inward and outward griefs, and is accounted good in wounds, bruises, or the like. The decoction to be drunk, or boiled into an ointment of oil, as a balsam or balm, and is good against bruises, and bones broken, or out of joint, and giveth much ease to the colic and splenetic diseases; and also for ruptures. The decoction of the root in white wine provoketh urine, and cleanseth the bladder and passages of urine.

FEVER-FEW, OR FEATHER-FEW.

Description.—Common feather-few hath large, fresh, green leaves, much torn or cut on the edges. The stalks are hard and round, set with many such like leaves, but smaller, and at the tops stand many single flowers upon small foot-stalks, consisting of many small white leaves round about a yellow thrum in the middle. The root is rather hard and short, with many strong fibres about it. The scent of the whole plant is very strong and stifling, and the taste very bitter.

Place.—It grows wild in some places, but it is for the most part cultivated in gardens.

Time.—It flowereth in the month of June and July.

Government and Virtues.—Venus governs this herb, and hath commended it to succour her sisters, women, and to be a general strengthener of their wombs, if the herb be boiled in white wine, and the decoction drunk ; it cleanseth the womb, expels the after-birth, and doth a woman all the good she can desire of an herb. If the herb cannot be got in winter ; a syrup of it may be made in summer ; it is chiefly used for the diseases of the mother, whether it be the hardness or inflammations of the same, applied outwardly, or a decoction of the flowers in wine, with a little nutmeg or mace put therein, and drunk often in a day, is an approved remedy to bring down women's courses speedily. For a woman to sit over the hot fumes of the decoction of the herb made in water or wine, is effectual for the same ; and some cases to apply the boiled herb warm to the privy parts. The decoction made with some sugar or honey is used by many to cure a cough and stuffing of the chest by colds, also to cleanse the reins and bladder, and to expel the stone.

The powder of the herb taken in wine with some oxymel, purgeth both choler and phlegm, and is available for those that are short-winded, and are troubled with melancholy and heaviness of spirits. It is very effectual for all pains in the head coming of a cold cause, the herb being bruised and applied to the crown of the head ; as also for the vertigo. The decoction drunk warm, and the herb bruised with a few corns of bay-salt, and applied to the wrists before the coming on of ague fits, do take them away The distilled water taketh away freckles and other spots and deformities of the face. The herb bruised and heated on a tile, with some wine to moisten it, or fried with a little wine and oil, and applied warm outwardly to the places, removes wind and colic in the lower part of the belly. It is an especial remedy against opium taken too liberally.

FENNEL.

MOST gardens grow it, and it needs no description.

Government and Virtues.—One good old custom is not yet left off, viz., to boil fennel with fish, for it consumes the phlegmatic humour which fish most plentifully afford and annoy the body with, though few that use it know wherefore they do it. It benefits this way, because it is an herb of Mercury, and under Virgo, and therefore bears antipathy to Pisces. Fennel expels wind, provokes urine, and eases the pains of the stone, and helps to break it. The leaves or seed boiled in barley water and drunk, are good for nurses, to increase their milk, and make it more wholesome for the child ; the leaves or rather the seeds, boiled in water, stayeth the hiccup, and taketh away nausea, or inclination to sickness. The seed and the roots much more help to open obstructions of the liver, spleen, and gall, and thereby relieve the painful and windy swellings of the spleen, and the yellow jaundice, as also the gout and cramp. The seed is of good use in medicines for shortness of breath and wheezing, by stopping of the lungs ; it helpeth also to bring down the courses, and to cleanse the parts after delivery. The roots are of most use in physic, drinks and broths, that are taken to cleanse the blood, to open obstructions of the liver, to provoke urine, and amend the ill colour of the face after sickness, and to cause a good habit through the body ; both leaves, seeds, and roots thereof, are much used in drink, or broth, to make people more lean that are too fat. A decoction of the leaves and root is good for serpent bites, and to neutralise vegetable poison, as mushrooms, &c. The distilled water of the whole herb, or the condensed juice dissolved, but especially the natural juice, that in some counties issueth out thereof of its own accord, dropped into the eyes, cleanseth them from mists and films. The sweet fennel is much weaker in physical uses than the common fennel. The wild fennel is stronger and hotter than the tame, and therefore most powerful against the stone, but not so effectual to increase milk, because of its dryness.

SOW FENNEL, OR HOG'S FENNEL.

BESIDES the commmon name in English, hog's fennel, and the Latin name pencidanum, it is called hoar-strange, and hoar-strong, sulphur-wort, and brimstone-wort.

Description.—The common sow-fennel hath several branched stalks of thick and rather long leaves, three for the most part joined together at a place, among which ariseth a crested straight stalk, less than fennel, with some joints thereon, and leaves growing thereat, and towards the top some branches issuing from thence ; on the tops of the stalks and branches stand divers tufts of yellow flowers, whereafter grows somewhat flat, thin, and yellowish seed, bigger than fennel-seed : the roots grow great and deep, with many other parts and fibres about them, of a strong scent like hot brimstone, and yield forth a yellowish milk, or clammy juice almost like a gum.

Place.—It groweth plentifully in the salt low marshes near Feversham, in Kent.

Time.—It flowereth plentifully in July and August.

Government and Virtues.—It is under Mercury. The juice of the sow-fennel (saith Dioscorides and Galen) used with vinegar and rose-water, or the juice with a little euphorbium put to the nose, benefits those that are troubled with the lethargy, frenzy, or giddiness of the head, the falling-sickness, long and inveterate head-ache, the palsy, sciatica, and the cramp, and generally all the diseases of the sinews, used with oil and vinegar. The juice dissolved in wine, or put into an egg, is good for a cough, or shortness of breath, and for those that are troubled with wind. It also purgeth gently, softens hardness of the spleen, giveth ease to women that have sore travail in child-birth, and easeth the pains of the reins and bladder. A little of the juice dissolved in wine and dropped into the ears, or into a hollow tooth, easeth the pains thereof. The root is less effectual to all the aforesaid disorders ; yet the powder of the root cleanseth foul ulcers, being put into them, and taketh out splinters of broken bones, or other things in the flesh, and healeth them perfectly; it drieth old running sores, and is of admirable virtue in all green wounds, and prevents gangrene.

FIG-WORT, OR THROAT-WORT.

Description.—Common great fig-wort sendeth many great, strong, hard, square brown stalks, three or four feet high, whereon grow large, hard, and dark green leaves, two at a joint, harder and larger than nettle leaves, but not stinging; at the tops of the stalks stand many purple flowers set in husks, which are sometimes gaping and open, somewhat like those of water betony; after which come hard round heads, with a small point in the middle, wherein lie small brownish seed. The root is large, white, and thick, with many branches, growing aslope under the upper crust of the ground, which abideth many years, but keepeth not its green leaves in winter.

Place.—It groweth in moist and shady woods, and in the lower parts of the fields and meadows.

Time.—It flowereth about July, and the seed will be ripe about a month after the leaves are fallen.

Government and Virtues.—Some Latin authors call it cervicaria, because it is appropriated to the neck; and we throatwort, because it is appropriated to the throat. Venus owns the herb, and the celestial Bull will not deny it; therefore a better remedy cannot be for the king's evil, because the moon that rules the disease is exalted there. The decoction of the herb taken inwardly and the bruised herb applied outwardly, dissolveth clotted and congealed blood within the body, coming by any wounds, bruise, or fall; and is no less effectual for the king's evil, or any other knobs, kernels, or wens growing in the flesh; and for the piles. An ointment made hereof may be used at all times when the fresh herb is not to be had. The distilled water of the whole herb, roots and all, is used for the same purposes, and drieth up the virulent moisture of hollow and corroding ulcers; it taketh away all redness, spots, and freckles in the face; as also the scurf, and any foul deformity therein, and the leprosy.

FILIPENDULA, OR DROP-WORT.

Description.--This sendeth forth many leaves, some large, some less, set on each side of a middle rib, and each of them dented about the edges, somewhat resembling wild tansy, or agrimony, but harder in handling ; among which rise up one or more stalks, two or three feet high, with the leaves growing thereon, and sometimes also divided into other branches, spreading at the top into many white, sweet smelling flowers, consisting of five leaves a-piece, with some threads in the middle of them, standing together, in a pith or umbel, each upon a small foot-stalk, which, after they have been blown upon a good while, do fall away, and in their places appear small, round, chaffy heads like buttons, wherein are the chaffy seeds set and placed. The root consists of many small, black, tuberous pieces, fastened together by many small, long, blackish strings, which run from one to another.

Place.— It groweth in many places of this land in the corners of dry fields and meadows, and the hedge sides.

Time.— They flower in June and July, and their seed is ripe in August.

Government and Virtues.— It is under the dominion of Venus. It effectually opens the passages of the urine, helpeth the strangury, the stone in the kidneys and bladder, the gravel, and all other pains of the bladder, the gravel, and all other pains of the bladder and reins, by taking the roots in powder, or a decoction of them in white wine, with a little honey. The roots in powder, mixed with honey as an electuary, doth help those whose stomachs are swollen, expelling the wind as the cause thereof ; and is also very effectual for all the diseases of the lungs, as shortness of breath, wheezing, hoarseness of the throat, and cough ; and to expectorate tough phlegm. It is called dropwort because it benefits those who urinate by drops.

THE YELLOW WATER-FLAG, or FLOWER-DE-LUCE.

Description.— This groweth like the flower-de-luce, but hath much longer and narrower sad green leaves joined together in that fashion; the stalk also growing often as high, bearing small yellow flowers shaped like the flower-de-luce, with three falling leaves, and other three arched, that cover their bottoms; but instead of the three upright leaves, as the flower-de-luce hath, this hath only three short pieces standing in their places, after which succeed thick and long three square heads, containing in each part flat seed, like those of the flower-de-luce. The root is long and slender, of a pale brownish colour on the outside, and of a horse-flesh colour inside, with many hard fibres, and very harsh in taste.

Place.—It usually grows in watery ditches, ponds, lakes, and moor sides overflowed with water.

Time. — It flowereth in July, and the seed is ripe in August.

Government and Virtues.—It is under the dominion of the Moon. The root of this water-flag is very astringent, cooling, and drying, and thereby restrains lasks and fluxes, whether of blood or humours, as bleeding at the mouth, nose or other parts, bloody-flux, and women's courses. The distilled water of the whole herb, flowers, and roots, is a sovereign remedy for watering eyes, both to be dropped into them, and to have cloths or sponges wetted therein and applied to the forehead; it also removeth spots and blemishes about the eyes or any other parts. This distilled water fomented on swellings, inflammations of women's breasts, upon cankers, and those spreading ulcers called *noli me tangere,* do much good. It cureth also foul ulcers in the privities of men or women; but an ointment made of the flowers is better for external applications.

FLAX-WEED, or TOAD-FLAX.

Description.—Our common flax-weed hath several stalks full fraught with long and narrow ash-coloured leaves, and from the middle of them almost upward, stored with a number of pale yellow flowers, of a strong unpleasant scent, with deeper yellow mouths, and blackish flat seed in round heads. The root is rather woody and white, especially the main downright one, with many fibres, abiding

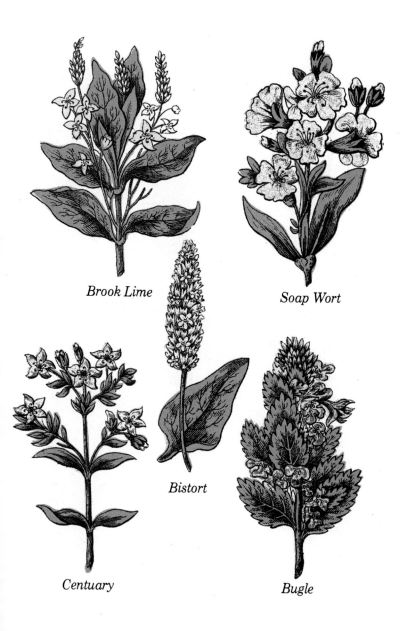

Brook Lime

Soap Wort

Bistort

Centuary

Bugle

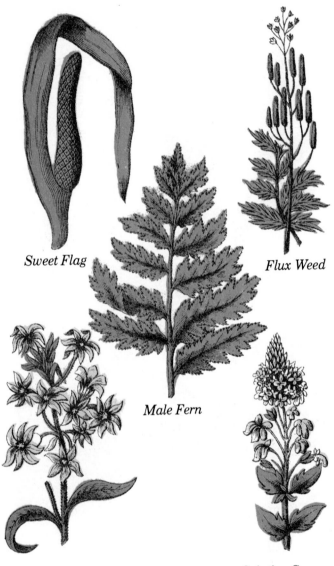

Sweet Flag

Flux Weed

Male Fern

Golden Rod

Sciatica Cress

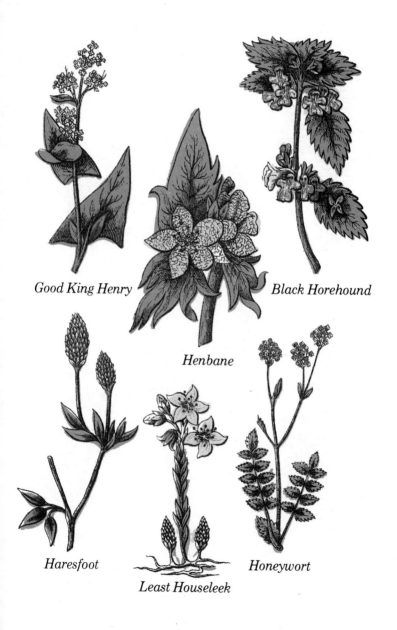

Good King Henry

Black Horehound

Henbane

Haresfoot

Least Houseleek

Honeywort

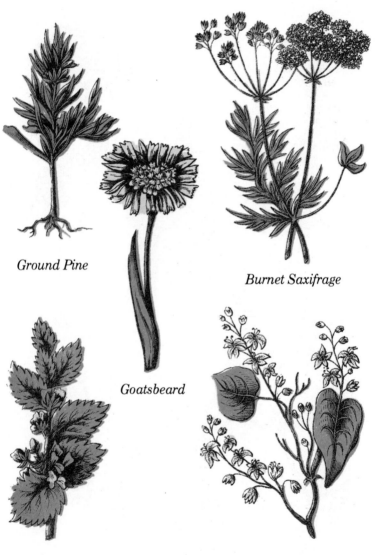

Ground Pine

Burnet Saxifrage

Goatsbeard

White Horehound

Bryony

many years, shooting forth roots, every way round about, and new branches every year.

Place.—This groweth by the way sides and in meadows, as also by hedge sides, and on banks and borders of fields.

Time.—It flowereth in summer, and the seed is ripe usually before the end of August.

Government and Virtues.—Mars owns this herb. In Sussex we call it gallwort, and lay it in our chicken's water to cure them of the gall ; it relieves them when they are drooping. It is often used to expel watery humours by urine which cause the dropsy. The decoction of the herb, both leaves and flowers, taken in wine and drunk, gently purges, and removes obstructions of the liver, cures the yellow jaundice ; expelleth poison, and provoketh women's courses. The distilled water of the herb and flowers is effectual for all the same purposes; being drunk with a drachm of the powder of the seeds or bark, or the roots of wall-wort and a little cinnamon for certain days together, it is held a singular remedy for the dropsy. The juice of the herb, or the distilled water, dropped into the eyes, is a certain remedy for inflammation, and redness in them. The juice or water put into foul ulcers, whether they be cancerous or fistulous, with tents rolled therein, or parts washed and injected therein, cleanseth them thoroughly from the bottom, and healeth them. The same juice or water also cleanseth the skin from mor-phew, scurf, wheals, pimples or spots, applied of itself, or used with some powder of lupins.

FLEA-WORT.

Description.—Ordinary flea-wort riseth up with a stalk two feet high or more, full of joints and branches on every side up to the top, and at every joint two small, long, and narrow whitish green leaves, somewhat hairy. At the top of every branch stand small, short, scaly, or chaffy heads, out of which come forth small whitish yellow threads, like those of the plantain herbs, which are the bloomings of flowers. The seed inclosed in these heads is small and shining while it is fresh, very like unto fleas both for colour and size, but turning black when it groweth old.

I

The root is not long, but white, hard, and woody, perishing every year, and rising again of its own seed, if it be suffered to shed. The whole plant is somewhat whitish and hairy, smelling like resin.

There is another sort differing not from the former in the way of growing, but only that this stalk and branches being somewhat greater do a little more bow down to the ground. The leaves are somewhat larger, the heads somewhat lesser, the seed alike ; and the root and leaves abide all the winter, and perish not as the former.

Place.—The first groweth only in gardens, the second plentifully in fields that are near the sea.

Time.—They flower in July, or thereabouts.

Government and Virtues.—The herb is cold, dry, and Saturnine. I suppose it obtained the name of flea-wort because the seeds are like fleas. The seed fried, and taken, stayeth the flux or lask of the belly, and the corrosions that come by reason of hot, choleric, or malignant humours, or by too much purging of any violent medicine, as scammony, or the like. The mucilage of the seed made with rose water, and a little sugar-candy, is very good in all hot agues and burning fevers, and other inflammations, to cool the thirst and lenify the dryness and roughness of the tongue and throat. It cures hoarseness, and diseases of the breast and lungs caused by heat, or sharp salt humours, and the pleurisy also. The mucilage of the seed made with plantain water, to which the yolk of an egg or two, and a little populeon are put is a most safe and sure remedy to ease the sharpness, pricking, and pain of the piles, if it be laid on a cloth and bound thereto. It is good for inflammations in any part of the body, and the pains that come thereby, as the headache and megrims, imposthumes, swellings, or breaking out of the skin, as blains, weals, pushes, purples, and the like ; as also the joints of those that are out of joint, the pains of the gout and sciatica, the ruptures of young children, and the swellings of the navel, applied with oil of roses and vinegar. It is also good to heal the nipples and sore breasts of women, being often applied thereunto. The juice of the herb, with a little honey, put into the ears, stays the running of them, the same also mixed with hog's lard, and applied to corrupt and filthy ulcers, cleanseth and healeth them.

FLUXWEED.

Description.—It riseth with a round, upright hard stalk, four or five feet high, spread into sundry branches, whereon grow many greyish green leaves, very finely cut and severed into a number of short and almost round parts. The flowers are very small and yellow, growing spike fashion, after which come small long pods with small yellowish seed in them. The root is long and woody, perishing every year.

There is another sort differing only in having rather broader leaves : they have a strong scent, and are of a drying taste.

Place.— They grow wild in the fields by hedge-sides and highways, and among rubbish and other places.

Time.—They flower and seed in June and July.

Government and Virtues.—This herb is Saturnine. Both the herb and seed of fluxweed are of excellent use to stay the flux or lask of the belly, being drunk in water wherein gads of steel heated have been often quenched ; and it is no less effectual for the same purpose than plantain or comfrey, and to restrain any other flux of blood in man or woman, as also to consolidate bones broken or out of joint. The juice drunk in wine, or the decoction of the herb drunk, kills worms in the stomach or belly, or the worms that grow in putrid ulcers ; and made into a salve doth quickly heal all old sores. The distilled water of the herb worketh the same effects, although somewhat weaker, yet it is a fair medicine, and more acceptable to be taken. It is called fluxweed because it cures the flux, and for its uniting broken bones, &c. Paracelsus extols it to the skies. It is fitting that syrup, ointment, and plasters of it were kept in your houses.

FLOWER-DE-LUCE.

It is so well known, being nourished in most gardens, that I shall not give any description.

Time. —The flaggy kinds thereof have the most physical uses : the dwarf kinds thereof flower in April, the greater sorts in May.

Government and Virtues. —The herb is Lunar.   The juice or the decoction of the green root of the flaggy kind of flower-de-luce, with a little honey drunk, doth purge and cleanse the stomach of gross and tough phlegm and choler, it cures the jaundice and dropsy, evacuating those humours both upwards and downwards, because it rather hurts the stomach, it is not to be taken without honey or spikenard. The same being drunk, eases the pains and torments of the belly and sides, the shaking of agues, the diseases of the liver and spleen, worms, the stone, convulsions and cramps that come of old humours : it is good for those whose seed passes from them unawares : it is a remedy against the bitings and stingings of venomous creatures, being boiled in water and vinegar and drunk, it provoketh urine, help-eth the colic, bringeth down women's courses ; and made into a pessary with honey, and put into the body, draweth forth the dead child.   It is much commended for cough, to expectorate tough phlegm ; it easeth pains in the head, and procureth sleep ; being put into the nostrils it pro-cureth sneezing, and thereby purgeth the head of phlegm ; the juice of the root applied to the piles it giveth much ease ; the decoction of the roots gargled in the mouth easeth the toothache, and cures a stinking breath.   Oil called oleum irinum, if it be right made of the great broad flag flower-de-luce (and not of the great bulbous blue flower-de-luce, as is used by some apothecaries) and the roots of the flaggy kind, is very effectual to warm and comfort all cold joints and sinews, and the gout and sciatica, and molli-fieth, dissolveth, and consumeth tumours and swellings in any part of the body, as also of the matrix ; it relieves cramp or convulsions of the sinews : the head and temples anointed therewith is good for catarrh, or thin rheum dis-tilled from thence ; and is used upon the breast or stomach, helpeth to extenuate the cold tough phlegm ; it cures also pains and noise in the ears, and the stench of the nostrils : the root itself, either green or in powder, tends to cleanse, heal, and to cover the naked bones with flesh again that ulcers have made bare ; and is also very good to cleanse and heal fistulas and cankers, that are hard to be cured.

FLUELLIN, or LLUELLIN.

Description.— It shooteth forth many long branches, partly lying upon the ground and partly standing upright, set with almost red leaves, yet a little pointed and sometimes more long than round, without order thereon, somewhat hairy, and of an evil greenish white colour ; at the joints all along the stalks and with the leaves come forth small flowers, one at a place, upon a very small short foot-stalk, gaping like snap-dragons, or rather like toadflax, with the upper jaw of a yellow colour, and the lower of a purplish, with a small heel or spur behind ; after which come forth small round heads, containing small black seed. The root is small and thready, dying every year, and raiseth itself again of its own sowing.

There is another sort of lluellin which hath longer branches, wholly trailing upon the ground, two or three feet long and somewhat more thin, set with leaves thereon upon small foot-stalks. The leaves are a little larger and somewhat round, and cornered sometimes in some places on the edges ; but the lower part of them being the broadest hath on each side a small point, making it seem as if they were ears, sometimes hairy, but not hoary, and of a better green colour than the former. The flowers come forth like the former ; but the colours therein are more white than yellow, and the purple not so fair ; it is a large flower, and so are the seed and seed vessels. The root is like the other, and perisheth every year.

Place.—They grow in corn-fields, and in borders about them, and in fertile grounds, &c.

Time.—They are in flower about June, and July, and the whole plant is dry and withered before August is over.

Government and Virtues.—It is a Lunar herb. The leaves bruised and applied with barley meal to watering eyes that are hot and inflamed by defluctions from the head, do very much help them, as also the fluxes of blood or humours, as the lask, bloody-flux, women's courses ; and stayeth all manner of bleeding at the nose, mouth or any other place, or that cometh by any bruise or hurt, or bursting a vein, it wonderfully helpeth all those inward parts that need consolidating or strengthening, and is no less effectual both to heal and close green wounds than to heal all foul ulcers, or it may be made into an ointment with hog's lard, and spermaceti, for the same purpose.

When simples were in use, men's bodies were better in health than now they are under the care of some physicians. The truth is this herb is of a fine cooling, drying quality, and an ointment or plaster of it might do a man a courtesy that hath any hot virulent sores ; it is admirable for ulcers of the French pox—if taken inwardly may cure the disease. It was first called female speedwell, but a gentleman of Wales, whose nose was almost eaten off with the pox, and so near the matter that the doctors commanded it to be cut off, being cured only by the use of this herb, and to honour the herb for saving his nose, gave it one of the country's names, Fluellin.

FOX-GLOVES.

Description.—It hath many long and broad leaves lying upon the ground dented about the edges, a little soft or woolly, and of a hoary green colour, among which rise up sometimes sundry stalks, but one very often, bearing such leaves thereon from the bottom to the middle, from whence to the top it is stored with large and long hollow reddish purple flowers, bell-shaped, with some white spots with them one above another, with small green leaves at every one, but all of them turning their heads one way, and hanging downwards, having some threads also in the middle, from whence rise round heads pointed sharp at the ends, wherein small brown seed lieth. The roots are so many small fibres, and some greater strings among them ; the flowers have no scent, but the leaves have a bitter hot taste.

Place.—It groweth on dry sandy ground for the most part, and on the higher as the lower places under hedge-sides, and on some banks.

Time.—It seldom flowereth before July, and the seed is ripe in August.

Government and Virtues.—The plant is under the dominion of Venus, being of a gentle cleansing nature, and very friendly to nature. The herb is familiarly and frequently used by the Italians to heal any fresh or green wounds, the leaves being but bruised and bound thereon, and the juice thereof is also used in old sores, to cleanse, dry, and heal them. The decoction made up with some sugar or honey, is available to purge and cleanse the body both upward and downward, sometimes of tough phlegm and clammy humours, and to open obstructions of the liver and spleen. It hath been found by experience to be available for the king's evil, the herb bruised and applied, or an ointment made with the juice thereof and so used : and a decoction of two handfuls thereof with four ounces of polypody in ale, hath been found by late experience to cure a person of the falling sickness, who had been troubled with it above twenty years. I am confident that an ointment of it is one of the best remedies for a scabby head that is.

FUMITORY

Description. — Our common fumitory is a tender sappy herb, sending forth from one square a slender weak stalk, and leaning downwards on all sides many branches two or three feet long, with finely cut and jagged leaves of whitish, or rather bluish sea-green colour ; at the tops of the branches stand many small flowers, in a long spike one above the other, made like little birds, of a reddish purple colour, with whitish bellies, after which come small round husks containing small black seeds. The root is yellow, small, and not very long, full of juice while it is green, but quickly perishing with the ripe seed. It beareth white flowers.

Place. — It groweth in corn-fields almost everywhere, as well as in gardens.

Time. — It flowereth in May for the most part, and the seed ripeneth shortly after.

Government and Virtues. — Saturn owns the herb, and presents it to the world as a cure for his own disease, and strengthener of the parts of the body he rules. If you find Saturn author of the disease, or if by direction from a nativity you fear a Saturnine disease approaching, you may by this herb prevent it in the one, and cure it in the other, and therefore it is fit that you should keep a syrup always by you. The juice or syrup made thereof, or the decoction made in whey by itself, with some other purging or opening herbs and roots to cause it to work the better, (itself being but weak) is very effectual for the liver and spleen, opening the obstructions thereof, and clarifying the blood from saltish and choleric humours, which cause leprosy, scabs, tetters, and itches, and such like breakings out of the skin, and after the purgings doth strengthen all the inward parts. It is also good against the yellow jaundice, and spendeth it by urine, which it procureth in abundance. The powder of the dried herb given for some time, cureth melancholy, but the seed is strongest in operation for all the former diseases. The distilled water of the herb is also of good effect in the aforesaid diseases. The distilled water also, with a little water and honey of roses, cureth sore mouths, or sore throats, being gargled often therewith. The juice dropped into the eyes cleareth the sight, and taketh away redness and other defects in them. The juice of fumitory and docks mingled with vinegar and the places gently washed or wet therewith, cureth all sorts of scabs, pimples, blotches, wheals and pushes, which arise on the face or hands, or any other parts of the body.

THE FURZE BUSH.

It is as well known by this name, as it is in some counties by the name of gorz or whins; it is so well known that a description is unnecessary.

Place.—They are known to grow on dry barren heaths, and other waste, gravelly, or sandy grounds in all counties of this land.

Time.—They also flower in the summer months.

Government and Virtues.—Mars owns the herb. It is hot and dry, and opens obstructions of the liver and spleen. A decoction made with the flowers thereof hath been found effectual against jaundice, and also to provoke urine, and cleanse the kidneys from gravel or stone engendered in them. Mars doth also this by sympathy.

GARLICK.

THE offensiveness of the breath of him that hath eaten garlick, will lead by the nose to the knowledge hereof, and instead of a description, direct you to the places where it groweth in gardens, which kinds are the best and most physical.

Government and Virtues.—Mars owns this herb. This was anciently accounted a remedy for all diseases and hurts except those which itself breeds. It provoketh urine and women's courses, curing the biting of mad dogs and other venomous creatures; it killeth worms in children, cutteth and voideth tough phlegm, purgeth the head, cureth lethargy, is a good preservative against and a remedy for any plague, sore, or foul ulcer; taketh away spots and blemishes in the skin, easeth pains in the ears, ripeneth and breaketh imposthumes and other swellings; and for all these diseases the onions are nearly as effectual. But the garlic hath some more peculiar virtues, viz., it hath a special quality to discuss inconveniences coming by corrupt agues or mineral vapours, or by drinking impure water. It is an antidote against poisonous or dangerous herbs. It is held good in dropsy, the jaundice, falling sickness, cramps, convulsions, and piles. Many authors quote many diseases garlic is good for, but conceal its vices. Its heat is very vehement, and all vehement hot things send up ill-favoured vapours to the brain. In choleric men it will add fuel to the fire; in men oppressed by melancholy, it will attenuate the humour, and send up strong fancies, and as many strange visions to the head; therefore let it be taken inwardly with great moderation-- outwardly you may make more bold with it.

GENTIAN, FELWORT, OR BALDMONY.

IT is confessed that gentian which is most used amongst us is brought from beyond the sea, yet we have two sorts of it growing in our nation, which, besides the reasons so frequently alleged why English herbs should be fittest for English bodies, hath been proved by the experience of physicians to be not a whit inferior in virtue to the foreign.

Description.—The greater of the two hath many small long roots striking deep into the ground, and abiding all the winter. The stalks are sometimes more, sometimes fewer, of a brownish green colour, which is sometimes two feet high if the ground be fruitful, having many long, narrow dark green leaves set by couples up to the top; the flowers are long and hollow, of a purple colour, ending in fine corners. The smaller sort which is to be found in our land, groweth up with sundry stalks not a foot high, parted into several small branches, whereon grow divers small leaves together, very like those of the lesser centaury, of a whitish green colour; on the tops of these stalks grow perfect blue flowers standing in long husks, but not so large as the other; the root is small and full of threads.

Place.—The first groweth in several places of both the east and west countries, and as well in wet as in dry grounds, as near Longfield by Gravesend, and also divers places in Kent, Bedfordshire, and other warm counties.

Time.—They flower in August.

Government and Virtues.—They are under the dominion of Mars, and one of the chief herbs he is ruler of. It resists putrefaction, poison, and a surer remedy cannot be found to prevent the pestilence than it is; it strengthens the stomach exceedingly, helps digestion, comforts the heart, and preserves it against faintings and swoonings. The powder of the dry roots cures the biting of mad dogs and venomous beasts, opens obstructions of the liver, and restoreth lost appetite. The herb steeped in wine, and the wine drunk, refresheth such as be over weary with travel, and those who are lame in their joints by cold; it cures stitches and pains in the sides : is an excellent remedy for such as are bruised by falls; it provokes urine and the terms; the same is very effectual for cramps and convulsions, to drink the decoction; it breaks the stone, and cures ruptures most certainly; it is excellent in all cold diseases, and for voiding tough phlegm, and curing scabs, itch, or any fretting sores and ulcers; it effectually kills worms, by taking half a drachm of the powder in a morning in any convenient liquor; the same is good taken inwardly for the king's evil. It helpeth agues of all sorts, and the yellow jaundice, as also the bots in cattle : when kine are bitten on the udder by any venomous beast, rub the place with the decoction of any of these, and it will instantly heal them.

CLOVE GILLIFLOWERS.

It is in vain to describe an herb so well known

Government and Virtues.—They are gallant, fine, temperate flowers, under the dominion of Jupiter ; yea, so temperate, that no excess neither in heat, cold, dryness, nor moisture can be perceived in them ; they are great strengtheners both of the brain and heart, and will therefore do either for cordials or cephalics, as your occasion will serve. There is both a syrup and a conserve made of them alone, commonly to be had of any apothecary. To take now and then a little of either, strengthens nature much in such as are in consumptions ; they are good in hot pestilent fevers, and expel poison.

GERMANDER.

Description.—Common Germander shooteth forth sundry stalks with small and somewhat round leaves, dented about the edges ; the flowers stand at the tops of a deep purple colour ; the root is composed of divers sprigs, which shoot forth a great way round about, quickly overspreading a garden.

Place.—It groweth usually with us in gardens.

Time.—And flowereth in June and July.

Government and Virtues.—It is an herb of Mercury, and strengthens the brain exceedingly. Taken with honey, (saith Dioscorides) it is a remedy for coughs, hardness of the spleen, and difficulty of making urine, and helpeth those that are fallen into a dropsy, especially at the beginning of the disease, a decoction being made thereof when it is green, and drunk : it also promotes women's courses, and expelleth the dead child. It is most effectual against the poison of all serpents, being drunk in wine, and the bruised herb outwardly applied. Used with honey it cleanseth old and foul ulcers : and made into an oil and the eyes anointed therewith, taketh away dimness and moistness : it is also good for pains in the sides and cramps. The decoction taken for four days, driveth away and cureth tertian and quartan agues. It is also good against all diseases of the brain, as continual head-ache, falling sickness, melancholy, drowsiness, and dulness of spirits, convulsions and palsies. A drachm of the seed taken in powder promotes urine, and is good against the yellow jaundice : the juice of the leaves dropped into the ears killeth worms in them. The tops thereof, when they are in flower, steeped twenty-four hours in a draught of white wine, and drunk, killeth worms.

STINKING GLADWIN.

Description.—This is one of the kinds of flower-de-luce having divers leaves arising from the roots very like a flower-de-luce, but that they are sharp-edged on both sides, and thicker in the middle, of a deeper green colour, narrower and sharper pointed, and a strong ill scent, if they be bruised between the fingers. In the middle riseth up a strong stalk, a yard high, bearing three or four flowers at the top, made somewhat like the flowers of the flower-de-luce, with three upright leaves, of a dead purple ash colour, with some veins discoloured in them : the other three do not fall down, nor are the three other small ones so arched nor cover the lower leaves as the flower-de-luce doth, but stand loose or asunder from them. After they are past, there cometh up three square hard husks, opening wide into three parts when they are ripe, wherein lie reddish seed, turning black when it hath abiden long. The root is like that of the flower-de-luce, but reddish on the outside, and whitish within, very hot in taste, of a bad scent.

Place.—This groweth as well in upland grounds as in moist places, woods, and shadowy places by the sea-side in many places of this land, and in some gardens.

Time.—It flowereth in July, and the seed is ripe in August or September ; yet the husks after they are ripe, opening themselves, will hold their seed with them for two or three months.

Government and Virtues.—It is under the dominion of Saturn. It is used by many country people to purge corrupt phlegm and choler, by drinking the decoction of the roots ; and some infuse the sliced roots in ale ; and some take the leaves, which serve well for weaker stomachs. The juice snuffed up the nose, causeth sneezing, and draweth from the head much corruption ; and the powder doth the same. The powder in wine, and drunk, relieves those that are troubled with cramps and convulsions, or with the gout and sciatica, and giveth ease in griping pains, and it cures the strangury. It is given with much profit to those that have had long fluxes by the sharp and evil quality of humours which it stayeth, having first cleansed and purged them by the drying and binding property therein. The root boiled in wine and drunk, procures women's courses ; and used as a pessary, worketh the same effect ; but causeth abortion in women with child. Half a drachm of the seed beaten into powder, and taken in wine, promotes urine. Taken with vinegar it dissolveth the swelling of the spleen. The root is very effectual in all wounds, especially of the head : as also to draw forth any splinters, thorns, or to heal broken bones, or any other thing sticking in the flesh without causing pain, being used with a little verdigrease and honey, and the great centaury root ; the same boiled in vinegar, and laid upon any tumour or swelling, doth very effectually dissolve and consume them ; yea, even the swellings of the throat called king's evil. The juice of the leaves or roots cures the itch, and all running or spreading scabs, sores, blemishes.

GOLDEN ROD.

Description.—This riseth up with brownish small round stalks, two feet high and sometimes more, having thereon many narrow and long dark green leaves, very seldom with any dents about the edges, or any stalks or white spots therein, yet they are sometimes so found divided at the top into many small branches, with divers small yellow flowers on every one of them, all which are turned one way, and being ripe do turn into down, and are carried away by the wind. The root consists of many small fibres, which grow not deep into the ground, but abideth all the winter therein, shooting forth new branches every year.

Place.—It groweth in the open places of woods and

copies, both moist and dry grounds, in many places of this land.

Time.—It flowereth about the month of July.

Government and Virtues.—It is governed by Venus. Arnoldus de Villa Nova commends it much against the stone in the reins and kidneys, and to provoke urine in abundance, whereby also the gravel and stone may be voided. The decoction of the herb, green or dry, or the distilled water thereof, is very effectual for inward bruises ; as also to be outwardly applied it stayeth bleeding in any part of the body, and of wounds ; also the fluxes of humours, the bloody flux and women's courses ; and is no less prevalent in ruptures, being drunk and outwardly applied. It is a sovereign wound herb, inferior to none both for inward and outward hurt ; green wounds, old sores, and ulcers, are quickly cured therewith. It is also of especial use in all lotions for sores or ulcers in the mouth, throat, or privy parts in man or woman. The decoction fasten teeth that are loose in the gums.

GOUTWORT, or HERB GERRARD.

Description.—It is a low herb, seldom rising above half a yard high, having sundry leaves standing on brownish green stalks by threes, snipped about, and a strong unpleasant savour ; the umbels of the flowers are white, and the seed blackish ; the root runneth in the ground, quickly taking a great deal of room.

Place.—It groweth by edges and wall-sides, and often in corners of fields, and in gardens.

Time.—It flowereth and seedeth about the end of July.

Government and Virtues.—Saturn rules it. Goutwort is effectual to cure gout and sciatica ; as also joint aches and other cold griefs.

GROMEL.

THERE are several kinds, which I will describe.

Description. — The greater gromel groweth up with slender, hard, and hairy stalks, trailing and taking root in the ground as it lieth thereon, and parted into many other small branches, with hairy dark green leaves thereon. At the joints with the leaves come forth very small blue flowers, and then hard stony roundish seed. The root is long and woody, abiding the winter, and shooteth forth fresh stalks in the spring.

The smaller wild gromel sendeth forth divers upright hard branched stalks two or three feet high, full of joints, at every one of which groweth small, long, hard, and rough leaves like the former, but lesser ; among which leaves come forth small white flowers, and after them greyish round seed like the former. The root is not large, but hath many strings.

The garden gromel hath divers upright, slender, woody, hairy stalks, blown and cressed, very little branched, with leaves like the former, and white flowers ; after which, in rough brown husks, is contained a white, hard, round seed, shining like pearls, and greater than either of the former : the root is like the first described, with divers branches and sprigs thereat, which continueth all the winter.

Place.—The two first grow wild in barren or untilled places, by way-sides, and in gardens.

Time.—They all flower from Midsummer until September, and in the meantime the seed ripeneth.

Government and Virtues.—The herb is under Venus ; and therefore if Mars cause the colic or stone, as usually he doth if in Virgo, this is your cure. These are most effectual to break the stone and to void it, and the gravel ; also to provoke urine being stopped, and to help the strangury. The seed is of greater use, being bruised and boiled in white wine or in broth, or the like, or the powder of the seed taken therein. Two drachms of the seed in powder taken with women's breast milk, is very effectual to procure a speedy delivery to such women as have sore pains in their travail, and cannot be delivered. The herb itself (when the seed is not to be had) either boiled, or the juice thereof drunk, is effectual to all the purposes aforesaid, but not so powerful and speedy in operation.

GOOSEBERRY-BUSH.

CALLED also feadberry, and, in Sussex, dewberry-bush, and in some counties wineberry.

Government and Virtues.—They are under the dominion of Venus. The berries, while they are unripe, being scalded or baked, are good to stir up a fainting or decayed appetite, especially for stomachs afflicted by choleric humours : they are good to stay the longings of women with child : you may keep them preserved with sugar all the year long. The decoction of the leaves of the tree cools hot swellings, and inflammations, and St. Anthony's fire. The ripe gooseberries are an excellent remedy to allay the violent heat both of the stomach and liver. The young tender leaves break the stone, and expel gravel.

WINTER-GREEN.

Description. — This sends forth seven, eight, or nine leaves, from a small brown creeping root, every one standing upon a long foot-stalk, which are almost as broad as long, round pointed, of a sad green colour, and like the leaf of a pear-tree ; from whence arises a slender stalk, yet standing upright, bearing at the top many small white sweet-smelling flowers like a star, consisting of five round pointed leaves, with many yellowish threads standing in the middle about a green head, and a long stalk with them, which groweth to be the seed-vessel, which being ripe is found five square, with a small point at it, wherein is contained seed as small as dust.

Place.—It groweth frequently in the woods northwards, viz. in Yorkshire, Lancashire, and Scotland.

Time.—It flowereth about June and July.

Government and Virtue.—It is under the dominion of Saturn, and is a first-rate wound remedy, to heal green wounds speedily, the green leaves being bruised and applied, or the juice of them. A salve made of the green herb stamped, or the juice boiled with hog's lard, or with salad oil and wax, and a little turpentine, is a sovereign salve, and highly extolled by the Germans who use it to heal all manner of wounds and sores. The herb boiled in wine and water, and drunk by those who have any inward ulcers in their kidneys or neck of the bladder, doth wonderfully help them. It stayeth all fluxes, as the lask, bloody fluxes, women's courses, and bleeding of wounds, and taketh away inflammations and pains of the heart ; it cures obstinate ulcers, and cankers or fistulas. The distilled water of the herb effectually performs the same.

GROUNDSEL.

Description. —Our common groundsel hath a round green and brownish stalk spreading towards the top into branches, set with long narrow green leaves cut in on the edges, like oak leaves, but lesser, and round at the end. At the tops of these branches stand many small green heads, out of which grow small yellow flowers, which are followed by downy seed. The plant is well known.

Place.—This groweth almost every where, amongst rubbish and untilled grounds, and in gardens.

Time.—It flowereth almost in every month in the year.

Government and Virtues.—This herb is under Venus, and is as gallant and universal a medicine for all diseases coming of heat, in any part of the body, it is very safe and friendly to the body of man, yet causeth vomiting if the stomach be weak, or gentle purging; it is moist and cold, thereby causing expulsion, and repressing the heat caused by the motion of the internal parts in purges and vomits. This herb preserved in a syrup, in a distilled water, or in an ointment, is a remedy in all hot diseases and will do it, 1.—safely, 2.—speedily.

The decoction of the herb, said Dioscorides, made with wine and drunk, helpeth the pains in the stomach, proceeding of choler, (which it may do well by a vomit) as daily experience showeth. The juice thereof taken in drink, or the decoction of it in ale gently performeth the same. It is good against the jaundice and falling sickness, taken in wine ; and for difficulty in making water. It expels gravel in the reins or kidneys, a drachm given in oxymel after some walking and stirring of the body. It relieves sciatica, griping, and colic ; defects of the liver, and provoketh women's courses. The fresh herb boiled and made into a poultice, applied to the breasts of women that are swollen with pain and heat, as also the privy parts of man or woman, the seat or fundament, or the arteries, joints, and sinews when they are inflamed or swollen,

J

will ease them; and used with salt, dissolves knots or kernels in any part of the body. The juice of the herb, or as Dioscorides saith, the leaves and flowers, with some frankincense in powder, used in wounds of the body, nerves, or sinews, help to heal them. The distilled water of the herb performeth well all the aforesaid cures, but especially for inflammations or waterings of the eyes, by reason of the defluction of rheum into them.

HEART'S EASE.

THIS herb is also called by some pansies.

Place.—Besides growing in gardens, they grow wild in the fields, especially in such as are very barren: sometimes you may find it on the tops of high hills.

Time.—They flower in the spring and summer.

Government and Virtues.—The herb is Saturnine, something cold, viscous, and slimy. A strong decoction of the herb and flowers (or made into syrup) is an excellent remedy for the French-pox, the herb being a gallant antivenerian; and that anti-venerians are the best cure for that disease, far better and safer than to torment them with the flux, as some foreign physicians have confessed. The spirit of it is good for convulsions in children, as also for falling sickness, and a capital remedy for the inflammation of the lungs and breast, pleurisy, scabs, itch, &c.

ARTICHOKES.

Government and Virtues.—They are under the dominion of Venus, and therefore provoke lust: they are rather windy meat: yet they stay the involuntary course of natural seed in man, called nocturnal pollutions. Galen says they contain plenty of choleric juice, of which he saith is engendered melancholy juice, and of that melancholy juice, thin choleric blood. But this is certain, that the decoction of the root boiled in wine, or the root bruised, and distilled in wine in an alembic, and being drunk, purgeth by urine exceedingly.

HART'S TONGUE.

Description.—This hath divers leaves arising from the root, every one severally, which fold themselves in their first springing and spreading; when full grown, they are about a foot long, smooth and green above, but hard and with but little sap in them, streaked on the back, thwart on both sides of the middle rib, with small, and long brownish marks; the bottoms of the leaves are a little bowed on each side of the middle rib, rather narrow with the length, and small at the end. The root is of many black threads interlaced together.

Time.—It is green all the winter, but new leaves spring every year.

Government and Virtues.—Jupiter claims dominion over this herb, therefore it is a good remedy for the liver, both to strengthen it when weak, and ease it when afflicted; you shall do well to keep in a syrup all the year. Hart's tongue is much commended against the hardness and stoppings of the spleen and liver, and against the heat of the liver and stomach, and against lasks and bloody-flux. The distilled water is very good against the passions of the heart, and to stay the hiccup, to help the falling of the palate, and to stay bleeding of the gums, being gargled.

HAZEL-NUT.

HAZEL-NUTS are well known to every body.

Government and Virtues.—They are under the dominion of Mercury. The parted kernels made into an electuary, or the milk drawn from the kernels with mead or honeyed water, is very good to help an old cough, and being parched and a little pepper put to them and drunk, digesteth the distillations of rheum from the head. The dried husks and shells to the weight of two drachms, taken in red wine, stayeth lasks and women's courses, and so doth the red skin that covers the kernels, which is more effectual.

And why should the vulgar affirm, that eating nuts causeth shortness of breath? than which nothing is falser. For how can that which strengthens the lungs cause shortness of breath? I confess the opinion is far older than I am; I knew tradition was a friend to error before, but never that he was the father of slander. If anything of the hazel-nut be binding, it is the husks and shells, and nobody is so mad to eat them unless physically.

HAWK-WEED.

Description.—It hath many large leaves lying upon the ground, much rent or torn on the sides into gashes like dandelion, but with greater parts, more like the smooth sow thistle, from among which riseth a hollow rough stalk, two or three feet high, branched from the middle upward, whereon are set at every joint longer leaves, little or nothing rent or cut, bearing on their top sundry pale yellow flowers, consisting of many small narrow leaves, broad pointed, and nicked in at the ends, set in a double row or more, the outermost being larger than the inner, which form most of the hawk-weeds (for there are many kinds of them) which turn into down, and with the small brownish seed is blown away with the wind. The root is long and somewhat greater, with many small fibres thereat. The whole plant is full of bitter milk.

Place.—It groweth in field sides, and the path-ways in dry grounds.

Time.—It flowereth and flies away in the summer months.

Government and Virtues.—Saturn owns it. Hawk-weed, saith Dioscorides, is cooling, rather drying and binding, and therefore good for the heat of the stomach and gnaw-ings therein; for inflammations and the hot fits of agues. The juice in wine promotes digestion, expels wind, prevents crudities in the stomach, and helpeth to make water, the biting of venomous serpents, if the herb be applied to the place, and is good against all other poisons. A scruple of the dried root given in wine and vinegar, cures the dropsy. The decoction of the herb taken with honey, digesteth the phlegm in the chest or lungs, and with hyssop cures cough. The decoction and of wild succory, made with wine and taken, cures windy colic, and hardness of the spleen; it procureth sleep, hindereth venery and venerous dreams, cooling heats, purgeth the stomach, increaseth blood, and helpeth the diseases of the reins and bladder. Outwardly applied, it is good for all the defects and diseases of the eyes, used with new milk; and is used with good success in fretting ulcers, especially in the beginning. The green leaves bruised, and with a little salt applied to any place burnt with fire before blisters arise, helpeth them ; also inflammations, St. Anthony's fire, and all pushes and eruptions, hot and salt phlegm. The same applied with meal and water, as a poultice, to any place affected with cramp, such as are out of joint, gives ease. The distilled water cleanseth the skin, and taketh away freckles, spots, morphew, or wrinkles in the face.

HAWTHORN.

IT is well known to all.

Government and Virtues.—It is a tree of Mars. The seeds in the berries beaten to powder, being drunk in wine, are good against the stone and the dropsy : the distilled water of the flower stayeth the lask. The seed bruised and boiled in wine, and drunk, is good for inward tormenting pains. If cloths and sponges be wet in the distilled water, and applied to any place wherein thorns and splinters, or the like, do abide in the flesh, it will notably draw them forth. And thus you see the thorn gives a medicine for its own pricking, and so doth almost everything else.

HEMLOCK.

Description.—The common great hemlock groweth up with a green stalk four or five feet high or more, full of red spots sometimes, and at the joints very large winged leaves set at them, which are divided into many other winged leaves, one set against the other, dented about the edges, of a sad green colour, branched towards the top, where it is full of umbels of white flowers, and afterwards with whitish flat seed ; the root is long, white, and somewhat crooked, and hollow within. The whole plant and every part hath a strong, heady, and a bad scent.

Place.—It groweth by walls and hedge-sides, in waste grounds and untilled places.

Time.—It flowereth and seedeth in July, or thereabouts.

Government and Virtues.—Saturn has dominion over it. Hemlock is very cold, and very dangerous, especially to be taken inwardly. It may be applied to inflammations, tumours, and swellings in any part of the body, (save the privy parts) as also to St. Anthony's fire, wheals, pushes, and creeping ulcers that arise of hot sharp humours, by cooling and repelling the heat : the leaves bruised and laid to the brow or forehead are good for the eyes that are red and swollen, as also to take away the pin and web growing in the eye ; this is a tried medicine. Take a small handful of this herb and half so much bay salt beaten together, and applied to the contrary wrist of the hand for twenty-four hours, it removes it in thrice dressing. If the roots thereof be roasted under the embers, wrapped in double wet paper until it be soft and tender, and then applied to the gout in the hands and fingers, it will quickly help this evil. If any through mistake eat the herb hemlock instead of parsley, or the root instead of parsnip (both of which it is very like) whereby happeneth a frenzy or perturbation of the senses, as if they were stupid and drunk, the remedy is as Pliny saith, to drink of the best and strongest pure wine, before it strikes to the heart, or gentian put in wine, or a draught of vinegar, wherewith Tragus doth affirm that he cured a woman that had eaten of the root.

HEMP.

It is well known, and needs not describing.

Time.—It is sown in the end of March or April, and is ripe in August or in September.

Government and Virtues.—It is a plant of Saturn, and good for something else than to make halters only. The seed of hemp consumeth wind, and by too much use disperseth it so much that it drieth up the natural seed for procreation ; yet being boiled in milk and taken, relieves such as have a hot dry cough. The Dutch make an emulsion of the seed and give it with good success in jaundice, especially in the beginning of the disease, if there be no ague accompanying it, for it openeth obstructions of the gall, and causeth digestion of choler. The emulsion or decoction of the seed stayeth lasks and continual fluxes, easeth the colic, and allayeth troublesome humours in the bowels, and stayeth bleeding at the mouth and nose, or other places, some of the leaves boiled and so given them to eat. It kills worms in men or beasts; and the juice dropped into the ears killeth worms in them, and draweth forth any insect gotten into them. The decoction of the root allayeth inflammations of the head or any other parts; the herb itself, or the distilled water thereof, doth the like. The decoction of the roots easeth pains of gout, the hard humours or knots in the joints, the pain and shrinking of the sinews and pains of the hips. The fresh juice mixed with a little oil and butter, is good for any place that hath been burnt with fire, being thereto applied.

HENBANE.

Description.—Our common henbane hath very large thick, soft woolly leaves lying on the ground, much cut in or torn on the edges, of a dark ill greyish green colour, among which rise up thick and short stalks two or three feet high, spread into small branches with less leaves on them, and many hollow flowers, scarcely appearing above the husks, and usually torn on one side, ending in five round points, growing one above another, of a deadish yellow colour, somewhat pale, towards the edges, with many purplish veins therein, and of a dark yellowish purple in the bottom of the flowers, with a small point of the same colour in the middle, each of them standing in a hard close husk, which, after the flowers are past, groweth very like the husk of assarabacca, and somewhat sharp at the top points, wherein is contained much small seed very like poppy seed, but of a dusky greyish colour. The root is great, white, and thick, branching forth divers ways under ground, so like a parsnip root (but not so white) that it hath deceived others. The plant hath a very ill, soporiferous, offensive smell.

Place.—It groweth by the way-sides, and under hedge-sides and walls.

Time.—It flowereth in July, and springeth again yearly of its own seed.

Government and Virtues.—Some astrologers make this an herb of Jupiter; Mezaldus, a man of a penetrating brain, was of that opinion. But the herb is under the dominion of Saturn, and I prove it by this argument :—All the herbs which delight most to grow in Saturnine places are Saturnine herbs ; but the henbane delights most to grow in Saturnine places, and whole cart loads of it may be found near places where they empty the common jacks, and scarce a ditch is to be found without it growing by it ; ergo, it is an herb of Saturn. The leaves of henbane do cool all inflammations in the eyes, or any other part of the body ; and are good to assuage swellings of the testicles, or women's breasts, if they be boiled in wine, and either applied themselves, or the fomentation warm ; it also assuageth the pains of the gout, the sciatica, and other pains in the joints, which arise from a hot cause : and applied with vinegar to the forehead and temples, helpeth the head-ache and want of sleep in hot fevers. The juice of the herb or seed, or the oil drawn from the seed doth the like. The oil of the seed is good for deafness, noise, and worms in the ears, being dropped therein : the juice of the herb or root doth the same. The decoction of the herb or seed, or both, killeth lice in man or beast. The fume of the dried herb, stalks and seed, burned, quickly healeth swellings, chilblains or kibes in the hands or feet, by holding them in the fumes thereof. The remedy to help those that have taken henbane is to drink goat's milk, honeyed water, or pine kernels, with sweet wine ; or, in the absence of these, fennel-seed, nettle-seed, the seed of cresses, mustard, or radish ; as also onions or garlick taken in wine help to free them from danger, and restore them to their due temper again.

Take notice, that this herb must never be taken inwardly ; outwardly, an oil, ointment or plaster of it is effectual for gout, and to cure French pox ; to stop the tooth-ache, being applied to the aching side ; to allay all inflammations, and to help the diseases before premised.

HEDGE HYSOP.

Description.—There are several sorts of this plant ; the first of which is an Italian by birth, and occasionally cultivated here in gardens. Two or three sorts are found growing wild here. The first is a smooth, low plant, not a foot high, very bitter in taste, with many square staks diversely branched from the bottom to the top, with divers joints, and two small leaves at each joint, broader at the bottom than they are at the end, a little dented about the edges, of a sad green colour, and full of veins. The flowers stand at the joints, being of a fair purple colour, with some white spots in them, in fashion like those of dead nettles. The seed is small and yellow, and the roots spread much under ground.

The second seldom groweth half a foot high, sending up many small branches, whereon grow many small leaves set one against the other, somewhat broad but very short. The flowers are like those of the other in fashion, but of a pale reddish colour. The seeds are small and yellowish. The root spreadeth like the other, neither will it yield to its fellow one ace of bitterness.

Place.—They grow in low wet grounds, and by the water-sides : the last in boggy lands.

Time.—They flower in June and July, and the seed is ripe presently after.

Government and Virtues.—They are herbs of Mars, and are choleric and churlish, being most violent purges, especially of choler and phlegm. It is not safe taking them inwardly, unless they be well rectified by the art of the alchymist, and only the purity of them given ; so used they are good for dropsy, gout, and sciatica ; outwardly used in ointments they kill worms, the belly anointed with it, and are excellent to cleanse old and filthy ulcers.

BLACK HELLEBORE.

IT is also called setter-wort, setter-grass, bear's foot, Christmas herb, and Christmas flower.

Description.—It hath green leaves rising from the root, each of them standing about an hand-breadth high from the earth ; each leaf is divided into seven, eight, or nine parts, dented from the middle of the leaf to the point on both sides, abiding green all winter : about Christmas-time, if the weather be temperate, the flowers appear upon footstalks, having five large, round, white leaves a-piece, which sometimes are purple towards the edges, with many pale yellow thrums in the middle ; the seeds are divided into several cells like those of columbines, only greater; the seeds are black, long, and round; the root consisteth of numberless blackish strings united into one head.

There is another black hellebore which groweth in the woods very like this, only the leaves are smaller and narrower, and perish in the winter, which this doth not.

Place.—The first is maintained in gardens. The second is commonly found in woods.

Time.—The first flowereth in December, or January, the second in February or March.

Government and Virtues.—It is an herb of Saturn. If any have taken any harm by taking it, the common cure is to take goat's milk; if you cannot get it, use cow's milk. The roots are very effectual against all melancholy diseases, such as are of long standing, as quartan agues, and madness; it helps the falling sickness, leprosy, yellow and black jaundice, gout, sciatica, and convulsions, and this was found out by experience; the root of that which groweth wild in our country, is superior to those which are brought from beyond the sea. The root used as a pessary, provokes the terms exceedingly; also strewed in powder upon foul ulcers, consumes the dead flesh, and instantly heals them; nay, it will help gangrenes in the beginning. Twenty grains taken inwardly is a sufficient dose for one time, and let that be corrected with half as much cinamon; country people used to rowel their cattle with it. If a beast be troubled with a cough, or have taken any poison, they bore a hole through his ear and put a piece of the root in it, and they say it cured.

HERB ROBERT.

Description.—It riseth up with a reddish stalk two feet high, having leaves thereon upon long reddish foot-stalks, divided at the ends into three or five divisions, each of them cut in on the edges, some deeper than the others, and all dented about the edges, which sometimes turn reddish. At tops of the stalks come forth flowers of five leaves much larger than the dove's foot, and a more reddish colour; after which come black heads, as in others. The root is small and thready, and smelleth badly.

Place.—It grows by the way-sides, upon ditch banks and waste grounds.

Time.—It flowereth in June or July chiefly, and the seed is ripe shortly after.

Government and Virtues.—It is under the dominion of Venus. Herb Robert is a cure for the stone, and to stay the flow of blood; it is a cure for all green wounds, and is effectual in old ulcers in any part of the body.

TRUE-LOVE, OR ONE-BERRY.

Description.—This herb hath a small creeping root running under the uppermost crust of the ground, somewhat like couch-grass root, but not so white, shooting forth stalks with leaves, some whereof carry no berries, the others do; every stalk smooth, without joints, and blackish green, rising half a foot high, if it bear berries, otherwise seldom so high, bearing at the top four leaves, set directly one against another, in manner of a cross or ribbon tied (as it is called) in a true-lover's knot, which are each of them apart, somewhat like unto a night-shade leaf, having sometimes three leaves, sometimes five, sometimes six; in the middle of the four leaves riseth up one small slender stalk, about an inch high, bearing at the tops one flower like a star, consisting of four small and long narrow-pointed leaves of a yellowish green colour, and four others lying between them less than they; in the middle whereof stands a round dark purplish button or head, compassed about with eight small yellow mealy threads with three colours, making it the more conspicuous and lovely to behold. This button or head in the middle, becometh a blackish purple berry full of juice, of the size of a grape, having within it many white seeds.

Place.—It groweth in woods and copses, and in the corners or borders of fields and waste grounds in very many places of this land, and abundantly in the woods, copses, and other places in Kent.

Time.—They spring up in the middle of April or May, and are in flower soon after. The berries are ripe in the end of May, and in some places in June.

Government and Virtues.—Venus owns it. The leaves

or berries hereof are effectual to expel poison especially that of the aconites : as also the plague and other pestilen tial disorders. Matthiolus saith, that some that have lain long in a lingering sickness, and were become half foolish, by taking a drachm of the seeds or berries hereof in pow-der every day for twenty days together, were restored to their former health. The roots in powder taken in wine, easeth the colic. The leaves are very effectual for green wounds as to cleanse and heal sores and ulcers : and are very powerful to discuss old tumours and swellings in the testicles, privy parts, the groin, and speedily allay all in-flammations. The juice of the leaves applied to felons, or those nails of the hands or toes that have imposthumes or sores at the roots of them, healeth them in a short space. This herb is fit to be nourished in every garden.

HOPS.

THESE need no description.

Description.—The wild hop groweth up as the other doth, climbing trees and edges that stand next to them, with rough branches and leaves like the former, but it giveth smaller heads, and in far less plenty.

Place.—They delight to grow in low moist grounds, and are found in all parts of this land.

Time.—They spring not up until April, and flower not until the latter end of June ; the heads are not gathered until the middle or latter end of September.

Government and Virtues.—It is under the dominion of Mars. It opens obstructions of the liver and spleen, cleanses the blood, opens the bowels, cleanses the reins from gravel and provokes urine. The decoction of the tops of hops, as well of the tame as the wild, worketh the same effects. In cleansing the blood they help to cure scabs, itch, and other breakings out of the body ; as also all tetters, ring-worms, and spreading sores ; the morphew, and all discolourings of the skin. The decoction of the flowers and tops expels poison that any one hath drunk. Half a drachm of the seed in powder taken in drink, kill-eth worms in the body, bringeth down women's courses, and expelleth urine. A syrup made of the juice and sugar

cureth yellow jaundice, easeth the headache, and tempereth the heat of the liver and stomach, and is profitably
given in long and hot agues that riseth in choler and blood.
Both the wild and the manured are of one property, and
alike effectual in all the aforesaid diseases.

HOREHOUND.

Description. — Common horehound groweth up with
square hairy stalks, half a yard or two feet high, set at the
joints with two round crumpled rough leaves of a hoary
green colour, of a good scent, but very bitter taste.   The
flowers are small, white, and gaping, set in a rough, prickly husk round about the joints, with the leaves in the
middle of the stalk upwards, wherein afterwards is found
small round blackish seed.   The root is blackish, hard, and
woody, with many strings, and abideth many years.

Place.—It is found in many parts of this land in dry
grounds and waste green places.

Time.—It flowereth in July, and the seed is ripe in
August.

Government and Virtues.—It is an herb of Mercury.   A
decoction of the dried herb, with the seed, or the juice of
the green herb taken with honey, is a remedy for asthma,
for coughs, or for consumption, either through long sickness or thin distillations of rheum upon the lungs.   It expectorates tough phlegm, taken as a decoction.   It promotes the menses ; it is an antidote to poison, and to the
bites or stings of serpents.   The leaves used with honey,
heal foul ulcers, stay running sores, and the growing of
the flesh over the nails ; it also eases pains of the sides.
The juice with wine and honey, cleares the eye-sight ; and
snuffed up purgeth away the yellow jaundice ; and with a
little oil of roses dropped into the ears, easeth pain there.
Galen saith, it openeth obstructions of the liver and spleen,
and purgeth the breast and lungs of phlegm ; and used outwardly it both cleanseth and digesteth.   A decoction made
of horehound (saith Matthiolus) is available for those that
have hard livers, and for such as have itches and running
tetters.   The powder hereof taken, or the decoction, killeth worms.   The green leaves bruised and boiled in old

hog's lard, into an ointment, healeth the bitings of dogs, abateth the swellings and pains that come by any pricking of thorns, or such like means ; and used with vinegar, cleanseth and healeth tetters. The syrup of horehound is very good for old coughs, to rid phlegm ; to expectorate from the lungs of old people. It is good in asthma.

HORSETAIL.

OF this there are many kinds, but all the kinds thereof being nothing else but knotted rushes, some with leaves and some without.

Description.—The great horsetail at the first springing hath heads somewhat like those of asparagus, and grow after to be hard, rough, hollow stalks, jointed at sundry places up to the top, a foot high, so made as if the lower parts were put into the upper, where grow on each side a bush of small long rush-like hard leaves each part resembling a horse-tail. At the tops of the stalks come forth small cat-kins like those of trees. The root creepeth under ground, have joints at sundry places.

Place.—It groweth in wet grounds.

Time.—They spring up in April, and their blooming cat-kins in July, seeding for the most part in August, and after perish down to the ground.

Government and Virtues.—The herb belongs to Saturn, yet it is very harmless. Horsetail, the smoother rather than the rough, and the leaved rather than the bare, is most physical. It is very powerful to staunch bleeding, either inward or outward, the juice or the decoction being drunk, or the juice, decoction, or distilled water applied outward-ly. It also stayeth all sorts of fluxes in man or woman, and voiding of blood ; healeth inward ulcers and excoriation of the entrails, bladder, &c. and foul, moist, and running ulcers, and soon closes the tops of green wounds : it cures ruptures in children. The decoction in wine being drunk, provoketh urine, and relieves the stone and strangury ; the distilled water drunk two or three times in a day, and a small quantity at a time, easeth the bowels, and is effec-tual against a cough that comes by distillation from the head. The juice or distilled water being warmed, and hot inflammations, pustules, or red wheals, and other breakings out in the skin being bathed therewith, cures them, and doth no less ease the swelling heat and inflammations of the fundament, or privy parts in men and women.

HOUSELEEK, or SENGREEN.

BOTH these are so well known to my countrymen, that I shall not need to write any description of them.

Place.—It groweth commonly upon walls and housesides, and flowereth in July.

Government and Virtues.—It is an herb of Jupiter ; and it is reported by Mezaldus to preserve what it grows upon from fire and lightning. Our ordinary houseleek is good for all inward heats, as well as outward, and in the eyes or other parts of the body : a posset made of the juice of houseleek, is singular good in all hot agues, for it cooleth and tempereth the blood and spirits, and quencheth the thirst ; and is also good to stay all defluctions or sharp and salt rheums in the eyes, the juice being dropped into them. If the juice be dropped into the ears, it easeth pain. It helpeth also other fluxes of humours in the bowels, and the immoderate courses of women. It cooleth and restraineth all hot inflammations, St. Anthony's fire, scaldings and burnings, the shingles, fretting ulcers, cankers, tetters, ringworms, and the like ; and much easeth the pain of the gout. The juice also taketh away warts and corns in the hands and feet, and being often bathed therewith, and the skin and leaves being laid on them afterwards : it easeth also the headache, and the distempered heat of the brain in frenzies, or through want of sleep, being applied to the temples and forehead. The leaves bruised and laid upon the crown or seam of the head, stayeth bleeding at the nose very quickly. The distilled water of the herb is profitable for all the purposes aforesaid. The leaves being gently rubbed on any place stung with nettles or bees, doth quickly take away the pain.

HOUND'S TONGUE.

Description.—The great ordinary hound's tongue hath many long and narrow, soft, hairy, darkish green leaves, lying on the ground, like unto bugloss leaves, from amongst which riseth up a rough hairy stalk about two feet high, with some smaller leaves thereon, and branched at the tops into divers parts, with a small leaf at the foot of every branch, which is somewhat long, with many flowers set along the same, which branch is crooked or turned inwards before it flowereth, and openeth by degrees as the flowers do blow, which consist of small purplish red leaves of a dead colour, rising out of the husks wherein they stand with some threads in the middle : it hath sometimes a white flower. After the flowers are past, there cometh rough flat seed with a small pointal in the middle, easily cleaving to any garment that it toucheth, and not so easily pulled off again. The root is black, thick, and long, hard to break, and full of clammy juice, smelling somewhat strong of an evil scent, as the leaves also do.

Place. —It groweth in most places of this land, in waste grounds and untilled places, by high-way sides, lanes, and hedge-sides.

Time.—It flowereth about May or June, and the seed is ripe shortly after.

Government and Virtues.—It is a plant under the dominion of Mercury. The root is very effectual used in pills, as well as the decoction or otherwise, to stay all sharp and thin defluxions of rheum from the head into the eyes or nose, or upon the stomach or lungs, as also for coughs and shortness of breath. The leaves boiled in wine (saith Dioscorides, but others advise it to be made with water, and add oil and salt) mollifieth or openeth the belly downwards. It helpeth to cure the biting of a mad dog, the leaves being applied to the wound. The leaves bruised, or the juice of them boiled in hog's lard, and applied restores the hair, and for a scald or burn : the leaves bruised and laid to any green wound heals it quickly ; the root baked under the embers, wrapped in paste or wet paper, or in a wet double cloth, and thereof a suppository made, and put up into or applied to the fundament, cures painful piles. The distilled water of the herb and root is very good to all the purposes aforesaid, to be used as well inwardly to drink, as outwardly to wash any sore place ; for

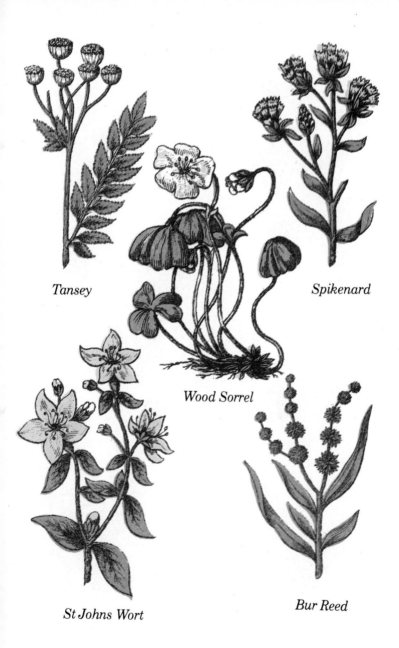

Tansey

Spikenard

Wood Sorrel

St Johns Wort

Bur Reed

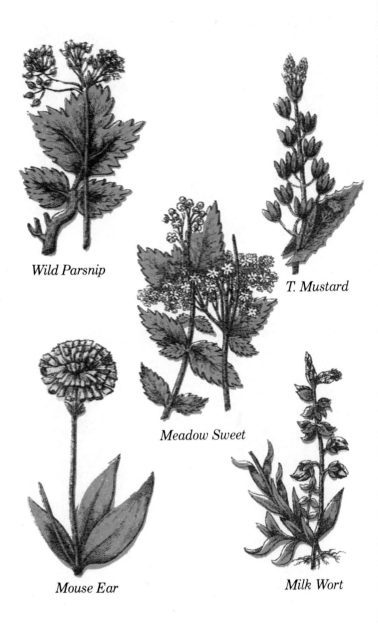

Wild Parsnip

T. Mustard

Meadow Sweet

Mouse Ear

Milk Wort

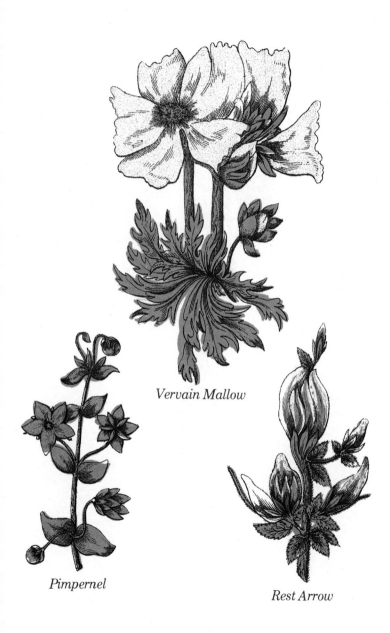

Vervain Mallow

Pimpernel

Rest Arrow

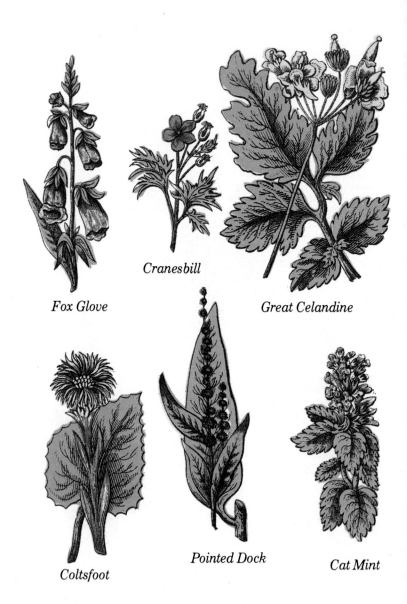

Fox Glove

Cranesbill

Great Celandine

Coltsfoot

Pointed Dock

Cat Mint

it healeth all manner of wounds and punctures. It is called hound's-tongue, because it ties the tongues of hounds ; whether true or not I never tried ; yet I cured the biting of a mad dog with this only medicine.

HOLLY, HOLM, HULVER BUSH.

To describe a tree so well known is needless.

Government and Virtues.—The tree is Saturnine. The berries expel wind, and therefore are curative in colic. The berries have a strong faculty with them ; for if you eat a dozen in the morning fasting, when they are ripe, they purge the chest of gross and clammy phlegm ; but if you dry the berries and beat them into powder, they bind the body, and stop fluxes, bloody-fluxes, and the terms in women. The bark of the tree, and also the leaves, are good used as fomentations for broken bones, and such members as are out of joint. Pliny saith the branches of the tree defend houses from lightning, and men from witchcraft.

HYSSOP.

Hyssop is so well known to be grown in every garden, that it is needless to describe it.

Government and Virtues.—The herb is Jupiter's, and the sign Cancer. It strengthens all the parts of the body under Cancer and Jupiter ; Dioscorides saith, that hyssop boiled with rue and honey, and drunk, relieves those that are troubled with coughs, shortness of breath, wheezing and rheumatic distillations upon the lungs : taken with oxymel, it purgeth gross humours by stool ; and with honey, killeth worms ; and with fresh and new figs bruised cureth costiveness, and more forcibly if the root of flower-de-luce and cresses be added thereto. It amendeth the native colour of the body affected by yellow jaundice ; and being taken with figs and nitre, cures the dropsy and spleen ; being boiled with wine, it is good to wash inflammations, and taketh away the black and blue spots and marks that come by strokes, bruises, or falls, being applied with warm water. It is an excellent medicine for the quinsy, or swelling in the throat, to wash and gargle it,

K

being boiled in figs : it helpeth the tooth-ache, being boiled in vinegar and gargled therewith. The hot vapours of the decoction taken by a funnel in at the ears, easeth the inflammation and singing noise of them. The oil thereof (the head being anointed) killeth lice, and taketh away itching of the head. It helpeth those that have the falling sickness. It helpeth to expectorate tough phlegm, and is effectual in all cold griefs or diseases of the chest or lungs, being taken either in syrup or as an electuary. The green herb bruised, and a little sugar applied thereto, quickly heals any cut or green wounds.

ST. JOHN'S WORT.

Description.—Common St. John's wort shooteth forth brownish, upright, hard round stalks, two feet high, spreading branches from the sides up to the tops of them, with two small leaves set one against another at every place, of a deep green colour, like the leaves of the lesser centaury, but narrow, and full of small holes in every leaf, which may be seen when they are held up to the light ; at the tops of the stalks and branches stand yellow flowers of five leaves a-piece, with many yellow threads in the middle, which being bruised, yield a reddish juice blood ; after which come small round heads, wherein is contained small blackish seed, smelling like rosin. The root is hard and woody, with strings and fibers of a brownish colour, which abideth in the ground many years, shooting anew every spring.

Place.—This groweth in woods and copses, and in those that are shady, as open to the sun.

Time.—They flower about midsummer and July, and the seed is ripe at the end of July or August.

Government and Virtues.—It is under the sign of Leo, and the dominion of the Sun. A papist will tell you, especially if he be a lawyer, that St. John made it over to him by a letter of attorney. It is a singular wound herb : boiled in wine and drunk it healeth inward hurts or bruises ; made into an ointment, it opens obstructions, dissolves swellings, and closes up the lips of wounds. The decoction of the herb and flowers, especially of the seed being drunk in wine with the juice of knot grass, it prevents vomiting and spitting of blood; it is good for bites or stings of venomous creatures and for retention of water. Two drachms of the seed of St. John's wort made into a powder, and drunk in a little broth, doth gently expel choler or congealed blood in the stomach. The decoction of the leaves and seed drunk somewhat warm before the fits of agues, alter the fits, and by often using, prevents them. The seed is much commended being drunk for forty days together for sciatica, falling sickness, and palsy.

IVY.

It is well known to grow in woods upon trees, and upon walls of churches, houses, &c.

Time.—It flowereth in July, and the berries are ripe at Christmas when they have felt the winter frosts.

Government and Virtues.—It is under the dominion of Saturn. A pugil of the flowers, which may be about a drachm, drunk twice a day in port wine, stays the lasks and bloody-flux. It is an enemy to the nerves and sinews taken inwardly, but excellent if outwardly applied. Pliny saith, the yellow berries are good against jaundice; and they are good for those who spit blood; and the white berries being taken inwardly, or applied outwardly, killeth worms. The berries prevent the plague, and cure it, by drinking a decoction of the berries made into a powder, for two or three days together: taken in wine, they help to break the stone, provoke urine, and women's courses. The fresh leaves of ivy boiled in vinegar, and applied warm to the sides of those that are troubled with the spleen, ache, or stitch in the sides, give ease: the same applied with rose water and oil of roses to the temples and forehead, easeth a long head-ache. The leaves boiled in wine, and obstinate ulcers washed therewith, wonderfully cleanses them: it quickly healeth green wounds, and all burnings and scaldings, and all kinds of exulcerations coming thereby. The juice of the berries or leaves snuffed up into the nose, purgeth the head and brain of rheum that maketh defluctions into the eyes and nose, and curing the ulcers and stench therein; the same dropped into the ears, healeth the old and running sores of them ; those that are troubled with the spleen, will find much ease by continual drinking of a cup of tea made of ivy, the leaves being sufficiently infused.

There seems to be a very great antipathy between wine and ivy ; for if one hath got a surfeit by drinking wine, his speediest cure is to drink a draught of the same wine wherein a handful of ivy leaves being first bruised, have been boiled.

JUNIPER BUSH.

For to give a description of a bush so commonly known is needless.

Place.—They grow plentifully in various woods in Kent, in Essex, Buckinghamshire, and other counties.

Time.—The berries are not ripe the first year, but continue green two summers and one winter before they are ripe, at which time they are all of a black colour, and therefore you may always find upon the bush green berries ; the berries are ripe about the fall of the leaf.

Government and Virtues.—This admirable solar shrub is scarce to be paralleled for its virtues. The berries are hot in the third degree, and dry but in the first, being a most admirable counter poison, and a great resister of the pestilence ; they are good against the bitings of venomous beasts : they provoke urine copiously, and therefore are very available to dysuries and stranguries. It is so powerful a remedy against the dropsy, that the very lye made of the ashes of the herb being drunk, cures the disease : it provokes the terms, strengthens the stomach exceedingly, and expels wind ; indeed there is scarce a better remedy for wind in any part of the body, or the colic, than the chemical oil drawn from the berries. Such country people as know not how to draw the chemical oil, may content themselves by eating ten or a dozen of the ripe berries every morning fasting. They are very good for cough, shortness of breath, consumptions, pains in the belly, ruptures, cramps, and convulsions. They give safe and speedy delivery to women with child : they strengthen the brain, help the memory, and fortify the sight by strengthening the optic nerves : are good in all agues, relieve gout and sciatica, and strengthen the limbs of the body. The ashes of the wood is a speedy remedy for scurvy, to rub their gums with. The berries stay all fluxes, cure piles, and kill worms in children. A lye made of the ashes of the wood, and the body bathed therewith, cures the itch, scabs, and leprosy. The berries break the stone, procure appetite when it is lost, and are good for all palsies, and falling sickness.

KIDNEYWORT, OR WALL PENNYROYAL, OR WALL PENNYWORT.

Description.—It hath many thick, flat, and round leaves growing from the root, each having a long foot-stalk, fastened underneath about the middle of it, and a little unevenly waved sometimes about the edges, of a pale green colour, and rather yellow on the upper side of it ; from among which arise one or more tender, smooth, hollow stalks, half a foot high, with two or three small leaves thereon, usually not round as those below, but somewhat long and divided at the edges ; the tops are divided into long branches bearing a number of flowers, set round about a long spike one above another, which are hollow like a little bell, of a whitish green colour, after which come small heads containing small brownish seed. The root is round, and smooth, greyish without, and white within, having small fibres at the head of the root and bottom of the stalk.

Place.—It groweth upon stone and mud walls, upon rocks, and in stony places upon the ground, at the bottom of old trees, and sometimes on the bodies of them that are decayed and rotten.

Time.—It flowereth in the beginning of May, and the seed ripeneth quickly after, shedding itself, so that about the end of May the leaves and stalks are withered, and gone until September, when the leaves spring up again, and abide all winter.

Government and Virtues.—Venus challengeth the herb under Libra. The juice or the distilled water being drunk, is very effectual for all inflammations, to cool a fainting hot stomach, a hot liver, or the bowels; the herb, juice, or distilled water outwardly applied, healeth pimples, St. Anthony's fire, and other outward heats. The said juice or water helpeth to heal sore kidneys, torn or fretted by the stone, or ulcerated within; it also provoketh urine, is available for the dropsy, and breaks the stone. Being used as a bath, or made into an ointment, it cooleth painful piles. It gives ease to pains of the gout, sciatica, and inflammations and swellings of the testicles, it cures kernels or knots in the neck or throat, called the king's evil; healing kibes or chilblains if they be bathed with the juice, or anointed with ointment made hereof, and some of the skin of the leaf upon them : it is used in green wounds to stay the blood, and to heal them quickly.

KNAPWEED.

Description.—The common sort hereof hath many long and rather broad dark green leaves, rising from the root, dented about the edges, and sometimes a little rent or torn on both sides in two or three places, and rather hairy ; amongst which ariseth a long round stalk four or five feet high, divided into many branches, at the tops whereof stand great scaly green heads, and from the middle of them thrust forth a number of dark purplish red thrums or threads, which after they are withered, there are found black seeds lying in a great deal of down, like thistle seed, but smaller ; the root is white, hard, and woody, and divers fibres annexed thereunto, which perisheth not, but abideth with leaves thereon all the winter, shooting out fresh every spring.

Place.—It groweth in most fields and meadows, and about their borders and hedges, and in waste grounds.

Time.—It usually flowereth in June or July, and the seed is ripe shortly after.

Government and Virtues.—Saturn governs it. The knapweed helpeth to stay fluxes of blood at the mouth, nose, or other outward parts, and those veins that are inwardly broken, or inward wounds, as also the fluxes of the belly ; it stayeth distillations of thin and sharp humours from the head upon the stomach and lungs : it is good for those that are bruised by falls, blows, or otherwise, and is good in ruptures, by drinking the decoction of the herb and roots in wine, and applying the same outwardly to the place. It is very good in all running sores, cancerous and fistulous, drying up the moisture, and healing them gently : it doth the like to running sores or scabs of the head or other parts. It is of special use for soreness of throat, swelling of the uvula and jaws, and very good to stay bleeding, and heal up all green wounds.

KNOTGRASS.

THIS is generally known so well, that it needeth no description.

Place.—It groweth in most fields and meadows, by the high-way sides, and by foot-paths in fields ; as also by the sides of old walls.

Time.—It springeth up late in the spring, and abideth until the winter, when all the branches perish.

Government and Virtues.—Saturn owns the herb, and yet some hold the Sun ; but Saturn governs it. The juice of the common kind of knotgrass is most effectual to stay bleeding of the mouth, being drunk in steeled port wine ; and the bleeding at the nose, to be applied to the forehead or temples, or to be squirted up into the nostrils. It is no less effectual to cool and temper the heat of the blood and stomach, and to stay any flux of the blood and humours, as lasks, bloody-flux, women's courses, and running of the reins. It is very good to provoke urine, help the strangury, and allayeth the heat that cometh thereby ; and is powerful by urine to expel the gravel or stone in the kidneys and bladder, a drachm of the powder of the herb being taken in wine for many days together ; being boiled in wine and drunk, it is good for stings and bites of venomous creatures, and very effectual to stay all defluctions of rheumatic humours on the stomach, and killeth worms, quieteth inward pains that arise from the heat, sharpness and corruption of blood and choler. The distilled water taken by itself, or with the powder of the herb or seed, is very effectual in all the purposes aforesaid, and is accounted one of the most sovereign remedies to cool all inflammations, breaking out through heat, hot swellings and imposthumes, gangrene and cankers, or foul ulcers, being applied or put in them; but especially for ulcers or sores happening in the privy parts of men or women. It heals fresh and green wounds. The juice dropped into the ears cleanseth them, being foul, and having running matter in them. It is also good for broken joints and ruptures.

LADIES' MANTLE.

Description.—It hath many leaves rising from the root standing upon long hairy foot-stalks, being almost round and a little cut on the edges into eight or ten parts, making it seem like a star with so many corners or points, and dented round about, of a light colour, rather hard in handling, and folded or plaited at first, and then crumpled in divers places, and a little hairy, as the stalk is also, which riseth up among them to the height of two or three feet; and being weak, is not able to stand upright, divided at the top into two or three branches, with small yellowish green heads, and flowers of a whitish colour, which being past there cometh a small yellowish seed like poppy seed: the root is rather long and black, with many strings and fibres.

Place.—It groweth in pastures and woodsides in Hertfordshire, Wiltshire, Kent, &c.

Time.—It flowereth in May and June, abiding after seed time green all the winter.

Government and Virtues.—Venus governs it. Ladies' mantle is very proper for inflamed wounds, and to stay bleeding, vomitings, fluxes of all sorts, bruises by falls, and ruptures: and such women or maids as have over great flagging breasts, causing them to grow less and hard, being both drunk and outwardly applied: the distilled water drunk for 20 days together, helpeth conception, and to retain the birth, and by sitting in a bath made of the decoction of the herb. It is one of the most singular wound herbs, and therefore highly prized and praised by the Germans, who use it in all wounds inward and outward, to drink a decoction thereof, and wash the wounds therewith, or dip tents therein and put them into the wounds, which wonderfully drieth up all humidity of the sores, and abateth all inflammations therein. It quickly healeth green wounds, not suffering any corruption to remain behind, and cureth old sores, though fistulous and hollow.

LAVENDER.

It is so well known that it needeth no description.

Time.—It flowereth about the end of June, and beginning of July.

Government and Virtues.—Mercury owns the herb, and it carries his effects very potently. Lavender is of special good use for all the griefs and pains of the head and brain that proceed of a cold cause, as apoplexy, falling sickness, the dropsy, or sluggish malady, cramps, convulsions, palsies, and often faintings. It strengthens the stomach, and freeth the liver and spleen from obstructions, provoketh women's courses. The flowers of lavender steeped in wine, effectually promotes urine, and cures flatulency and colic, if the place be bathed therewith. A decoction made with the flowers of lavender, horehound, fennel, and asparagus root, and a little cinnamon, cures the falling sickness, and giddiness or turning of the brain ; to gargle the mouth with the decoction, is good for tooth-ache. Two spoonfuls of the distilled water of the flowers taken, restores a lost voice, and also the tremblings and passions of the heart, and faintings and swoonings, being drunk, and applied to the temples, or nostrils by smell ; but it is not safe to use it where the body is replete with blood and humours, because of the hot and subtle spirits wherewith it is possessed. The chemical oil drawn from lavender, usually called oil of spike, is of so fierce and piercing a quality, that it is cautiously to be used, some few drops being sufficient, to be given with other things, either for inward or outward griefs.

LAVENDER COTTON

It being a common garden herb, I shall forbear giving a description, only take notice, that it flowereth in June and July.

Government and Virtues.—It is under the dominion of

Mercury. It resisteth poison, putrefaction, and heals the biting of venomous beasts; a drachm of the powder of the dried leaves taken every morning fasting, stops the running of the reins in men, and whites in women. The seed beaten into powder, and taken as worm-seed, kills worms in children, and adults; the like doth the herb itself, being steeped in milk and the milk drunk; the body bathed with the decoction cures scabs and the itch.

LADIES' SMOCK, OR CUCKOW-FLOWERS.

Description.—The root is composed of many small white threads, from whence spring up long stalks of winged leaves, with round, tender, dark green leaves set one against another upon a middle rib, the greatest being at the end, amongst which rise up weak, round, green stalks, streaked, with longer and smaller leaves upon them; on the tops of which stand flowers, almost like the stock gilliflowers, but rounder and not so long, and of a blushing white colour; the seed is reddish, and groweth in small bunches, being of a sharp biting taste, and so hath the herb.

Place.—They grow in moist places, and near brook-sides.

Time.—They flower in April and May, and the lower leaves continue green all the winter.

Government and Virtues.—They are under the dominion of the Moon, and very little inferior to water-cresses in all their operations; they are good for scurvy; they provoke urine and break the stone, and warm a cold and weak stomach, restoring lost appetite, and promote digestion.

LETTUCE.

It is well known, being used as a salad.

Government and Virtues.—The Moon owns them, and that is the reason they cool and moisten what heat and dryness Mars causeth, because Mars hath his fall in Cancer; and they cool the heat because the sun rules it. The juice of lettuce mixed or boiled with oil of roses, applied to the forehead and temples, procureth sleep, and easeth the headache proceeding from heat. Being eaten boiled, it opens the bowels; promotes digestion, quencheth thirst, increaseth milk in nurses, easeth griping pains in the stomach and bowels that come of choler; it abateth bodily lust, outwardly applied to the testicles with a little camphire. Applied to the region of the heart, liver, or reins, or by bathing the place with the juice in distilled water, wherein some white sanders, or red roses are put, represseth the heat and inflammations therein, and strengthens and comforts those parts, and also tempereth the heat of urine. Galen adviseth old men to use it with spice; and where spices are wanting, to add mints, and such like hot herbs; or else citron, lemon, or orange seeds, to abate the cold of one, and heat of the other. The seed and distilled water of lettuce work the same effects in all things; but the use of the lettuce is chiefly forbidden to those that are short-winded, or have any imperfection in the lungs, or spit blood.

WATER LILY.

Of these there are two principally noted kinds, viz.— the white and the yellow.

Description.—The white lily hath large and thick dark green leaves lying on the water, sustained by long and thick foot-stalks, that rise from a great, thick, round, and long tuberous black root, spongy or loose, with many knobs thereon, like eyes, and whitish within; from amidst which rise other thick, green stalks, and sustaining one large flower, green on the outside, but white as snow within, consisting of rows of long and thick and narrow leaves, encompassing a head with many yellow threads or thrums in the middle; where, after they are past, stand round poppy-like heads, full of broad, oily, and bitter seed.

The yellow kind is little different from the former, save only that it hath fewer leaves on the flowers, greater and more shining seed, and a whitish root both within and without. The root of both is somewhat sweet in taste.

Place.—They are found growing in great pools and standing waters, and sometimes in slow running rivers and ditches of water, in sundry places of this land.

Time.—They flower more commonly about the end of May, and their seed is ripe in August.

Government and Virtues.—The herb is under the dominion of the Moon, and therefore cools and moistens like the former. The leaves and flowers are cold and moist, but the roots and seeds are cold and dry ; the leaves cool inflammations, both outward and inward heats of agues ; and so do the flowers, either by syrup or by conserve : the syrup helpeth to procure rest, and to cool the brain of frantic persons. The seed, as well as the root, is effectual to stay fluxes of blood or humours, either of wounds or of the belly : but the roots are most used, and more effectual to cool, bind, and restrain all fluxes in men or women : also running of the reins, and passing away of the seed when asleep. The root is good for those whose urine is hot and sharp, to be boiled in wine and water, and the decoction drunk. The distilled water of the flowers is very effectual for all the diseases aforesaid, both inwardly taken and outwardly applied ; and is much commended to take away freckles, spots, sunburn, and morphew from the face, or other parts of the body. The oil made of the flowers is profitably used to cool all hot tumours, and to ease the pains and heal the sores.

LILY OF THE VALLEY.

CALLED also conval lily, male lily, and lily constancy.

Description.—The root is small, and creepeth far in the ground, as grass roots do. The leaves are many, against which riseth up a stalk half a foot high, with many white flowers, like little bells with turned edges, of a strong though pleasing smell ; the berries are red, not much unlike these of asparagus.

Place.—They grow upon warm heaths, in gardens, and in warm places, where the soil is good.

Time.—They flower in May, and the seed is ripe in September.

Government and Virtues.—It is under the dominion of Mercury, and therefore strengthens the brain, and recruits a weak memory. The distilled water dropped into the eyes, cures inflammations, and that infirmity which they call a pin and web. The spirit of the flowers distilled in wine, restoreth lost speech, cures palsy, and is very good in apoplexy, comforteth the heart and vital spirits. Gerrard saith, that the flowers being close stopped up in a glass, put into an ant-hill, and taken away again a month after, ye shall find a liquor in the glass, which being outwardly applied, cures the gout.

WHITE LILIES.

It were in vain to describe a plant so commonly known in gardens.

Government and Virtues.—They are under the dominion of the Moon, and by antipathy to Mars expel poison ; they are good in pestilential fevers, the roots being bruised and boiled in wine, and the decoction drunk, for it expels the venom to the exterior parts of the body ; the juice of it being tempered with barley-meal, baked, and so eaten for ordinary bread, is an excellent cure for the dropsy. An ointment made of the root and hog's lard, is excellent for scald heads, unites the sinews when they are cut, and cleanseth ulcers. The root boiled in any convenient decoction, gives speedy delivery to women in travail, and expels the after-birth. The root roasted, and mixed with hog's lard, makes a gallant poultice to ripen plague sores. The ointment is good for swellings in the privities, and will cure burnings and scaldings without a scar, and deck a blank place with hair.

LIQUORICE.

Description.—Our English liquorice riseth up with divers woody stalks, wherein are set at several distances many narrow, long, green leaves, set together on both sides of the stalk, and an odd one at the end, very well resembling a young ash tree sprung up from the seed. This by many years' continuance in a place without moving, and not else will bring forth flowers, many standing together, spike fashion, one above another upon the stalk, of the form of pea blossom, but of a very pale blue colour, which turn into long somewhat flat and smooth cods, wherein is contained a small, round, hard seed : the roots run deep into the ground, with other small roots and fibres growing with them, and shoot out suckers from the main root all about, whereby it is much increased, of a brownish colour on the outside, and yellow within.

Place.—It is planted in fields and gardens in divers places of this land, and thereof good profit is made.

Government and Virtues.—It is under the dominion of Mercury. Liquorice boiled in pure water, with some maiden hair and figs, is a good drink for a dry cough or hoarseness, wheezing, shortness of breath, and for all diseases of the breast and lungs, phthisic, or consumptions. It is good in all pains of the reins, the strangury, and heat of urine. The fine powder of liquorice blown through a quill into the eyes that have a pin-and-web, or rheumatic distillations in them, it cleanses and heals them; the juice of liquorice is as effectual in diseases of the breast and lungs, the reins and the bladder, as the decoction; the juice distilled in rose-water, with some gum tragacanth, is a fine licking medicine for hoarseness, wheezing, &c.

LIVERWORT.

Description.—Common Liverwort groweth close, and spreadeth much upon the ground in moist and sandy places, with many small green leaves, or rather sticking flat to one another, very unevenly cut in on the edges, and crumpled; from among which arise small slender stalks an inch or two high at most, bearing small star-like flowers at the top; the roots are very fine and small.

Government and Virtues.—It is under the dominion of Jupiter, and the sign Cancer. It is a rare herb for all diseases of the liver, to cool and cleanse it, and subdue inflammations in any part, and to cure yellow jaundice; bruised and boiled in small beer, and drunk, it cooleth the liver and kidneys and cures the running of the reins in men, and whites in women; stays the spreading of tetters, ringworms, and other running sores or scabs, and is a first-rate remedy for such whose livers are corrupted by surfeits, which cause their bodies to break out, for it fortifieth the liver exceedingly, and makes it impregnable.

LOOSESTRIFE, OR WILLOW-HERB.

Description.—Common yellow loosestrife groweth to be four or five feet high, or more, with great round stalks a

little crested, diversely branched from the middle of them
to the tops into great and long branches, on all which at
the joints grow long and narrow leaves, but broader below,
and usually two at a joint, yet sometimes three or four,
somewhat like willow leaves, smooth on the edges, and of
a fair green colour, and at the tops of them also stand
many yellow flowers of five leaves a-piece, with divers yellow threads in the middle, which turn into small round
heads containing small cornered seeds : the root creepeth
under-ground like couch-grass, but greater, and shooteth
up every spring brownish heads, which grow up into stalks.
It is astringent.

Place.—It groweth in many places of this land, in moist
meadows, and by water-sides.

Time.—It flowereth from June to August.

Government and Virtues.—This herb is good for bleeding
at the mouth, nose, or wounds, and fluxes of the belly, and
the bloody flux, given either to drink, or taken by clyster;
it stays profuse menstruation ; it is a singular good wound
herb for green wounds, to stay the bleeding, and closing
the lips of the wound, if the herb be bruised, and the juice
applied. It is often used in gargling for sore mouths, as
also for the secret parts. The smoke hereof being burned,
driveth away flies and gnats, which in the night time molest people in marshes and fenny countries.

LOOSESTRIFE,

WITH SPIKED HEADS OF FLOWERS.

Description.—This groweth with many woody, square
stalks, full of joints, three feet high at least; at every one
whereof stand two long leaves, shorter, narrower, and a
larger green colour than the former, and some brownish ;
the stalks are branched into many long stems of spiked
flowers half a foot long, growing in bundles one above another out of small husks, like the spiked heads of lavender,
each of which flowers have five round-pointed leaves of a
purple violet colour, inclining to red ; in which husks stand
small round heads after the flowers are fallen, wherein is
contained small seed. The root creepeth under ground

like to the yellow, but is larger, and so are the heads of the leaves when they first appear out of the ground, and browner than the other.

Place.—It groweth by river and ditch-sides in wet grounds, and in many places.

Time.—It flowereth in the months of June and July.

Government and Virtues.—It is an herb of the Moon, and under the sign Cancer. It is a great preserver of the sight when it is well, and a cure for sore eyes, with eyebright taken inwardly, and this used outwardly—it is cold in quality. This herb has some peculiar virtues of its own ; as, the distilled water is a remedy for hurts and blows on the eyes, and for blindness, so as the chrystalline humours be not perished or hurt ; and this hath been proved true by the experience of a man of judgement, who kept it long as a great secret. It cleareth the eyes of dust or any other particle, and preserveth the sight. It is very good for wounds and thrusts, made thus into an ointment :—To every ounce of water add two drachms of May butter without salt, and the same of sugar and wax ; let them boil gently together ; let tents dipped in the cold liqour be put into the wounds, and the place covered with a linen cloth doubled and anointed with the ointment ; this is an approved medicine. It cleanseth and healeth ulcers and sores, and stayeth their inflammations by washing them with the water, and laying on them a green leaf or two in summer, or dry leaves in winter. This water gargled warm in the mouth and sometimes drunk cures quinsey, or king's evil in the throat. The said water applied warm, taketh away spots, marks, and scabs in the skin ; and a little of it drunk, quencheth thirst when it is extraordinary.

LOVAGE.

Description.—It hath many long green stalks of large winged leaves, divided into many parts like smallage, but cut much larger and greater, every leaf being cut about the edges, broadest forward, and smallest at the stalk, of a sad green colour, smooth and shining, from among which rise up sundry strong, hollow, green stalks, five or six, sometimes seven or eight feet high, full of joints, but less

leaves set on them than grow below; and with them towards the tops come forth large branches, bearing at their
tops large umbels of yellow flowers, and after them flat
brownish seed. The root groweth thick, great, and deep,
spreading much, and enduring long, of a brownish colour
on the outside, and whitish within. The whole plant and
every part of it smelling strong and aromatically, and is of
a hot, sharp, biting taste.

Place.—It is usually planted in gardens, where, if it be
suffered, it groweth large.

Time.—It flowereth in the end of July, and seedeth in
August.

Government and Virtues.—It is an herb of the Sun, under
the sign Taurus. It openeth, cureth, and digesteth humours, and mightily provoketh women's courses, and urine.
Half a drachm at a time of the dried root in powder taken
in wine, wonderfully warms a cold stomach, helpeth digestion, and consumeth all raw and superfluous moisture
therein; easeth all gripings and pains, expels wind and resisteth poison and infection. It is highly recommended to
drink the decoction of the herb for agues, and to relieve
pains of the body and bowels coming of cold. The seed is
very effectual to all the purposes aforesaid, and worketh
more powerfully. The distilled water is good for quinsey,
if the mouth and throat be gargled and washed therewith,
and relieveth pleurisy being drunk three or four times.
Being dropped into the eyes it taketh away their redness
or dimness; it removes spots or freckles in the face. The
leaves bruised and fried with a little hog's lard, and laid
hot to any blotch or boil, will quickly break it.

LUNGWORT.

Description.—This is a kind of moss that groweth on
sundry sorts of trees, especially oaks and beeches, with
broad, greyish, tough leaves diversly folded, crumpled, and
gashed in on the edges, and some spotted also with many
small spots on the upper side. It bears no stalk or flower.

Government and Virtues.—Jupiter owns this herb. It
is of great use to physicians to cure diseases of the lungs,

L

and for coughs, wheezings, and shortness of breath, which it cureth both in man and beast. It is profitable to put into lotions taken to stay the moist humours that flow to ulcers and hinder their healing, as also to wash ulcers in the privy parts of man or woman. It is an excellent remedy boiled in beer for broken-winded horses.

MADDER.

Description. — Garden madder shooteth forth many very long, weak, four-square, reddish stalks, trailing on the ground a great way, very rough and hairy, and full of joints ; at every one of these joints come forth long and narrow leaves, standing like a star about the stalks, rough also and hairy, towards the tops whereof come forth many small pale yellow flowers, after which come small round heads, green at first and reddish afterwards, but black when they are ripe, wherein is contained the seed. The root is not very great, but long, running deep into the ground, red and clear while it is fresh.

Place. — It is only manured in gardens or large fields for the profit that is made thereof.

Time. — It flowereth towards the end of summer, and the seed is ripe quickly after.

Government and Virtues. — It is an herb of Mars. It is an aperient, but afterwards binds and strengthens. It is a sure remedy for yellow jaundice, by opening the obstructions of the liver and gall, and cleansing those parts : also the obstructions of the spleen, and diminisheth the melancholy humour ; it is good for palsy and sciatica, and effectual for bruises inward and outward, and is much used in vulnerary drinks. The root for all such purposes is to be boiled in wine or water, and some honey and sugar put thereunto afterwards. The seed hereof taken in vinegar and honey, mollifies swelling and hardness of the spleen. The decoction of the leaves and branches is a good fomentation for women to sit over that have not their courses. The leaves and roots beaten and applied to any part that is discoloured with freckles, morphew, the white scurf, or any such deformity of the skin, cleanseth thoroughly and taketh them away.

MAIDEN HAIR.

Description.—Our common maiden-hair doth, from a number of hard black fibres, send forth a great many blackish shining brittle stalks, hardly a span long, in many not half so long, on each side set very thick with small, round, dark green leaves, and spitted on the back of them like a fern.

Place.—It groweth upon old stone walls in Kent, and other places in this land ; it grows by springs, wells, and rocky and shady places, and is always green.

Its *medicinal virtues* are similar to other Maiden Hairs, which follow.

WALL RUE, OR WHITE MAIDEN HAIR.

Description.—It has very fine pale, green stalks, almost as fine as hairs, set confusedly with pale green leaves on very short foot-stalks, nearly the colour of garden rue, and not much differing in form, but more diversely cut in on the edges, and thicker, smooth on the upper part, and spotted finely underneath.

Place.—It groweth in many places of this land, in Kent, Buckinghamshire, Huntingdonshire, Suffolk, Sussex, Somersetshire, and is green in winter as well as summer.

Government and Virtues.—Both this and the former are under the dominion of Mercury, and so is that also which followeth after, and the virtues of both these are so near alike, that I shall in writing their virtues, join them both as followeth.

The decoction of the herb being drunk, helpeth those that are troubled with cough, shortness of breath, yellow jaundice, diseases of the spleen, stopping of urine, and very good for stone in the kidneys. It provoketh women's courses, and stays bleedings and fluxes of the stomach and belly, especially when the herb is dry ; for being green, it is purgative, and voideth choler and phlegm from the stomach and liver ; it cleanseth the lungs, and by rectifying the blood, improves the complexion. The herb boiled in oil of camomile, dissolveth knots, allayeth swellings, and drieth up moist ulcers. The ley made thereof is good to cleanse the head from scurf, and from dry and running sores, stayeth the shedding of the hair, and causeth it to grow thick, fair, and well coloured ; for which purpose some boil it in wine, putting some smallage seed thereto, and afterwards some oil.

The wall rue is as effectual as maiden hair in all the diseases of the head, or falling and recovering of the hair again, and generally for all the afore-mentioned diseases. And the powder of it taken in drink for forty days, cureth ruptures in children.

GOLDEN MAIDEN HAIR.

Description.—It hath many small, brownish red hairs to make up the form of leaves growing on the ground from the root ; and in the middle of them, rise small stalks of the same colour, set with very fine yellowish green hairs, bearing a small, gold yellow head, less than a wheat corn, standing in a great husk. The root is small and thready.

Time.—It groweth in bogs and moorish places ; also on dry and shady places.

Its medicinal virtues are same as the other maiden hairs.

MALLOWS AND MARSHMALLOWS.

COMMON mallows are generally so well known, that they need no description. Our common marshmallows have divers soft, hairy white stalks, rising to be three or four feet high, spreading forth many branches, the leaves whereof are soft and hairy, less than the other mallow leaves, but longer pointed, cut, for the most part, into some few divisions, but deep. The flowers are many, but smaller also than the other mallows, and white, or tending to a bluish colour; after which come such long round cases and seeds as in the other mallows. The roots are many and long, shooting from one head, of the size of a finger, very pliant, tough, and like liquorice, of a light yellow on the outside, and white within, full of slimy juice, which being laid in water, will thicken it like a jelly.

Place.—The common mallows grow almost everywhere ; and marshmallows are almost to be got everywhere.

Time.—They flower all the summer months, even until the winter doth pull them down.

Government and Virtues.—Venus owns them both. The leaves of mallows, and the roots boiled in wine and water, or in broth with parsley or fennel roots, open the body, and are very convenient in agues, or other distempers of the body, to apply the leaves warmed to the belly. It not only voideth choleric, and other offensive humours, but easeth the pains of the belly, and are therefore used in all clysters conducing to those purposes : the same used by nurses procureth them stores of milk. The decoction of the seed of mallows made in milk or wine, marvelously cures excoriations, phthisic, pleurisy, and other diseases of the chest and lungs, if it be taken constantly.

The leaves and roots work the same effects ; they help much in the excoriations of the bowels, and hardness of the mother, and in all hot and sharp diseases thereof. The juice drunk in wine, or the decoction of them therein promotes speedy and easy delivery. Pliny saith, that whosoever shall take a spoonful of any of the mallows, shall that day be free from all threatened diseases, and it is good for falling sickness. The syrup and conserve made of the flowers, are very effectual for the same diseases, and to open the body. The leaves bruised and laid to the eyes with a little honey, take away the imposthumes of them; the leaves bruised or rubbed upon the place stung with bees, or wasps, and take away pain, and swellings. Dioscorides saith the decoction of the roots and leaves are an antidote to poisons. A poultice made of the leaves boiled and bruised with some bean or barley flour, and oil of roses added, is an especial remedy against all hard tumours and inflammations, or imposthumes, or swelling of the testicles ; it softens the hardness of the liver and spleen. The juice of mallows boiled in oil and applied, taketh away all roughness of the skin, scurf, dandriff, or dry scabs in the head or other parts, if they be anointed therewith, or washed with the decoction, and it preserveth the hair from falling off. It is also effectual against scaldings and burnings, St. Anthony's fire, and all hot, red, and painful swellings in any other part of the body.

The flowers boiled in oil or water whereunto a little honey and alum are put, is an excellent gargle to wash, cleanse, or heal any sore mouth or throat in a short time. If the feet be washed with the decoction of the leaves, roots, and flowers, it helpeth heat and rheum from the head : if the head be washed therewith, it stayeth shedding of the hair.

Marshmallows are a gentle purge, and in decoctions for clysters to ease all pains of the body, opening a straight passage and making it slippery, whereby the stone may descend more easily and without pain, out of the kidneys and bladder, and to ease the torturing pains. But the roots are of special use for those purposes, and coughs, hoarseness, shortness of breath, and wheezings, being boiled in wine or water, are with good success used for excoriations in the bowels, or the bloody flux, easing the pains, and healing the soreness. It is profitably taken for rupture, cramp, or convulsions of the sinews ; and boiled in white wine for the imposthumes of the throat, in the king's evil, and inflammations and swellings in women's breasts. The dried roots boiled in milk and drunk, are good for the hooping cough. Hippocrates used to give the decoction of the roots, or the juice thereof, to drink, to those that are wounded and ready to faint through loss of blood, and applied the same mixed with honey and rosin to the wounds ; as also the roots boiled in wine, to those that have received any hurts by bruises, falls, or blows, or had any bone or member out of joint, or any swelling pain or ache in the muscles, sinews, or arteries. The mucilage of the roots, and of linseed and fenugreek put together, is much used in poultices, ointments, and plasters, to mollify and digest all hard swellings, and the inflammation of them, and to ease pains in any part of the body. The seed either green or dry, mixed with vinegar, cleanseth the skin of morphew, and all other discolourings, being boiled therewith in the sun.

A young man, related to me, had the bloody flux, and the excoriation of his bowels was very grea⁴ ; myself being in the country, was sent for, the only thing I gave him was mallows, bruised and boiled in milk and drunk ; in two days (the blessing of God being upon it) it cured him.

MAPLE TREE.

Government and Virtues.—It is under the dominion of Jupiter. The decoction either of the leaves or bark must needs strengthen the liver much. It is very good to open obstructions of the liver and spleen, and easeth pains of the sides thence proceeding.

WILD MARJORAM.

CALLED also origane, origanum, eastward marjorum, wild marjoram, and grove marjoram.

Description.—Wild or field marjoram hath a root which creepeth much underground, which continueth a long time sending up sundry brownish, hard square stalks, with small dark green leaves, like those of sweet marjorum, but harder, and somewhat broader; at the top of the stalks stand tufts of flowers, of a deep purplish red colour. The seed is small and blacker than that of sweet marjoram.

Place.—It groweth plentifully in the borders of cornfields, and in some copses.

Time.—It flowereth towards the latter end of summer.

Government and Virtues.—It is under the dominion of Mercury. It strengthens the stomach and head much, there being scarce a better remedy growing for such as are troubled with acidity in the stomach; it restores a lost appetite; it relieves coughs and consumption of the lungs; it cleanseth the body of choler, expelleth poison, and remedieth the infirmities of the spleen; cures the bitings of venomous beasts, and such as are poisoned by eating hemlock, henbane, or opium. It promotes urine and the terms in women, relieves dropsy, scurvy, scabs, itch, and yellow jaundice. The juice being dropped into the ears, cures deafness, pains and noise in the ears. And thus much for this herb, between which and adders there is a deadly antipathy.

SWEET MARJORAM.

THIS is well known, being an inhabitant in every garden.

Place.—They grow mostly in gardens; some sorts grow

wild in the borders of corn-fields and pastures ; but the garden kind are most used and useful.

Time.—They flower in the end of summer.

Government and Virtues.—It is an herb of Mercury and under Aries, and is an excellent remedy for the brain, and other parts of the body and mind under the dominion of the same planet. Our common sweet marjoram is warming and comfortable in cold diseases of the head, stomach, sinews, and other parts, taken inwardly, or outwardly applied. The decoction thereof being drunk, helpeth all diseases of the chest with shortness of breathing, and is also profitable for the obstructions of the liver and spleen. It relieves the cold griefs of the womb, and the windiness thereof ; and the loss of speech. The decoction thereof made with some pelitory of Spain and long pepper, or with a little acorns or origanum, being drunk is good for persons falling into a dropsy, for those that cannot make water, and for pains in the belly : it provoketh women's courses if it be used as a pessary. Being made into powder and mixed with honey, it taketh away the black marks of blows or bruises, it is good for inflammations and watering of the eyes, mixed with fine flour and laid upon them. The juice dropped into the ears easeth the pains and singing noise in them. It is profitably put into those ointment and salves that are warm, and it comforts the joints and sinews ; for swellings also, and places out of joint. The powder thereof snuffed up into the nose, provoketh sneezing, and purgeth the brain ; and chewed draweth forth much phlegm. The oil made thereof is very warm and comfortable to stiff joints, and the sinews that are hard, to mollify and supple them. Marjoram is much used in all odoriferous waters, powders, &c. that are for ornament or delight.

MARIGOLDS.

THESE being so plentiful in every garden, are so well known that they need no description.

Time.—They flower all the summer long, and sometimes in winter if it be mild.

Government and Virtues.—It is an herb of the Sun, and

under Leo. They strengthen the heart exceedingly, and are very expulsive, and little less effectual in the small pox and measles than saffron. The juice of marigold leaves mixed with vinegar, and any hot swellings bathed with it, instantly giveth ease, and assuageth it. The flowers, either green or dried, are much used in possets, broths, and drink, as a comforter of the heart and spirits, and to expel any malignant quality which may annoy them. A plaster made with the dried flowers in powder, hog's lard, turpentine, and rosin, applied to the breast, strengthens and succours the heart in fevers.

MASTERWORT.

Description.—Common masterwort hath divers stalks of winged leaves divided into sundry parts, three standing together at small foot-stalks on both sides of the greater, and three likewise at the end of the stalk, somewhat broad, and cut in on the edges into three or four divisions, all of them dented about the brims, of a dark green colour, resembling the leaves of angelica, but growing lower to the ground, and on lesser stalks ; among which rise up two or three short stalks about two feet high, and slender, with such like leaves at the joints which grow below, but with less and fewer divisions, bearing umbels of white flowers, and thin, flat, blackish seeds. The root grows rather sideways than deep in the ground, shooting forth sundry heads, which taste sharp, biting on the tongue, and is the hottest and sharpest part of the plant.

Place.—It is usually grown in gardens.

Time.—It flowereth and seedeth about the end of August.

Government and Virtues.—It is an herb of Mars. The root of Masterwort is hotter than pepper, and very available in cold griefs and diseases both of the stomach and body, dissolving very powerfully both upwards and downwards. It is also used in a decoction with wine against all cold rheums, distillations upon the lungs, or shortness of breath, to be taken morning and evening. It promotes urine, and breaks the stone, and expels the gravel in the kidneys ; provoketh women's courses, and expelleth the

dead birth. It is very good for strangling of the mother
and other such like feminine diseases.   It is effectual also
in dropsy, cramps, and falling sickness ; for the decoction
in wine being gargled in the mouth, draweth down much
water and phlegm from the brain, purging and easing it
of what oppressed it.   It is of a rare quality against all
sorts of cold poison, to be taken as there is a cause; it
provoketh sweat.   But lest the taste hereof, or of the seed,
should be too offensive, the best way is to take the water
distilled both from the herb and root.   The juice hereof
dropped, or tents dipped therein and applied either to
green wounds or rotten ulcers, and those that come by en-
venomed weapons, doth soon cleanse and heal them.   The
same is also very good in gout coming of a cold cause.

SWEET MAUDLIN.

Description. — Common maudlin hath somewhat long
and narrow leaves, snipped about the edges.   The stalks
are two feet high, bearing at the tops many yellow flowers
set around together, and all of an equal height, in umbels
or tufts like unto tansy, after which followeth small whitish seed.

Place and Time. — It groweth in gardens, and flowereth
in June and July.

Government and Virtues. — The virtues hereof being the
same with costmary or alecost, I shall not make any re-
petition thereof, lest my book grow too big, but rather
refer you unto costmary for satisfaction.

THE MEDLAR.

Description. — The tree groweth near the size of the
quince tree, spreading branches reasonably large, with
longer and narrower leaves than either the apple or quince,
and not dented about the edges.   At the end of the sprigs
stand the flowers, made of five white, great, broad-pointed
leaves, nicked in the middle with some white threads
also ; after which cometh the fruit, of a brownish green
colour being ripe, bearing a crown as it were on the top,
which were the five green leaves ; and being fallen away,
the head of the fruit is seen to be rather hollow.   The

fruit is harsh before it is mellowed, and has five hard kernels within it. There is another kind like the former, but that it hath some thorns in several places, which the other hath not, and the fruit is small, and not so pleasant.

Place and Time.—They grow in this land, and flower in May, and bear fruit in September.

Government and Virtues.—The fruit is Saturn's, and there is not a better medicine to strengthen the retentive faculty. A plaster made of the fruit dried, and other convenient things, and applied to the reins of the back prevent miscarriage. They stay fluxes of blood or humours; and the leaves also have this quality. The fruit eaten by women with child, stayeth their longing after unusual meats, and prevents miscarriage. The decoction of them is good to gargle and wash the mouth, throat, and teeth, when there is any defluctions of blood to stay it, or humours which causeth pains and swellings. It is a good bath for women to sit over that have their courses flowing too abundant; or for the piles. If a poultice or plaster be made with dried medlars, and mixed with the juice of red roses, and a few cloves and nutmegs added, and a little red coral also, and applied to the stomach that is given to casting or loathing of meat, it cureth. The dried leaves in powder strewed on fresh bleeding wounds restraineth the blood and healeth the wound quickly. The medlar-stones made into powder, and drunk in wine, in which parsley roots have been infused all night, or a little boiled, breaks and expels stone in the kidneys.

MELLILOT, OR KING'S CLAVER.

Description.—This hath many green stalks two or three feet high, rising from a tough, long, white root, set round about at the joints with small and rather long, well-smelling leaves, set three together, unevenly dented about the edge. The flowers are yellow, made like other trefoil, but small, standing in long spikes one above another, for an hand-breadth long, which turn into long crooked cods, containing flat brownish seed.

Place.—It groweth plentifully in Suffolk, Essex, and in

Huntingdonshire and other places; but most usually in corn-fields, and in corners of meadows.

Time.—It flowereth in June and July, and the seed is ripe quickly after.

Government and Virtues.—Mellilot boiled in wine and applied mollifieth hard tumours and inflammations in the eyes, or other parts of the body, as the fundament or privy parts; and sometimes the yolk of a roasted egg, or fine flour, or poppy-seed, or endive is added to it. It cures spreading ulcers in the head, used as a wash or ley. It relieves pains of the stomach being applied fresh, or boiled with any of the afore-named things; also pains of the ears, being dropped into them; and steeped in vinegar or rose water, it mitigateth the head-ache. The flowers of mellilot and camomile are much used to be put together in clysters to expel wind, and ease pains; and also in poultices for the same purpose, and to assuage swelling tumours in the spleen or other parts and stayeth inflammations. The juice dropped into the eyes, is effectual to take away the film or skin that dimmeth the eye-sight. The head often washed with distilled water of the herb and flower, or a ley made therewith, is effectual in insanity; as also to strengthen the memory, to comfort the head and brain, and to preserve them from apoplexy.

FRENCH AND DOG MERCURY.

Description.—This riseth up with a square great stalk full of joints, two feet high or thereabouts, with two leaves at every joint, and the branches likewise from both sides of the stalk set with fresh green leaves, broad and long, about the size of the leaves of basil, finely dented about the edges; towards the tops of the stalks and branches come forth at every joint, in the male mercury, two small round green heads standing together upon a short footstalk, which growing ripe, are seeds not having flowers. The female stalk is longer, spike-fashion, set round about with small green husks, which are the flowers, made like small bunches of grapes, which have no seed, but abide long upon the stalks without shedding. The root is composed of many small fibres, which perisheth in winter, and riseth again of its own sowing.

Having described French mercury, I come now to show you a description of DoG MERCURY.

Description.—This is male and female, having many stalks slender and lower than mercury, without any branches; the root is set with two leaves at every joint, larger than the female, but more pointed and full of veins, and harder in handling, of a dark green colour, and less dented about the edges; at the joints with the leaves come forth longer stalks than the former, with two hairy round seeds upon them, twice as large as those on the former mercury. The female has much harder leaves standing upon longer foot-stalks, and the stalks are much longer; from the joints come forth spikes of flowers like the French female mercury. The roots of them both are many, and full of small fibres, which run underground and mat themselves very much, not perishing as the former mercuries do, but abiding all the winter, and shoot forth new branches every year.

Place.—The male and female French mercury are found wild in divers places of this land.

The dog mercury in sundry places of Kent also, and elsewhere; but the female more seldom than the male.

Time.—They flower in the summer months, and therein give their seed.

Government and Virtues.—Mercury owns the herb, but I think it is Venus's. The decoction of the leaves of mercury, or the juice in broth, or drunk with a little sugar, purgeth choleric and waterish humours. Hippocrates commended it wonderfully for women's diseases, and applied to the secret parts to ease the pains of the mother; and used the decoction of it to procure women's courses; and gave the decoction with myrrh or pepper, or applied the leaves outwardly against strangury and diseases of the reins and bladder. He used it for sore and watering eyes, and for deafness and pains in the ears, by dropping the juice into them, and bathing them afterwards in white wine. The decoction made with water and a cock chicken, is a most safe medicine for hot fits of agues. It cleanseth the breast and lungs of phlegm, but a little offendeth the stomach. The juice or distilled water snuffed up into the nostrils, purgeth the head and eyes of catarrhs and rheums. Some used to drink two or three ounces of the distilled water, with a little sugar, in the morning fasting, to purge the body of gross, viscuous, and melancholy humours. It is wonderful (if not fabulous) what Dioscorides and Theophrastus relate of it, viz.—That if women use these herbs either inwardly or outwardly, for three days together after conception, they shall bring forth male or female children, according to that kind of herb they use. Matthiolus saith, that the seed of mercury boiled with wormwood and drunk, soon cureth yellow jaundice. The leaves or the juice rubbed upon warts, taketh them away. The juice mingled with some vinegar, cures running scabs, tetters, ringworms, and the itch. Galen saith, that being applied as a poultice to any swelling or inflammation, it subdues both, and is given in clysters to evacuate offensive humours. The dog mercury, although less used, yet may serve in the same manner, to the same purposes, to purge waterish and melancholy and waterish humours.

MINT.

OF the kinds of mint, the spear mint, or heart mint, I shall only describe as follows :

Description.—Spear mint hath divers round stalks, and long but narrowish leaves set thereon, of a dark green colour. The flowers stand in spiked heads at the tops of the branches, being of a pale blue colour. The scent is nearly like that of bazil ; it increaseth by the root under ground, as all the others do.

Place.—It is much grown in gardens ; and as it seldom giveth any good seed, the defect is recompensed by the plentiful increase of the root, which being once planted, is difficult to get rid of.

Time.—It flowereth in the beginning of August.

Government and Virtues.—It is an herb of Venus. It hath an heating, binding, and drying quality, and therefore the juice taken in vinegar stayeth bleeding ; it stirreth up venery or bodily lust ; two or three branches thereof taken in the juice of four pomegranates stayeth the hiccup, vomiting, and allayeth choler. It dissolveth imposthumes being laid to with barley-meal. It is good to repress the milk in women's breasts, and for such as are swollen. Applied with salt, it cures the biting of a mad dog : with mead and honeyed water it easeth the pains of the ears, and taketh away the roughness of the tongue being rubbed thereupon. It suffereth not milk to curdle in the stomach, if the leaves be steeped or boiled in it before you drink it. The decoction is a powerful medicine to stay women's courses and the whites. Applied to the forehead and temples, it easeth headache, and is good to wash the heads of children with, for eruptions, sores, scabs, and healeth sores of the fundament. The distilled water is good for all the purposes aforesaid. But if a spirit thereof be chemically drawn, it is more powerful than the herb itself. Simeon Sethi saith, it helpeth a cold liver, strengtheneth the belly, causeth digestion, stayeth vomits and the hiccup ; it taketh away obstructions of the liver, and stirreth up bodily lust ; but too much must not be taken, as it maketh the blood thin, and turneth it into choler, therefore angry persons must abstain from it. It is a safe medicine for the biting of a mad dog, being bruised with salt and laid thereon. The powder taken after meat, helpeth digestion and those that are splenetic. Taken with wine, it helpeth women in travail. It is good for gravel and stone, and the strangury. Being smelled unto, it relieves the head and memory. The decoction gargled in the mouth, cureth sore gums and mouth, and ill-savoured breath. With rue and coriander, it causeth the palate of the mouth to turn to its place, being gargled with the decoction, and held in the mouth.

The virtues of the wild HORSE-MINT, such as grow in ditches, expel wind in the stomach, cure colic, and relieve short-winded, and are an especial remedy for pollutions in the night, being applied to the testicles. The juice dropped into the ears easeth their pains. They are good against venomous biting of serpents. The juice laid on warm is good for the king's evil. The decoction or distilled water cure a stinking breath, and snuffed up the nose, purgeth the head. Pliny saith, that eating the leaves hath cured the leprosy, applying some of them to the face, and to prevent scurf in the head, used with vinegar.

MISTLETOE.

Description.—This riseth up from the branch or arm of the tree whereon it groweth, with a woody stem, putting itself into sundry branches, and they again divided into smaller twigs interlacing themselves one within another, covered with a greyish green bark, having two leaves set at every joint, and at the ends, which are somewhat long and narrow, small at the bottom, but broader towards the end. At the knots or joints of the branches grow small yellow flowers, which run into small, round, white, transparent berries, three or four together, full of a glutinous moisture, with a blackish seed in each of them.

Place.—It groweth rarely on oaks with us ; but upon sundry other timber as fruit trees plentifully in woody groves, in this land.

Time.—It flowereth in the spring-time, but the berries are not ripe until October, and abideth on the branches all the winter.

Government and Virtues.—This is under the dominion of the Sun. That which grows upon oaks participates something of the nature of Jupiter, because an oak is one of his trees ; as also that which grows upon pear-trees and apple-trees participates something of his nature, because he rules the tree it grows upon, having no root of its own. But why that should have most virtues that grows upon oaks I know not. Clusius affirms that which grows upon pear-trees to be as prevalent, and gives order that it should not touch the ground after it is gathered. Both the leaves and berries of mistletoe do heat and dry, and are of subtle parts ; the birdlime doth mollify hard knots, tumours, and imposthumes ; ripeneth and discusseth them, and draweth forth the humours from the remote parts of the body. And being mixed with equal parts of rosin and wax, doth mollify the hardness of the spleen, and cures ulcers and sores. Being mixed with sandaric and orpiment. it helpeth to draw off foul nails ; and if quicklime and wine lees be add-

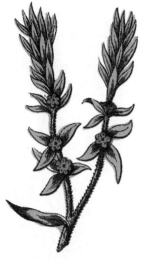

Glasswort

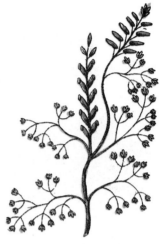

Fumitory

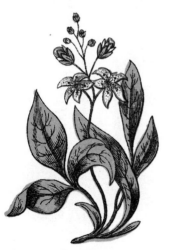

Buckbean

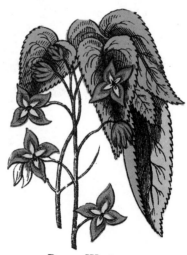

Baren Wort

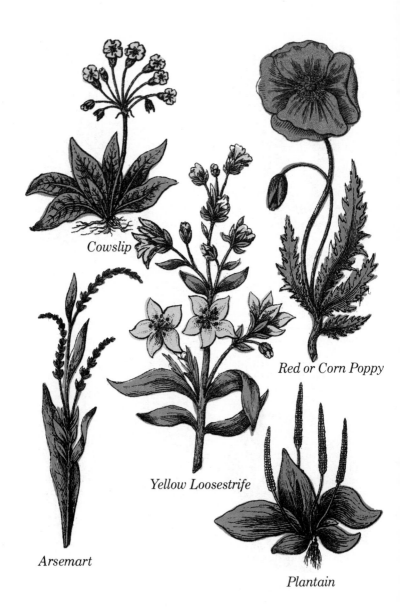

Cowslip

Red or Corn Poppy

Arsemart

Yellow Loosestrife

Plantain

ed thereunto, it worketh the stronger. The mistletoe itself of the oak, made into powder, and given in drink to
those that have the falling-sickness, effects a cure in a few
days. Some, for the virtues thereof, have called it *lignun
sanctæ crucis*, wood of the holy cross, as it cures falling
sickness, apoplexy, and palsy very speedily, not only to be
inwardly taken, but to be hung at their neck. Tragus
saith, that the fresh wood of any mistletoe bruised, and
the juice drawn forth and dropped into the ears, cures imposthumes in them.

MONEYWORT, or HERB TWOPENCE.

Description.—The common moneywort sendeth forth
from a small thready root, divers long, weak, and slender
branches, lying and running upon the ground two or three
feet long or more, set with leaves two at a joint one against
another at equal distances, which are almost round, but
pointed at the ends, smooth, and of a good green colour.
At the joints, with the leaves from the middle, forward,
come forth at every point sometimes on two yellow flowers
standing each on a small foot-stalk, and made of five
leaves, narrow-pointed at the ends, with some yellow
threads in the middle, and afterwards small round heads
of seed.

Place.—It groweth plentifully in most places, in moist
grounds by hedge-sides, and in the middle of grassy fields.

Time.—They flower in June and July, and their seed is
ripe quickly after.

Government and Virtues.—Venus owns it. Moneywort
is singularly good to stay all fluxes, whether lasks, bloody
fluxes, the flowing of women's courses, bleeding inwardly
or outwardly, and weak stomachs given to casting. It is
very good for the ulcers or excoriations of the lungs. It
is capital for wounds, either fresh or green, to heal them
speedily, and for ulcers of a spreading nature. For all
which purposes the juice of the herb, or the powder drunk
in water wherein hot steel has been often quenched ; or
the decoction of the green herb in wine or water drunk,
or applied to the outward place, as a wash, or tents dipped
therein and put into them. are effectual.

M

MOONWORT.

Description.—It riseth up usually but with one dark, green, thick and flat leaf, standing upon a short foot-stalk not above two fingers' breadth ; but when it flowers it bears a small slender stalk about five inches high, having but one leaf in the middle, which is much divided on both sides into sometimes five or seven parts on a side ; each of which parts is small like the middle rib, but broad forwards, pointed and round, resembling a half moon, from whence it took the name ; the uppermost parts or divisions being larger than the lower. The stalks rise above this leaf two or three inches, bearing many branches of small long tongues, like the spiky head of the adder's tongue, of a browish colour, which after they have continued a while, resolve into a mealy dust. The root is small and fibrous.

Place.—It groweth on hills and heaths, and where there is much grass, it delighteth to grow.

Time.—It is to be found only in April and May ; for in hot weather it withers and dies.

Government and Virtues. — The Moon owns the herb. Moonwort is cold and drying more than adder's tongue, and is therefore held to be more available for wounds both inward and outward. The leaves boiled in white wine, and drunk, stays the immoderate flux of women's courses, and the whites. It also stayeth bleeding, vomiting, and other fluxes. It is good for blows and bruises, and to consolidate all fractures and dislocations. It is good for ruptures, but it is chiefly used by most with other herbs to make oils or balsams to heal fresh or green wounds, for which it is lent.

Moonwort (they absurdly say,) will open locks and unshoe such horses as tread upon it ; but some country people call it *unshoe the horse.*

MOSSES.

I SHALL speak only of two kinds, as the principal, viz. *ground moss* and *tree moss*, both of which are very well known.

Place.—The ground moss groweth in moist woods, and

in the bottom of hills, in boggy grounds and in shady ditches, and many other such like places. The tree moss groweth only on trees.

Government and Virtues.—They are under the dominion of Saturn. The ground moss is said to be good to break the stone, and to expel it by urine, being boiled in wine and drunk. The herb being bruised, boiled in water, and applied, easeth pains coming from a hot cause, and is used to ease the pains of the gout.

The tree mosses are cooling and binding, and partake of a digesting and mollifying quality, as Galen saith. But each moss partakes of the nature of the tree from whence it is taken : therefore that of the oak is more binding, and is of good effect to stay fluxes, vomiting or bleeding, the powder being taken wine. The decoction thereof in wine is very good for women to sit in, that have profuse menstruation. The same being drunk prevents vomiting, and hiccup, and as Avicena saith, it comforteth the heart. The powder thereof taken in drink for some time is good in dropsy. The oil that has had fresh moss steeped therein for a time and afterwards boiled and applied to the temples and forehead, marvelously eases the headache caused by heat, as also the distillations of hot rheums or humours in the eyes or other parts. The ancients much used it in their ointments and other medicines against lassitude, and to strengthen the sinews, for which it was found good then, it may be found so still.

MOTHERWORT.

Description.—It has a hard, square, brownish, rough, strong stalk. rising three or four feet high, spreading into many branches, whereon grow leaves on each side with long foot-stalks two at every joint, which are rather broad and long, with many great veins therein of a sad green colour, and deeply dented about the edges, and almost divided. From the middle of the branches to the tops of them, grow the flowers round them at distances, in sharp-pointed, rough, hard husks, of a more red or purple colour than balm or horehound, but in the same manner or form as the horehounds, after which come many small, round, blackish seeds. The root sendeth forth long strings and small fibres, of a dark yellowish or brownish colour, and abideth.

Place.—It groweth only in gardens.

Government and Virtues.—Venus owns the herb, and it is under Leo. There is no better herb to take melancholy vapours from the heart, to strengthen it, and make a merry, cheerful soul than this herb. It may be kept in a syrup, or conserve; therefore the Latins called it *cardiaca.* Besides, it makes women joyful mothers of children, and settles their wombs; therefore they call it motherwort. It allays trembling of the heart, and faintings and swoonings; from whence it took the name *cardiaca.* The powder thereof, about a spoonful drunk in wine, is a wonderful help to women in their sore travail. It also provoketh urine and women's courses, cleanseth the chest of cold phlegm, and killeth worms. It is of good use to dry up the cold humours, to digest and disperse them from the veins, joints, and sinews; and to relieve cramps and convulsions.

MOUSE-EAR.

Description.—Mouse-ear is a low herb, creeping upon the ground by small strings like the strawberry plant, whereby it shooteth forth small roots, whereat grow many small and somewhat short leaves, set in round form together, and very hairy, which being broken give a whitish milk : from among these leaves spring up two or three small hoary stalks about a span high, with a few smaller leaves thereon ; at the tops whereof standeth usually but one flower, consisting of many pale yellow leaves broad at the point and a little dented in, set in three or four rows, very like a dandelion flower, and a little reddish underneath about the edges, especially if it grow in a dry ground ; which after they have stood long in flower, do turn into down, which with the seed is carried away with the wind.

Place.—It groweth on ditch banks, and sometimes in ditches if they be dry, and in sandy grounds.

Time.—It flowereth about June or July, and abideth green all the winter.

Government and Virtues.—The Moon owns this herb. The juice taken in wine, or the decoction drunk, cures the jaundice, though of long continuance, to drink thereof morning and evening, and abstain from other drink two or three hours after. It is a special remedy for the stone, and the tormenting pains thereof; and griping pains of the bowels. The decoction with succory and centaury, is very effectual in dropsy, and the diseases of the spleen. It stayeth fluxes of blood at the mouth or nose, and inward bleeding also; for it is a singular wound herb for wounds both inward and outward; it restrains the bloody-flux, and the abundance of women's courses. There is a syrup made of the juice and sugar, by the apothecaries of Italy, which is highly esteemed, and given to those that have a cough, and in phthisic, and for ruptures or burstings. The green herb bruised, and bound to any cut or wound, doth quickly close the lips thereof; and the decoction, or powder of the dried herb, wonderfully stays spreading and fretting cankers and ulcers in the mouth and other parts. The distilled water of the plant is applicable for the diseases aforesaid, and to wash outward wounds and sores, and apply tents of cloths wet therein.

MUGWORT.

Description.—Common mugwort hath divers leaves lying on the ground, very much divided, or cut deeply in about the brims, like wormwood, but much larger, of a dark green colour on the upper side, and hoary white underneath. The stalks rise four or five feet high, having on it such like leaves as those below, but somewhat smaller, branching forth very much towards the top, whereon are set very small, pale, yellowish flowers, like buttons, which fall away, and after them come small seeds inclosed in round heads. The root is long and hard, with many small fibres growing from it, whereby it taketh strong hold on the ground; but both stalks and leaves lie down every year, and the root shooteth anew in the spring.

Place.—It groweth plentifully by the water-sides, and by small water-courses.

Time.—It flowereth and seedeth in the end of summer.

Government and Virtues.—This is an herb of Venus, therefore maintaineth the parts of the body she rules, remedies the diseases of the parts that are under her signs Taurus and Libra. Mugwort is with good success put among other herbs that are boiled for women to sit over to draw down their courses, to help the delivery of their birth ; as also for the obstructions and inflammations of the mother. It breaketh the stone, and causeth one to make water where it is stopped. The juice thereof made up with myrrh, and put under as a pessary, worketh the same effects, and so do the roots. Being made with hog's lard into an ointment, it taketh away wens and hard knots, and kernels in the neck and throat, and easeth the pains about the neck more effectually if some field daisies be put with it. The herb being fresh, or the juice taken, is a special remedy upon the overmuch taking of opium. Three drachms of the powder of the dried leaves taken in wine, is a speedy and certain help for sciatica. A decoction made with camomile and agrimony, and the place bathed while it is warm, taketh away pains of the sinews and cramp.

THE MULBERRY TREE.

THIS is so well known where it groweth, that it needeth no description.

Time.—It beareth fruit in the months of July and of August.

Government and Virtues.—Mercury rules the tree. The mulberry is of different parts : The ripe berries by reason of their sweetness and slippery moisture, opening the body, and the unripe binding it, especially when they are dried, and they are good to stay fluxes, lasks, and profuse menstruation. The bark of the root killeth broad worms. The juice or the syrup made of the juice of the berries, cures inflammations or sores in the mouth or throat, and palate when it is fallen down. The juice of the leaves is a remedy againt the bitings of serpents, and for those that have taken aconite. The leaves beaten with vinegar are good for burns with fire. A decoction of the bark and leaves is good to wash the mouth and teeth when they ache. If the root be a little slit or cut, and a small hole made in the ground next thereunto in the harvest time, it will give out a certain juice, which being hardened the next day, is of good use for the tooth-ache, to dissolve knots, and to purge. The leaves of mulberries stay bleeding at the mouth or nose, or the bleeding of the piles or of a wound, being bound unto the places.

MULLEIN.

Description.—Common white mullein hath many fair, large, woolly, white leaves lying next the ground, somewhat larger than broad, pointed at the ends, and dented about the edges. The stalk riseth up five feet high, covered over with such like leaves, but less, so that no stalk can be seen for the multitude of leaves thereon up to the flowers, which come forth on all sides of the stalk, without any branches for the most part, and many are set together in a long spike, in some of a yellow colour, some paler, consisting of five round-pointed leaves, which afterwards have small round heads, wherein is small brownish seed. The root is long, white, and woody, perishing after it hath borne seed.

Place.—It groweth by way-sides and lanes in many places of this land.

Time.—It flowereth in July, or thereabouts.

Government and Virtues.—It is under the dominion of Saturn. A small quantity of the root given in wine, is commended by Dioscorides against lasks and fluxes of the belly. The decoction hereof drunk, is profitable for ruptures, and for cramps and convulsions, and for old coughs. The decoction gargled easeth tooth-ache; and the oil made by the often infusion of the flowers, is of good effect for piles. The decoction of the root in red wine or in water, (if there be an ague) wherein red hot steel hath been often quenched, doth stay the bloody-flux. The same also openeth obstructions of the bladder and reins when one cannot make water. A decoction of the leaves, and of sage, marjoram, and camomile flowers, and the places bathed therewith, that have sinews stiff with cold or cramps, gives much ease and comfort. Three ounces of the distilled water of the flowers drunk morning and evening for some days together, is a most excellent remedy for the gout. The juice of the leaves and flowers being laid upon rough warts, also the powder of the dried roots rubbed on, taketh them away, but doth no good to smooth warts. The powder of the dried flowers is an especial remedy for belly-ache, or colic. The decoction of the root, or the leaves, is of great effect to dissolve the tumours, swellings, or inflammations of the throat. The seed and leaves boiled in wine, and applied, draw forth speedily thorns and splinters in the flesh, and heal them also. The leaves bruised and wrapped in double papers, and covered with hot ashes and embers to bake awhile, and then taken and laid warm on any blotch or boil happening in the groin or share, heal them. The seed bruised and boiled in wine, and laid on any member that hath been out of joint, and set again, taketh away all swelling and pain.

MUSTARD.

Description.—Our common mustard hath large and broad rough leaves, very much jagged with uneven and unorderly gashes, somewhat like turnip leaves, but lesser and rougher. The stalk riseth a foot high, and sometimes more, being round, rough, and branched at the top, bearing such like leaves thereon as grow below, but less, and less divided, and divers yellow flowers one above another at the tops, after which come small rough pods, with small, lank, flat ends, wherein is contained round yellowish seed, sharp, hot, and biting upon the tongue.

Place.—This groweth with us in gardens only, and other manured places.

Time.—It is an annual plant, flowering in July, and the seed is ripe in August.

Government and Virtues.—It purifies the blood, and strengthens weak stomachs, being an herb of Mars, it is good for aged who are troubled with cold diseases. Aries claims something to do with it, therefore it strengthens the heart and resisteth poisons. Let such whose stomachs are weak and cannot digest their food, or relish it, take of mustard-seed a drachm, cinnamon as much, and having beaten them to powder, and half as much mastick in powder, and with gum arabic dissolved in rose water, make it up into troches, of which they may take one of about half a drachm weight an hour or two before meals ; let old men and women make much of this medicine, and they will give me thanks.

Mustard-seed hath the virtue of heat, discussing, rarifying. It is of good effect to bring down women's courses, for the falling sickness or lethargy, to use it both inwardly and outwardly, to rub the nostrils, forehead, and temples, to warm and quicken the spirits, for by the fierce sharpness it purgeth the brain by sneezing, and drawing down rheum and other humours, which by their distillations upon the lungs and chest, procure coughing ; and with some honey, doth much good therein. The decoction of the seed made in wine and drunk, provoketh urine, resisteth the force of poison, the malignity of mushrooms, and the venom of venomous creatures, if it be taken in time ; and taken before the cold fits of agues, it cureth them. The seed taken either by itself or with other things, either in an electuary or drink, stirs up bodily lust, and helpeth the spleen and pains in the sides, and gnawings in the bowels ; and used as a gargle, draweth up the palate of the mouth being fallen down ; and it dissolveth the swellings about the throat if it be outwardly applied. Being chewed it relieves the toothache. The outward application upon the pained place of sciatica, easeth the pains, as also the gout and other joint aches ; and is often used to ease pains in the sides or loins, the shoulder and other parts of the body, upon applying it as a plaster or poultice, till it raises blisters, and cureth the disease by drawing it to the outward parts of the body. It is also used to prevent the falling off of the hair. The seed bruised, mixed with honey, and applied, or made up with wax, taketh away the black and blue spots of bruises, the roughness or scabbiness of the skin, the leprosy and lousy evil. It relieves crick in the neck. The distilled water of the herb, when it is in flower, is drunk for any of the diseases aforesaid, or to wash the mouth when the palate is down, and for the diseases of the throat to gargle ; but outwardly for scabs, and itch, and cleanseth the face from morphew, spots freckles, and other deformities.

THE HEDGE MUSTARD.

Description. — This groweth up with one dark green stalk, tough, easy to bend, but not to break, branched into divers parts, and sometimes into stalks set full of branches, whereon grow long, rough, rugged leaves, much torn or cut on the edges in many parts, of a dirty green colour. The flowers are small and yellow, that grow on the tops of the branches in long spikes, flowering by degrees ; so that continuing long in flower, the stalk will have small round swads at the bottom, growing upright and close to the stalk, in which are contained small yellow seed, sharp and strong, as the herb is also. The root groweth down slender and woody, springing again every year.

Place.—This groweth frequently by the ways and hedge-sides, and sometimes in the open fields.

Time.—It flowereth most usually about July.

Government and Virtues.—Mars owns this herb also. It is good in all diseases of the chest and lungs, hoarseness, and by the use of the decoction for a little space, those have been recovered who had utterly lost their voice, and almost their spirits also. The juice made into a syrup or electuary with honey or sugar, is effectual for the same purpose, and for all coughs, wheezing, and shortness of breath. It cures the jaundice, pleurisy, pains in the back and loins, and torments in the belly, or colic, being also used in clysters. The seed is held to be a special remedy against poison and venom. It is good for sciatica, and in joint aches, ulcers, and cankers in the mouth, throat, or behind the ears, and for the hardness and swellings of the testicles, or women's breasts.

NAILWORT, or WHITLOW-GRASS.

Description.—This very small and common herb hath no roots, save only a few strings, it only grows to be above a hand's breadth high, the leaves are very small and somewhat long, not much unlike those of chickweed, among which rise up divers slender stalks bearing many small white flowers one above another, after which come small flat pouches containing small seed, of a sharp taste.

Place.—It grows upon old stone and brick walls, sometimes in dry gravelly grounds, especially if there be grass or moss near to shadow it.

Time.—They flower very early in the year, sometimes in January and February.

Government and Virtues.—It is very good for impostumes in the joints, and under the nails, which they call whitlows, felons, and nail wheals.

NEP, or CATMINT.

Description.—Common garden nep shooteth forth hard four-square stalks, with a hoariness on them, a yard high or more, full of branches, bearing at every joint two broad leaves like balm, but longer-pointed, softer, and more hoary, nicked about the edges, of a strong sweet scent. The flowers grow in large tufts at the tops of the branches, and underneath them likewise on the stalks, of a whitish purple colour. The roots are composed of many long strings or fibres, and abide with green leaves thereon all the winter.

Place.—It is only cultivated in gardens.

Time.—It flowereth in July, or thereabouts.

Government and Virtues.—It is an herb of Venus. Nep is generally used for procuring the courses, taken inwardly, or outwardly applied, either alone or with other herbs in a decoction as a bath, or sit over the vapour thereof ; and by the frequent use thereof it cureth barrenness, wind and pains of the mother. It is also used in pains of the head coming of any cold cause, catarrhs, rheums, and for swimming and giddiness thereof, and is of special use for colic and flatulency. It is effectual for cramps or cold aches, to disperse cold and wind that afflicteth the place, and is used for colds, coughs, and shortness of breath. The juice drunk in wine, is good for bruises. The green herb bruised and applied to the fundament, and lying there two or three hours, easeth and cureth piles ; the juice made into an ointment is effectual for the same purpose. The head washed with a decoction taketh away scabs, scurf, &c.

NETTLES.

NETTLES are well known by all.

Government and Virtues.—It is under the dominion of Mars. Mars is hot and dry, and winter is cold and moist; that is the reason why nettle tops eaten in the spring consume the phlegmatic superfluities in the body of man, that the coldness of winter hath left behind. The roots or leaves boiled, or the juice of either, or both made into an electuary with honey and sugar, is a safe and sure medicine to open the pipes and passages of the lungs, which is the cause of wheezing and shortness of breath, and expectorates tough phlegm, as also to raise the imposthumed pleurisy, and spend it by spitting; the same subdues the swelling of the almonds of the throat, the mouth and throat being gargled therewith. The juice is effectual to settle the palate of the mouth in its place, and to heal and temper the inflammations and soreness of the mouth and throat. The decoction of the leaves in wine being drunk, is good to provoke women's courses, and to settle the suffocation, strangling of the mother, and all other diseases thereof; also applied outwardly with a little myrrh. The same also, or the seed, provoketh urine and expelleth the gravel and stone, often proved to be effectual by many that have taken it. The same killeth worms in children, easeth pains in the sides, and dissolveth the windiness of the spleen. The juice of the leaves taken two or three days together, stayeth bleeding of the mouth. It is good for the bite of a mad dog. It is good in lethargy, especially to use it outwardly, to rub the forehead or temples in the lethargy, with a little salt. The distilled water of the herb is also effectual for the diseases aforesaid; as for outward wounds and sores to wash them, and cleanse the skin from morphew, leprosy, and other discolourings. The seed or leaves bruised and put into the nostrils, stayeth the bleeding of them, and taketh away the flesh growing in them called polypus. The juice of the leaves, or the decoction of them or the roots, is good to wash either old,

offensive sores, fistulas and gangrenes, and fretting or corroding scabs, manginess and itch in any part of the body,
as also green wounds, by washing them therewith, or applying the green herb bruised thereunto, though the flesh
were separated from the bones ; the same applied to those
that have been out of joint, being first set up again,
strengtheneth them ; as also gouty pains, and the defluction of humours upon the joints and sinews. An ointment
made of the juice, oil, and a little wax, is very good to rub
cold and benumbed members. A handful of the leaves of
green nettles, and another of wallwort, or deanwort,
bruised and applied to the gout, sciatica, or joint aches,
hath been found to be an admirable remedy.

NIGHTSHADE.

Description.— Common nightshade hath an upright,
round, green, hollow stalk, about a foot or half a yard high,
bushing forth in many branches, whereon grow many
green leaves somewhat broad, and pointed at the ends, soft
and full of juice like bazil, but longer, and unevenly dented about the edges ; at the tops of the stalks and branches
come forth three or four more white flowers, of five small
pointed leaves a-piece, standing on a stalk one above
another, with yellow pointels in the middle, composed of
four or five yellow threads set together, which afterwards
run into so many pendulous green berries, the size of small
peas, full of green juice, and small, whitish, round, flat
seed lying within it. The root is white, and a little woody
after its flower and fruit, with many small fibres at it.

Place.—It groweth wild under walls in rubbish, the common paths, and sides of hedges and fields, and in our gardens, without planting.

Time.—It lieth down every year, and riseth again of its
own sowing at the end of April.

Government and Virtues.—It is a cold Saturnine plant.
The common is used to cool hot inflammations either inwardly or outwardly, being no ways dangerous to any that
use it, as most other nightshades are, yet it must be used
moderately. The distilled water of the herb is safest to
be taken inwardly ; the juice also, clarified and taken, be-

ing mingled with a little vinegar, is good to wash the mouth and throat that is inflamed ; but outwardly the juice of the herb and berries, with oil of roses and a little vinegar, beaten in a mortar, is good to anoint all hot inflammations in the eyes. It is good for the shingles, ringworms, and in running and corroding ulcers, applied thereunto. A pessary dipped in the juice and dropped into the matrix, stayeth the immoderate menstruation ; a cloth wet therein, and applied to the testicles, upon any swelling therein, giveth much ease, also to the gout. The juice dropped into the ears easeth pains thereof, and Pliny saith it is good for hot swellings under the throat.

Do not mistake the deadly nightshade for this ; if you know it not, you may then let them both alone.

THE OAK.

Government and Virtues.—Jupiter owns the tree. The leaves and bark and the acorn cups bind and dry very much. The inner bark of the tree, and the thin skin that covereth the acorn, effectually stay spitting of blood and the bloody flux. The decoction of the bark and the powder of the cups, stay vomitings, spitting of blood, bleeding at the mouth, or other fluxes in men or women ; diarrhœa. The acorn in powder taken in wine, provoketh urine. The decoction of acorns and the bark made in milk is an antidote to poisonous herbs and medicines, and to the virulency of cantharides, when he hath his bladder ulcerated, and voideth blood. The distilled water of the oaken bud, before they break out into leaves, is good to be used either inwardly or outwardly to assuage inflammations, and stop all manner of fluxes. The same is very good in pestilential and hot burning fevers, for it resisteth the force of the infection, and allayeth heat ; it cooleth the heat of the liver, breaketh the stone, and stayeth women's courses. The decoction of the leaves worketh the same effects. The water that is found in the hollow places of old oaks, is very effectual against foul spreading scabs. The distilled water (or decoction, which is better) of the leaves, is one of the best remedies that I know of for the whites.

OATS.

Government and Virtues.—Oats fried with bay-salt and applied to the sides, take away the pains of stitches and wind in the sides of the belly, A poultice made of the meal of oats, and some oil of bays put thereunto, helpeth the itch and leprosy, also fistulas of the fundament, and dissolveth hard imposthumes. The meal of oats boiled with vinegar and applied, taketh away freckles and spots in the face.

ONE BLADE.

Description.—This small plant never beareth more than one leaf, but only when it riseth up with his stalk, which thereon beareth another, and seldom more, which are a blueish green colour, pointed with many ribs or veins therein, like plantain. At the top of the stalk grow many small white flowers star-fashion, smelling sweet; after which come small red berries, when they are ripe. The root is small, creeping under the upper crust of the earth, shooting forth in divers places.

Place.—It groweth in moist, shadowy, and grassy places of woods in many other places.

Time.—It flowereth about May, and the berries are ripe in June ; and then quickly perisheth, but springeth from the same root again.

Government and Virtues.—It is a precious herb of the Sun. Half a drachm or a drachm at most, in powder of the roots hereof taken in wine and vinegar, of each equal parts, and the party laid to sweat thereupon, is a sovereign remedy for the plague, and those who have a sore upon them; it expels the poison and infection, and defends the heart and spirits from danger. It is a singular good wound herb, is used in many compound balsams for curing of wounds, be they fresh and green, or old and malignant, and especially if the sinews be burnt.

ORCHIS.

IT hath almost as many several names attributed to the several sorts of it as would almost fill a sheet of paper ; as dog-stones, goat-stones, fool-stones, and fox-stones.

Description.—The roots are to be used with discretion. They have each of them a double root within, some of them are round, in others like a hand : these alter every year, when the one riseth and waxeth full the other perisheth : now it is that which is full which is to be used in medicines, the other being of no use.

Time.—One or other of them may be found in flower from the beginning of April to the end of August.

Government and Virtues.—They are hot and moist in operation. under the dominion of Venus, and provoke lust exceedingly, which, they say, the dried and withered roots do restrain. They kill worms in children · being bruised and applied they heal the king's evil.

ONIONS.

Government and Virtues.—Mars owns them, and they have this quality, to draw any corruption to them, for if you lay a pared one upon a dunghill, it will rot in half a day by drawing putrefaction to it : being bruised and applied to a sore, it will do the like. Onions are flatulent or windy, yet they somewhat promote appetite, increase thirst, ease the bowels, provoke women's courses, cureth the biting of a mad dog, and other venomous creatures, to be used with honey and rue. They kill worms in children if they drink the infusion fasting. Being roasted under the embers and eaten with honey or sugar and oil, they much conduce to relieve an inveterate cough, and expectorate tough phlegm. The juice being snuffed up into the nostrils, purgeth the head, and helpeth the lethargy ; yet often eating them procures pains in the head. By country people it is held as a great preservative against infection, to eat onions fasting with bread and salt ; to make a great onion hollow, and filling it with treacle, and then roast it well under the embers, which after removing the outermost skin, and beaten together, is a sovereign salve for sores, or any putrified ulcer. The juice of onions is good for either scalds or burnings by fire, water, or gunpowder, and used with vinegar, taketh away all blemishes, spots, and marks in the skin ; and dropped into the ears, easeth the pains and noise in them. Applied with figs beaten together, it ripens and break imposthumes and other sores.

Leeks are like them in quality, they are a remedy against surfeit baked under the embers and taken, and being boiled and applied very warm, cureth the piles. In all other things they have the same property as the onions, though not so effectual.

ORPINE.

Description. —Common orpine riseth up with round brittle stalks, thick set with flat and fleshy leaves, without any order, and little or nothing dented about the edges, of a green colour. The flowers are white, or whitish, growing in tufts, after which come small chaffy husks, with seeds like dust in them. The roots are thick, white, tuberous clogs.

Place.— It is plentiful in this land, and in gardens, where it groweth larger than that which is wild, it groweth in shady sides of fields, and in woods.

Time.—It flowereth about July, and the seed is ripe in August.

Government and Virtues.—The Moon owns the herb. Orpine is seldom used in inward medicines with us, though Tragus saith from experience in Germany, that the distilled water thereof is profitable for gnawings or excoriations in the stomach or bowels, for ulcers in the lungs, liver, or other inward parts, and cures those diseases, being drunk for days together. It slayeth the sharpness of humours in the bloody-flux, and other fluxes, or in wounds. The root performeth the like effects. It is used outwardly to cool inflammation upon any hurt or wound, and easeth the pains of them ; as also to heal scaldings and burnings, the juice thereof being beaten with some green salad oil and anointed. The leaf bruised and laid to any green wound in the hand or legs, doth heal them quickly, and being bound to the throat, cureth the quinsy ; and it reduceth ruptures. If you make the juice into a syrup with honey or sugar, you may safely take a spoonful or two at a time.

PARSLEY.

Government and Virtues.—It is under the dominion of Mercury ; and is very comfortable to the stomach ; pro-

N

motes urine and women's courses, expels wind from the stomach and bowels, and doth a little open the body, but the root much more. It openeth obstructions both of the liver and spleen, and is accounted one of the five opening roots. Galen commended it for the falling sickness, and to provoke urine mightily, especially if the roots be boiled and eaten like parsnips. The seed is effectual to provoke urine and women's courses, to expel wind, to break the stone, and ease the pains and torments thereof ; it is also effectual in lethargy, and is as good for coughs. The distilled water of parsley is a familiar medicine with nurses to give their children when are troubled with wind in the stomach and belly, and is good for the aged. The leaves of parsley laid to the eyes that are inflamed with heat, or swollen, relieves them if it be used with bread or meal ; and being fried with butter, and applied to women's breasts that are hard through the curdling of their milk, it abateth the hardness quickly, it taketh away black and blue marks caused by bruises and falls. The juice dropped into the ears with a little wine, easeth the pains. Tragus hath an excellent medicine for falling-sickness and jaundice, dropsy and stone in the kidneys, take of the seed of parsley, fennel, annise, and carraway, of each an ounce ; of the roots of parsley, burnet, saxifrage, and carraways, of each an ounce and a half ; let the seeds be bruised, and the roots washed and cut small ; let them lie all night in steep in a bottle of white wine, and in the morning be boiled until a third part or more is wasted ; strain and clear, take four ounces thereof morning and evening, first and last, abstaining from drink after it for three hours. This openeth obstructions of the liver and spleen, and expelleth the dropsy or jaundice by urine.

PARSLEY PIERT, OR PARSLEY BREAKSTONE.

Description. — The root, though it be small and thready, yet it continues many years, from whence arise many leaves lying upon the ground, each standing upon a long small foot-stalk, the leaves as broad as a man's nail, very deeply dented on the edges, somewhat like a parsley leaf, but of a very dusky green colour. The stalks are very weak and slender, about three or four fingers in length, set so full of leaves that they can hardly be seen, either having no foot-stalks at all, or but very short ; the flowers are so small they can hardly be seen, and the seed as small as may be.

Place.—It is a common herb throughout the nation, and rejoiceth in barren, sandy, and moist places.

Time.—It may be found all the summer time, even from the beginning of April to the end of October.

Government and Virtues.—It promotes urine, and expels the stone. It is a very good salad herb. And is a very wholesome herb. You may take a drachm of the powder of it in sherry wine : it will bring away gravel from the kidneys insensibly and without pain. It cures strangury.

PARSNIPS.

THE garden kind is so well known that I shall not give a description of it. But the wild being of more physical use, I shall now describe it unto you.

Description.—The wild parsnip differeth little from the garden, but groweth not so fair and large, nor hath so many leaves, and the root is shorter, more woody, and not so fit to be eaten, and therefore more medicinal.

Place.—The name of the first showeth the place of its growth. The other groweth wild in divers places, as in marshes, and flowereth in July ; the seed being ripe about the beginning of August the second year after the sowing.

Government and Virtues.—The garden parsnips are under Venus ; it nourisheth much, and is good and wholesome, but a little windy : but it fatteneth the body if much used. It is good for the stomach and reins, and provoketh urine.

The wild parsnip hath a cutting, attenuating, cleansing, and opening quality therein. It easeth the pains and stitches in the sides, and expels wind from the stomach and bowels, or colic, and provoketh urine. The root is often used, but the seed much more. The wild being better than the tame.

COW PARSNIP.

Description.—This groweth with three or four large spread-winged, rough leaves, lying often on the ground. or else raised a little from it, with long, round, hairy footstalks under them, parted usually into five divisions, the two couples standing each against the other ; and one at the end, and each being almost round, yet somewhat deeply cut in on the edges in some leaves, and not so deep in others, of a whitish green colour, smelling strongly ; among which riseth up a round, crusted, hairy stalk, two or three feet high, with a few joints and leaves thereon, and branched at the top, where stand large umbels of white, and sometimes of reddish flowers, and after them flat, whitish, thin, winged seed, two always joined together. The root is long and white, with two or three long strings smelling strong and unpleasant.

Place.—It groweth in moist meadows, the borders and corners of fields, and near ditches.

Time.—It flowereth in July and seedeth in August.

Government and Virtues.—Mercury hath the dominion over them. The seed thereof is of a sharp and cutting quality, and therefore is a fit medicine for a cough and shortness of breath, the falling sickness and jaundice. The root is available to all the purposes aforesaid, and is also of great use to take away the hard skin that groweth on a fistula, if it be but scraped upon it. A decoction of the seed being drunk, cleanseth the chest from tough phlegmatic matter therein, easeth them that are liver-grown, being drunk and the smoke thereof received underneath, it arouses such as are fallen into a deep sleep, called lethargy, or by burning it under their nose. The seed and root boiled in oil, and the head rubbed therewith, is good in frenzy, lethargy, and in head-ache, if it be used with rue. It cureth running scabs and shingles. The juice of the flowers dropped into the ears that run and are full of matter, cleanseth and healeth them.

THE PEACH TREE.

Description.—A peach-tree groweth not so great as the apricot tree, yet spreadeth branches, from whence spring smaller reddish twigs, whereon are set long and narrow green leaves dented about the edges ; the blossoms are greater than the plum, and of a light purple colour ; the fruit round, sometimes the size of a pippin, others smaller, as also differing in colour and taste, as russet, red, or yellow, waterish or firm, rather downy, with a cleft like an apricot, and a rugged, furrowed, great stone within it, and a bitter kernel.

Place.—They are nursed in gardens and orchards through this land.

Time. —They flower in spring, and fructify in autumn.

Government and Virtues.—Venus owns this tree ; and for children and others nothing is better to purge choler and the jaundice than the leaves or flowers of this tree, being made into a syrup or conserve ; let such as delight to please their lust regard this fruit ; but such as have lost their health or their children's, let them regard what I say ; they may safely give two spoonfuls of the syrup at a time. The leaves of peaches bruised and laid on the belly, kill worms : and so being boiled in ale and drunk, and open their bowels ; and being dried is a safer medicine to discuss humours. The powder strewed upon fresh bleeding wounds stayeth their bleeding and closeth them. The flowers steeped all night in a little wine standing warm, strained in the morning, and drunk fasting, gently opens the bowels. A syrup made of them, as the syrup of roses is made, worketh more forcibly than that of roses, for it promotes vomiting, and spendeth waterish and hydropic humours by the continuance thereof. The flowers made into a conserve, worketh the same effect. The liquor that droppeth from the tree, being wounded, is given in the decoction of colt's-foot to those that are troubled with cough or shortness of breath, by adding thereunto some sweet wine, and putting some saffron therein. It is good for hoarseness and loss of voice ; helpeth all defects of the lungs, and those that vomit and spit blood. Two drachms in the juice of lemons or of raddish, is good for the stone. The kernels of the stones do wonderfully ease the pains and wringings of the belly, through wind or sharp humours, and help to make an excellent medicine for the stone upon all occasions in this manner : *I take fifty kernels of peach stones, and one hundred of the kernels of cherry stones, a handful of elder flowers fresh or dried, and three pints of muscatel; set them in a close pot into a bed of horse dung for ten days, after which distil in a glass with a gentle fire,* and keep it for your use : you may drink three or four ounces at a time. The milk or cream of these kernels with some vervain water, and applied to the forehead and temples, procures rest and sleep to sick persons. The oil drawn from the kernels, the temples therewith anointed, doth the like. The said oil put into clysters, easeth the pains of the wind colic ; and so, if anointed on the lower parts of the belly ; and dropped into the ears easeth the pains in them : the juice of the leaves doth the like. Being also anointed on the forehead and temples it helpeth the megrim, and all other pains in the head. If the kernels be bruised and boiled in vinegar until they become thick, and applied to the head, it marvelously causes the hair to grow again upon any bald place, or where it is too thin.

THE PEAR-TREE.

Government and Virtues.—The tree belongs to Venus. For their physical use they are best discerned by their taste. All the sweet and luscious sorts, whether manured or wild, help to move the belly downwards more or less. Those that are hard and sour, bind the belly as much, and the leaves do so also : those that are moist do to some extent cool, but harsh or wild ones much more, and are very good in repelling medicines ; and if the wild sort be boiled with mushrooms, it makes them less dangerous. The said pears boiled with a little honey, helps much the oppressed stomach, as all sorts of them do, some more, some less ; but the harsher sorts do more cool and bind, serving well to be bound in green wounds to cool and stay the blood, and heal the wound without any further trouble or inflammation, as Galen saith he found it by experience. The wild pears sooner close the lips of green wounds.

PELLITORY OF SPAIN.

COMMON pellitory of Spain, if it be planted in our gardens, will prosper well ; yet there is one sort growing ordinarily here wild, which I esteem to be little inferior to the other, if at all.

Description. — Common pellitory is a very common plant, and will not be kept in our gardens without diligent looking to. The root goes down right into the ground, bearing leaves, being long and finely cut upon the stalk, lying on the ground, much larger than the leaves of camomile are. At the top it bears one single large flower at a place, having a border of many leaves, white on the upper side, and reddish underneath, with a yellow thrum in the middle, not standing so close as that of camomile doth.

The other common pellitory which groweth here, hath a root of a sharp biting taste, scarcely discernible by the taste from that before described, from whence arise brittle stalks a yard high, with narrow long leaves finely dented about the edges, standing one above another. The flowers are white, standing in tufts like those of yarrow, with a small yellowish thrum in the middle. The seed is small.

Place. — The last groweth in fields, by the hedge sides and paths almost every where.

Time. — It flowereth at the latter end of June and in July.

Government and Virtues. — It is under the government of Mercury, and it is one of the best purgers of the brain that grows. An ounce of the juice taken in a draught of muscatel wine an hour before the fit of the ague comes, will assuredly drive away the ague at the second or third time taking at the farthest. Either the herb or root dried and chewed in the mouth, purgeth the brain of plegmatic humours ; thereby easing pains in the head and teeth, hindereth the distilling of the brain upon the lungs and eyes, thereby preventing coughs, phthisics, and consumptions, apoplexy and falling sickness. It is an excellent approved remedy in lethargy. The powder of the herb or root snuffed up the nostrils, procureth sneezing, and easeth the headache ; being made into an ointment with hog's lard, it takes away black and blue spots occasioned by blows or falls, and helps both the gout and sciatica.

PELLITORY OF THE WALL.

Description. — It riseth with brownish, red, tender, weak, and almost transparent stalks about two feet high, upon which grow at the joints two leaves somewhat broad and long, of a dark green colour, which afterwards turn brownish, smooth on the edges, but rough and hairy, as the stalks are also. At the joints with the leaves from the middle of the stalk upwards, where it spreadeth into branches, stand many small, purplish flowers in hairy rough heads or husks, after which come small, black, rough seed, which will stick to any cloth or garment that shall touch it. The root is long, with small fibres, of a dark reddish colour, which abideth in winter, although the stalks and leaves perish and spring every year.

Place.—It groweth wild generally, about the borders of fields and by the sides of walls and among rubbish. It will endure well if cultivated in gardens, and, planted on the shady sides, where it will spring again of its own sowing.

Time.—It flowereth in June and July, and the seed is ripe soon after.

Government and Virtues.—It is under the dominion of Mercury. The dried herb pellitory made up into an electuary with honey, or the juice of the herb, or the decoction thereof made up with sugar or honey, is a singular remedy for an old dry cough, shortness of breath, and wheezing. Three ounces of the juice taken at a time, wonderfully cures stopping of urine, and to expel the stone or gravel in the kidneys or bladder, and is therefore usually put among other herbs used in clysters to mitigate pains in the back, sides, or bowels, proceeding of wind, stopping of urine, the stone or gravel, as aforesaid. If the bruised herb sprinkled with some muscatel, be warmed upon a tile, or in a dish upon a few quick coals in a chafing dish, and applied to the belly, it has the same effect. The decoction of the herb being drunk, easeth pains of the mother, promotes women's courses; it also easeth those griefs that arise from obstructions of the liver, spleen, and reins. The decoction with a little honey, is good to gargle a sore throat. The juice held awhile in the mouth, easeth pains in the teeth. The distilled water of the herb drunk with sugar, worketh the same effects, and cleanseth the skin from spots, freckles, purples, wheals, sunburn, morphew, &c. The juice dropped into the ears, easeth the noise in them, and taketh away the pricking and shooting pains therein : the same, or the distilled water, assuageth hot and swelling imposthumes, burnings, and scaldings by fire or water ; as also other hot tumours and inflammations, or breakings out of heat, being bathed often with wet cloths dipped therein ; the juice made into a liniment with ceruse and oil of roses, and anointed therewith, cleanseth rotten ulcers, and stayeth spreading ulcers, and scabs or sores in children's heads ; and keeps the hair from falling off.   The ointment or the herb applied to the fundament, is capital for the piles ; and being mixed with goat's tallow, cureth gout : the juice is very effectual to cleanse and heal fistulas ; or the herb bruised and applied with a little salt.   It is effectual to heal a green wound, if it be bruised and bound thereto for three days.   A poultice made with it and mallows, and boiled in wheat bran and bean flour, and some oil, and applied warm to any bruised sinews, tendon, or muscle, doth in a very short time restore them to their strength, taking away the pains of the bruises, and dissolveth the congealed blood coming from blows, or falls from high places.

The juice of pellitory of the wall clarified and boiled in a syrup with honey, and a spoonful of it drunk every morning by such as are subject to the dropsy, it is sure to cure them.

PENNYROYAL.

PENNYROYAL needs no description.

There is a greater kind than the ordinary sort found wild which so abideth being brought into gardens, and differeth not from it, but only in the largeness of the leaves and stalks, in rising higher, and not creeping upon the ground so much ; the flowers are purple, growing about the stalks like the other.

-*Place.*—The first is common in gardens, and groweth in many moist and watery places of this land.

Time.—They flower in the latter end of summer, about August.

Government and Virtues.—The herb is under Venus. Dioscorides saith, that pennyroyal maketh thin tough phlegm, warmeth the coldness of any part whereto it is applied, and digesteth raw or corrupt matter ; being boiled and drank, it provoketh women's courses, and stayeth the disposition to vomit being taken in water and vinegar. And being mingled with honey and salt, it voideth phlegm out of the lungs, and purgeth melancholy by stool. Drunk with with wine, it cures such as are bitten and stung by venomous beasts, and applied to the nostrils with vinegar, reviveth those that are fainting and swooning. Being dried and burnt, it strengthens the gums. It is excellent in gout, being applied to the place until it is red ; applied as a plaster it takes away spots or marks in the face ; applied with salt, it profiteth those that are splenetic or liver grown. The decoction cures the itch if washed therewith ; being put into baths for women to sit therein, it helpeth the swellings and hardness of the mother. The green herb bruised and put into vinegar, cleanseth foul ulcers, and taketh away the marks or bruises and blows about the eyes, and all discolourings of the face by fire ; and the leprosy, being drunk and outwardly applied. Boiled in wine with honey and salt, it relieveth the toothache, and the cold griefs in the joints, taking away the pains, being fast bound to the place, after a bathing or sweating in a hot-house. Pliny addeth, that pennyroyal and mints together, cure faintings, being put into vinegar and put into the nostrils or mouth. It easeth headaches, pains of the breast and belly, and gnawing of the stomach ; applied with honey, salt, and vinegar, it cureth cramps or convulsions of the sinews. Boiled in milk and drunk, it is effectual for coughs, and for ulcers and sores in the mouth ; drunk in wine it provoked women's courses, and expelleth the dead child and after-birth. Matthiolus saith, the decoction cureth jaundice, dropsy, pains of the head and sinews that come of a cold cause, and cleareth the eye-sight. It cureth lethargy, and applied with barley-meal, burnings, and put into the ears easeth pain.

MALE AND FEMALE PEONY.

Description.—Male peony riseth up with brownish stalks, whereon grow green and reddish leaves, upon a stalk without any particular division in the leaf. The flowers stand at the top of the stalks, consisting of five or six broad leaves of a purplish red colour, with many yellow threads in the middle, standing about the head, which after riseth up to be the seed vessels, divided into two, three or four crooked pods like horns, which being fully ripe, open and turn themselves down backward, showing within them round, black, shining seeds, having crimson veins intermixed with black. The roots are great, thick, and long, spreading and running down deep in the ground.

The ordinary female peony hath as many stalks and more leaves on them than the male, the leaves are not so large, but nicked on the edges, some with great and deep, others with smaller cuts and partitions, of a dead green colour. The flowers are of a strong scent, usually smaller, and of a more purple colour than the male, with yellow thrums about the head. The seed vessels are like horns, as in the male, but smaller; the seed is black, but less shining. The roots consist of many short tuberous clogs fastened at the end of long strings, and fall from the head of the roots, which is thick and short, and of the like scent with the male.

Place and Time.—They grow in gardens, and flower usually about May.

Government and Virtues.—It is an herb of the Sun, and under the Lion. Physicians say, male peony roots are best; but Dr. Reason told me male peony was best for men, and female peony for women, and he desires to be judged by his brother Dr. Experience. The roots are held to be of more virtue than the seeds; next the flowers, and last of all the leaves. The roots of the male peony fresh gathered, have been found by experience to cure the falling-sickness; but the surest way is, besides hanging it about the neck, by which children have been cured, to take the root of the male peony washed clean, and stamped small, and infused in wine for twenty-four hours, strain it, and take it first and last morning and evening, a good draught for some days together before and after full moon, and it will cure older persons if the disease be not grown too old and past cure, especially if there be a due and orderly preparation of the body with posset made of betony, &c. The root is effectual for women that are not sufficiently cleansed after child birth, and such as are troubled with the mother ; for which the black seed beaten to powder, and given in wine, is also available. The black seed also taken before bed-time and in the morning, is very effectual for such as in their sleep are troubled with Night-mare ; a disease which melancholy persons are subject unto ; it is also good against melancholy dreams. The distilled water or syrup made of the flowers, worketh the same effects that the root and the seed do, although more weakly. The female is often used for the purposes aforesaid, by reason the male is so scarce a plant that it is possessed by few, and those great lovers of rarities in this kind.

PEPPERWORT, or DITTANDER.

Description. — Our common pepperwort sendeth forth long and broad leaves, of a light bluish green colour, finely dented about the edges, and pointed at the ends, standing many branches on all sides, and having many small white flowers at the tops of them, after which follow small seeds in small heads. The root is slender, running much underground, and shooting up again in many places, and both leaves and roots are very hot and sharp of taste, like pepper, for which cause it took the name.

Place. — It groweth naturally in many places of this land ; but is usually kept in gardens.

Time. — It flowereth in the end of June and July.

Government and Virtues. — Pliny and Paulus Ægineta say, that pepperwort is beneficial for the sciatica, or gout or pain in the joints, or any other inveterate grief : the leaves hereof to be bruised and mixed with hog's lard, and applied to the place, and to continue thereon four hours in men, and two in women, the place being afterwards bathed with wine and oil mixed together, and then wrapped up with wool or skins after they have sweat a little. It also removes discolourings of the skin, and also marks, scars, and scabs, or the foul marks of burning with fire or iron. The juice is by some used to be given in ale to drink to women with child, to procure them a safe speedy deliverence in travail.

PERIWINKLE.

Description.—The common sort hath many branches running upon the ground, shooting out small fibres at the joints as it runneth, taking hold in the ground, and rooteth in divers places. At the joints of these branches stand two small dark green shining leaves like bay leaves, but smaller, and with them come forth also the flowers, one at a stalk, standing upon a tender foot-stalk, being rather long and hollow, parted at the brims sometimes into four, sometimes into five leaves ; the most ordinary sorts are of a pale blue colour : some are pure white, and some of a dark reddish purple colour. The root is rather larger than a rush, bushing in the ground and creeping with his branches far about, it is usually planted under hedges where it may have room to run.

Place.—Those with the pale blue, and those with the white flowers, grow in woods and orchards, by the hedge sides, in divers places of this land ; but those with the purple flowers in gardens ouly.

Time.—They flower in March and April.

Government and Virtues.—Venus owns this herb, and saith that the leaves eaten together by man and wife, causeth love between them. The periwinkle is a great binder, stayeth bleeding at the mouth and nose, if some of the leaves be chewed. The French use it to stay women's courses. ` Dioscorides, Galen, and Ægineta commended it against lasks and fluxes, to be drunk in wine.

ST. PETER'S WORT.

Description.—It riseth up with square upright stalks, somewhat higher than St. John's wort, but brown in the same manner, having two leaves at every joint, like, but larger than St. John's wort, a little rounder pointed, with a few or no holes to be seen thereon, and having some smaller leaves rising from the bottom of the greater, and sometimes a little hairy also. At the tops of the stalks stand many star-like flowers, with many threads in the middle, very like those of St. John's wort, and only to be known by its being larger and higher, but the seeds are alike. The root abideth long, sending forth new shoots every year.

Place.—It groweth in many groves and small low woods in many places of this land, near water-courses.

Time.—It flowereth in June and July, and the seed is ripe in August.

Government and Virtues.—There is not a straw to choose between this and St. John's wort, only St. Peter must have it lest he should want pot herbs ; it is of the same property as St. John's wort, but somewhat weak, and therefore more seldom used. Two drachms of the seed taken at a time in honeyed water, purgeth choleric humours, as saith Dioscorides, Pliny, and Galen, and cureth sciatica. The leaves are used as St. John's wort, for burns.

PILEWORT.—See CELANDINE, *Lesser.*

PIMPERNEL.

Description.—Common Pimpernel hath weak square stalks lying on the ground, beset all along with two small almost round leaves at every joint, one against another, very like chickweed, but hath no foot-stalks, for the leaves compass the stalk ; the flowers stand singly each by themselves, and the stalk, consisting of about five small round pointed leaves of a pale red colour tending to an orange, with many threads in the middle, in whose place succeed smooth round heads, wherein is contained small seed. The root is small and fibrous, perishing every year.

Place.—It groweth every where almost, as well in meadows and corn-fields, as by the way-sides and in gardens, arising of itself.

Time.—It flowereth from April until May, and the seed ripeneth in the mean time and falleth.

Government and Virtues.—It is a gallant Solar herb, of a cleansing attractive quality, whereby it draweth forth thorns and splinters gotten into the flesh, and put into the nostrils purgeth the head ; and Galen saith they have a drying faculty, whereby they are good to close the lips of wounds, and to cleanse foul ulcers. The distilled water or juice is much celebrated by French dames to cleanse the skin from any roughness, deformity, or discolourings thereof ; being boiled in wine and given to drink, it is a good remedy against the plague, and other pestilential fevers, if the party after taking it be warm in his bed, and sweat for two hours after, and use the same twice at the least. It helpeth also all stinging or biting of venomous beasts or mad dogs, being used inwardly, and applied outwardly. The same also openeth obstructions of the liver, and is very available against infirmities of the reins ; it provoketh urine, helpeth to expel the stone and gravel out of the kidneys and bladder, and helpeth much in all inward pains and ulcers. The decoction or distilled water is effectual, applied to all wounds that are fresh and green, or old and running ulcers, which it very effectually cures in a short space. A little honey mixed with the juice and dropped into the eyes, cleanseth them from cloudy mists or thick films which grow over them and hinder the sight. It easeth the tooth-ache, being dropped into the ear on the contrary side of the pain ; it is also effectual to ease the pains of the piles.

GROUND PINE, OR CHAMEPITYS.

Description.—Our common ground pine groweth low, seldom rising above a hand's breadth high, shooting forth divers small branches set with slender, small, long, narrow, greyish or whitish leaves, somewhat hairy, and divided into three parts, many bushing together at a joint, some growing scatteringly upon the stalks, smelling somewhat strong like unto rosin : the flowers are small, and of a pale yellow colour, growing from the joint of the stalk all along among the leaves ; after which come small and round husks.

Place.—It groweth more plentifully in Kent than in any other county of this land.

Time.—It flowereth and giveth seed in the summer.

Government and Virtues.—Mars owns the herb. The decoction drunk, cureth the strangury or any inward pains arising from the diseases of the reins and urine, and is special good for all obstructions of the liver and spleen, and it gently openeth the body ; for which purpose in former times they made pills with the powder thereof and the pulp of figs. It marvelously helpeth all diseases of the mother, inwardly or outwardly applied, procuring the courses ; yea, it is so powerful that it is utterly forbidden for women with child, for it will cause abortion or delivery before the time. The decoction of the herb in wine taken inwardly or applied outwardly, for some time together, is effectual in all pains and diseases of the joints, as gouts, cramps, palsies, sciatica and aches ; for which purpose the pills made with powder of ground pine, and of hermodactyls with Venice turpentine, are very effectual. The pills also, continued for some time, are special good for those that have the dropsy, jaundice, griping pains of the joints, belly, or inward parts. It helpeth all diseases of the brain, proceeding of cold and phlegmatic humours and distillations, as also for the falling sickness. It is a special remedy for the poison of the aconites and other poisonous herbs, as also against the stinging of any venomous creature. It is a good remedy for a cold, cough, especially in the beginning. For all the purposes aforesaid, the herb being tunned in new drink and drunk, is almost as effectual, but far more acceptable to weak and dainty stomachs. The distilled water of the herb hath the same effects, but more weakly. The conserve of the flowers doth the like, which Matthiolus much commendeth against the palsy. The green herb, or the decoction, being applied, cures the hardness of women's breasts, and all other hard swellings in any other part of the body. The green herb also applied, or the juice with some honey, cleanseth putrid and malignant ulcers and sores of all sorts, and closes the lips of green wounds in any part also.

PLANTAIN.

THIS groweth usually in meadows and fields, and by path sides, and is well known.

Time.—It is in its beauty about June, and the seed ripeneth shortly after.

Government and Virtues.—Mizaldus and other astrology-

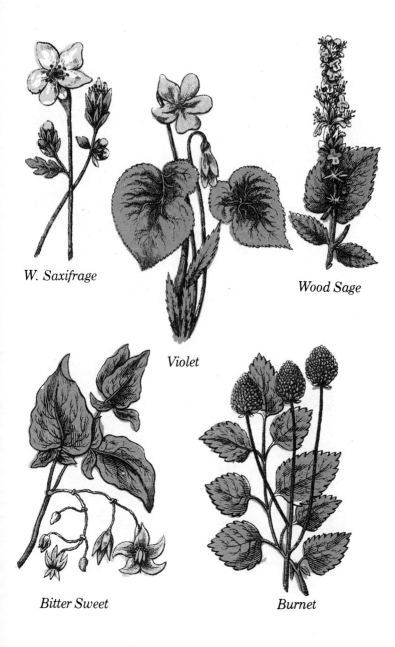

W. Saxifrage

Wood Sage

Violet

Bitter Sweet

Burnet

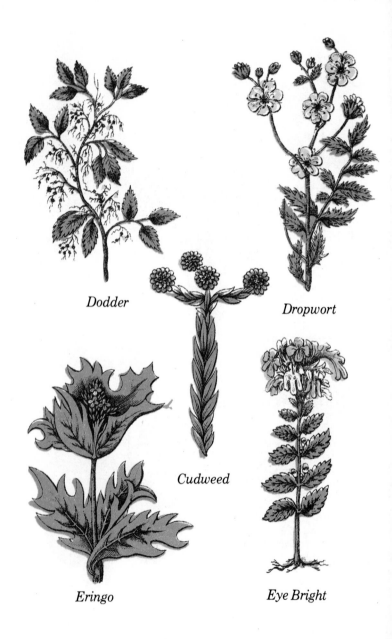

Dodder

Dropwort

Cudweed

Eringo

Eye Bright

physicians, say it is an herb of Mars, because it cureth the
diseases of the head and privities, which are under the
houses of Mars, Aries, and Scorpio ; the truth is, it is under Venus, and cures the head by antipathy to Mars, and
the privities by sympathy to Venus ; neither is there hardly
a martial disease but it cures.

The juice of plantain clarified and drunk for some days,
either of itself or in other drink, prevaileth wonderfully
against all torments or excoriations in the bowels, stayeth
the distillations of rheum from the head, and stayeth all
fluxes, and profuse menstruation. It is good to stay spitting of blood and other bleedings of the mouth, or the
making of bloody water, by reason of any ulcer in the
reins or bladder, and also the too free bleeding of wounds.
It is an especial remedy for those that are troubled with
consumption of the lungs, or ulcers of the lungs, or coughs
that come of heat. The decoction or powder of the roots
or seeds, is much more binding for the purposes aforesaid
than the leaves. Dioscorides saith, that three roots boiled
in wine and taken, helpeth the tertian ague, and for the
quartan ague, I conceive the decoction of divers roots may
be effectual. The herb, but especially the seed, is good
against dropsy, the falling-sickness, the yellow jaundice,
and obstructions of the liver and reins. The roots of plantain and pellitory of Spain, beaten into powder and put
into the hollow teeth, taketh away the pains. The clarified
juice, or distilled water dropped into the eyes, cooleth inflammations in them, and taketh away the pin and web ;
and dropped into the ears easeth the pains in them, and
removeth the heat. The same also with the juice of houseleek, is profitable against all inflammations and breakings
out of the skin, and against burnings and scaldings by
fire and water. The juice or decoction is of much use and
good effect for old hollow ulcers that are hard to be cured,
and for cankers and sores in the mouth and privy parts of
man or woman ; and helpeth also the pains of the piles in
the fundament. The juice mixed with oil of roses, and the
temples and forehead anointed therewith, easeth the pains
of the head caused by heat, and helpeth lunatic and frantic persons ; as also the biting of serpents or a mad dog.

O

The same also is profitably applied to gout in the feet and hands, especially in the beginning. It is also good to be applied where any bone is out of joint, to hinder inflammations, swellings, and pains that presently rise thereupon. The powder of the dried leaves taken in drink, killeth worms; and boiled in wine, killeth worms that breed in foul ulcers. One part of plantain water, and two parts of the brine of powdered beef, boiled together and clarified, is a sure remedy to heal scabs or itch in the head and body, and tetters, ringworms, the shingles, and all other running sores. The plantain is a very good wound herb to heal fresh or old wounds or sores, either inward or outward.

PLUMS

ARE so well known that they need no description.

Government and Virtues.—All plums are under Venus, and there are various kinds,—some that are sweet moisten the stomach and make the belly soluble; those that are sour quench thirst more and bind the belly; the moist and waterish sooner corrupt in the stomach, but the firm nourish more, and offend less. The dried fruit, called prunes, are aperient, and being stewed, are often used in health and sickness, to relish the mouth and stomach, to procure appetite, and a little to open the body, allay choler, and cool the stomach. Plum-tree leaves boiled in wine, are good to wash and gargle the mouth and throat, to dry the flux of rheum coming to the palate, gums, or almonds of the ears. The gum of the tree is good to break the stone. The gum or leaves boiled in vinegar and applied, kills tetters and ringworms. Matthiolus saith, the oil pressed out of the kernels of the stones, as oil of almonds is msde, is good against the inflamed piles, and tumours or swellings of ulcers, hoarseness, roughness of the tongue and throat, and pains in the ears. And that five ounces of the oil taken with one ounce of muscatel, driveth forth the stone, and cureth colic.

POLYPODY OF THE OAK.

Description.—This is a small herb consisting of nothing but roots and leaves. bearing neither stalk, flower, nor seed, as it is thought. It hath three or four leaves rising from the root, every one single by itself, of about a hand length, are winged, consisting of many small narrow leaves cut into the middle rib, standing on each side of the stalk, large below and smaller up to the top, not dented nor notched at the edges at all, of a sad green colour, and smooth on the upper side, but on the other side rough by reason of some yellowish spots set thereon. The root is small, lying aslope or creeping along under the upper crust of the earth, brownish on the outside and greenish within, of a sweetish harshness in taste, set with certain rough knags on each side thereof, having also much mossiness or yellow hairiness upon it, with fibres underneath it, whereby it is nourished.

Place.—It groweth as well upon old rotten stumps or trunks of trees, as oak, beech, hazel, willow, or any other, and upon old mud walls, in mossy, stony, and gravelly places near unto woods. That which groweth upon oak is accounted the best ; but the quantity is scarce sufficient for common use.

Time.—It being always green, may be gathered for use at any time.

Government and Virtues.—It is an herb of Saturn, and *generally* grows upon the ground. The fresh root is most used. Meuse (who is called the physician's evangelist, for the certainty of his medicines, and the truth of his opinion) saith, that it drieth up thin humours, and especially expectorates tough and thick phlegm, and thin phlegm also ; therefore it is good for those that have melancholy or quartan agues, especially if it be taken in whey or honeyed water, or in barley water, or the broth of a chicken with beets and mallows. It is good for hardness of the spleen, and for stitches in the sides, as also for the colic ; some add fennel seeds, anise seed, or ginger, to correct that loathing it bringeth to the stomach ; it is a safe and gentle medicine, fit for all persons, which daily experience confirmeth ; and an ounce of it may be given at a time in a decoction, if there be not senna or some other strong purgative put with it. A drachm or two of the powder of the dried roots taken fasting in a cup of honeyed water, worketh gently, and for the purposes aforesaid. The distilled water of roots and leaves, is much commended for the quartan ague, to be taken for many days together, as also against melancholy, or fearful and troublesome sleeps or dreams; and with some sugar-candy dissolved therein, is good against cough, shortness of breath. wheezings, and those distillations of thin rheum upon the lungs, which cause phthisic, and oftentimes consumptions. The fresh roots beaten small, or the powder of the dried roots mixed with honey, and applied to the member that is out of joint, doth much help it; and applied to the nose, cureth the disease called polypus, which is a piece of flesh growing therein, which in time stoppeth the passage of breath through that nostril; and it helpeth those clefts or chops that come between the fingers or toes.

THE POPLAR TREE.

THERE are two sorts of poplars which are most familiar with us, viz. black and white.

Description.—The white poplar groweth great, and high, covered with thick, smooth, white bark, especially the branches, having long leaves cut into several divisions almost like a vine leaf, but not of so deep a green colour on the upper side, and hoary white underneath, of a good scent, the whole form representing the form of colt's foot. The cat-kins which it bringeth forth before the leaves, are long and of a faint reddish colour, which fall away, bearing seldom good seed with them. The wood hereof is smooth, soft, and white, very finely waved, whereby it is much esteemed.

The black poplar groweth higher and straighter than the white, with a greyish bark, bearing broad green leaves somewhat like ivy leaves, not cut in on the edges like the white, but whole and dented, ending in a point, and not white underneath, hanging by slender long foot-stalks, which, with the air, are continually shaken as the aspen leaves are. The cat-kins hereof are greater than those of the white, composed of many round green berries, as if they were set together in a long cluster, containing much downy matter, which being ripe is blown away with the wind. The clammy buds hereof, before they spread into leaves, are gathered to make *unguentum populneum*, and are of a yellowish green colour, and small, somewhat sweet, but strong. The wood is smooth, tough, and white, and easy to be cloven. On both these trees groweth a sweet kind of musk, which in former times was used to put into sweet ointments.

Place.—They grow in moist woods, and by water-sides in sundry places of this land ; yet the white is not so frequent as the other.

Time.—Their time is also expressed before. The catkins coming forth before the leaves in the end of summer.

Government and Virtues.—Saturn hath dominion over both. White poplar, saith Galen, is of a cleansing property ; the weight of one ounce in powder of the bark thereof being drunk, saith Dioscorides, is a remedy for sciatica, the strangury. The juice of the leaves dropped warm into the ears, easeth pain. The young clammy buds before they break out into leaves, bruised and a little honey put to them, is a good medicine for a dull sight. The black poplar is more cooling than the white, and therefore the leaves bruised with vinegar is good for falling sickness. The water that droppeth from the hollow places of this tree, taketh away warts, pushes, wheals, and breakings out of the body. The young black poplar buds, saith Matthiolus, are much used by women to beautify their hair, bruising them with fresh butter, straining them after they have been kept for some time in the sun. The ointment called *populneum*, which is made of this poplar, is very good for inflammation in any part of the body, and tempereth the heat of wounds. It is much used to dry up the milk in women's breasts when they have weaned their children.

POPPY.

Of this I shall describe three kinds, viz. the white and black of the garden, and the erratic wild poppy, or corn rose.

Description.—The white poppy hath at first four or five whitish green leaves lying on the ground. which rise with the stalk, compassing it at the bottom of them, and are very large, much cut or torn on the edges, and dented also besides; the stalk, which is usually four or five feet high, hath sometimes no branches at the top, and usually but two or three at most, bearing every one but one head wrapped up in a thin skin, which boweth down before it is ready to blow, and then rising and being broken, the flower within it spreading itself open, and consisting of four very large white, round leaves, with many whitish round threads in the middle, set about a small, round, green head, having a crown or star-like cover at the head thereof, which growing ripe, becomes as large as an apple, wherein are contained a great number of small round seeds, in several partitions or divisions next unto the shell, the middle thereof remaining hollow and empty. The whole plant, both leaves, stalks, and heads, while they are fresh, young, and green, yield a milk when they are broken of an unpleasant bitter taste, which produces opium. The root is white and woody, perishing as soon as it hath given ripe seed.

The black poppy little differeth from the former, until it beareth its flower, which is somewhat less, and of a black purplish colour, but without any purple spots in the bottom of the leaf. The head of the seed is much less than the former, and openeth itself a little round about to the top, under the crown, so that the seed which is very black will fall out, if one turn the head thereof downward.

The wild poppy, or corn rose, hath long and narrow leaves, very much cut in on the edges, into many divisions, of a light green colour, sometimes hairy; the stalk is blackish and hairy also, but not so tall as the garden kind, having some such like leaves thereon as grow below, parted into three or four branches sometimes, whereon grow small hairy heads, bowing down before the skin break, wherein the flower is, which when it is full blown open, is of a fair yellowish red or crimson colour, in some much paler, without any spot in the bottom of the leaves, having many black soft threads in the middle, compassing a small green head, which, when it is ripe, is only small, wherein is contained much black seed, smaller by half than that of the garden. The root perisheth every year, and springeth again of its own sowing. Of this kind there is one less in all the parts thereof, and differeth in nothing else.

Place.—The garden kinds do not naturally grow wild in any place, but are sown in gardens where they grow.

The wild poppy, or corn rose, is very plentiful in corn fields, upon ditch banks and by hedge sides. The smaller wild kind is found in corn fields.

Time.—The garden kinds are usually sown in the spring, which then flower about the end of May, and earlier if they spring of their own sowing. The wild kind flower usually from May until July, and the seed of them is ripe soon after the flowering.

Government and Virtues.—The herb is Lunar, and of the juice of it is made opium. The garden poppy heads with seeds made into a syrup, is very good to procure sleep to the sick and weak, and to stay catarrhs and defluctions of thin rheums from the head into the stomach and lungs, causing a constant cough, the forerunner of consumption ; it relieveth hoarseness, loss of voice, which the seed doth likewise. The black seed boiled in wine and drunk, stays the flux of the belly, and women's courses. The empty shells or poppy heads boiled in water, procure rest and sleep ; so do the leaves ; and if the head and temples be bathed with the decoction warm, or with the oil of poppies, the green leaves or heads bruised and applied with a little vinegar, or made into a poultice with barley meal, or hog's lard, cooleth all inflammations, as Erysipelas, called St. Anthony's fire. It is generally used in treacle and mithridate, and in all other medicines to procure rest and sleep, and to ease pains in the head and other parts. It is also used to cool inflammations, agues, and frenzies, or to stay defluctions which cause a cough, or consumption, and also other fluxes of the belly or women's courses ; it is also put into hollow teeth to ease pain, and it relieves gouty pains.

The wild poppy, or corn rose, as Matthiolus saith, is good to prevent the falling sickness. The syrup made with the flowers, is with good effect given to those that have the pleurisy ; and the dried flowers also, either boiled in water, or made into powder and drunk, either in the distilled water or some other drink, worketh the same effect. The distilled water of the flowers is held to be of much use against surfeits, being drunk evening and morning; it is also more cooling than any of the other poppies, and therefore effectual in hot agues, frenzies, and other inflammations either inward or outward. Galen saith, the seed is dangerous to be used inwardly.

PURSLAINE.

GARDEN purslaine, being used as a salad herb, is so well known that it needeth no description.

Government and Virtues.—It is an herb of the Moon. It is good to cool heat in the liver, blood, reins, and stomach, and in hot agues nothing better; it stayeth hot and choleric fluxes of the bowels, women's courses, the whites and gonorrhœa, or running of the reins, the distillation from the head, and pains therein proceeding from heat, want of sleep, or frenzy. The seed is more effectual than the herb, to cool the heat and sharpness of urine, and bodily lust, or desire for procreation. The seed bruised and boiled in wine, and given to children, expelleth worms. The juice of the herb is effectual to all the purposes aforesaid; and to stay vomitings, and taken with sugar or honey, relieves an old dry cough, shortness of breath, and phthisic, and stayeth immoderate thirst. The distilled water of the herb is used as more pleasing, with a little sugar, to work the same effects. The juice also is good for inflammations and ulcers in the secret parts, as also the bowels and hæmorrhoids when ulcerous. The herb bruised and applied to the forehead and temples, allays excessive heat therein that hinders rest and sleep, and applied to the eyes taketh away the redness and inflammations in them, and those other parts where pushes, wheals, pimples, St. Anthony's fire, and the like, break forth; if a little vinegar be added, and laid to the neck with as much of galls and linseed together, it taketh away the pains therein, and the crick in the neck. The juice is used with oil of roses for the same causes, or for blastings by lightning, and burnings by gunpowder, or for women's sore breasts, and to allay the heat in all other sores or hurts; applied also to the navels of children that stick forth, it cureth them; it is good for sore mouths and gums that are swollen, and to fasten loose teeth. Camerarius saith, that the distilled water took away the pains in the teeth when all other remedies failed, and the thickened juice made into pills with the powder of gum tragacanth and arabic being taken, relieveth those that make bloody water. Applied to the gout it easeth pains, and softens the hardness of the sinews, if it come not of the cramp, or a cold cause.

PRIMROSES.

THEY are too well known to need description.

Of the leaves of primroses is made as fine a salve to heal wounds as any I know; do not see your poor neighbours go with wounded limbs when a halfpenny cost will heal them.

PRIVET.

Description.—Our common privet is carried up with many slender branches to a good height and breadth, to cover arbours, bowers, and banquetting houses, and brought, wrought, and cut into so many forms of men, horses, birds, &c. which though at first supported, groweth afterwards strong of itself. It beareth long and narrow green leaves by couples, and sweet smelling white flowers in tufts at the ends of the branches, which turn into small black berries that have a purplish juice with them, and some seeds that are flat on one side, with a hole or dent therein.

Place.—It groweth in woods, and garden hedges.

Time.—Our privet flowereth in June and July, and the berries are ripe in August and September.

Government and Virtues.—The moon governs it. It is used in lotions to wash sores and sore mouths, and to cool inflammations and dry up fluxes. Yet Matthiolus saith, it serveth to all the purposes for which cypress or the east privet is appointed by Dioscorides and Galen. He farther saith, that the oil that is made of the flowers of privet infused therein, and set in the sun, is good for the inflammations of wounds, and for the headache coming of a hot cause. There is a sweet water distilled from the flowers that is good for all those diseases that need cooling and drying, and therefore helpeth all fluxes of the belly or stomach, bloody fluxes and women's courses, either drunk or applied ; as also those that void blood at the mouth or any other place, and for distillations of rheum in the eyes, especially if it be used with tutty.

QUEEN OF THE MEADOWS, MEADOW SWEET, OR MEAD SWEET.

Description.—The stalks of this are reddish, from three feet to five feet, having at the joints large winged leaves one above another, consisting of many rather broad leaves set on each side of a middle rib, being hard, rough, or rugged, crumpled like elm leaves, having also smaller leaves with them, (as agrimony hath) rather deeply dented about the edges, of a sad green colour on the upper side, and greyish underneath, of a sharp scent and taste, somewhat like the burnet ; a leaf put into a cup of claret wine, giveth a fine relish to it. At the tops of the stalks and branches stand many tufts of small white flowers thick together, which smell much sweeter than the leaves ; and in their places, being fallen, some cornered seed. The root is rather woody, and blackish on the outside, and brownish within, with great strings and less fibres set thereat, of a strong scent, but nothing so pleasant as the flowers and leaves, and perishing not, but abideth for many years, and shooteth forth anew every spring-time.

Place.—It groweth in moist meadows that lie much wet, or near the courses of water.

Time.—It flowereth in some place or other all the three summer months, that is, June, July, and August, and the seed is ripe soon after.

Government and Virtues.—Venus governs the herb. It is used to stay all manner of bleedings, fluxes, vomitings, and women's courses, as also their whites. It is said to alter and take away the fits of the quartan agues, and to make a merry heart, for which purpose some use the flowers and some the leaves. It soon relieves the colic; being boiled in wine, and with a little honey taken warm, it openeth the bowels, but boiled in port wine and drunk, stayeth the flux of the belly. Outwardly applied it healeth old ulcers that are cancerous, hollow and fistulous, for which it is by many commended, and for sores in the mouth, or secret parts. The leaves when they are full grown being laid on the skin, will in a short time raise blisters, as Tragus saith. The water thereof subdues heat and inflammation in the eyes.

THE QUINCE TREE.

Description.—The ordinary quince tree groweth often to the height of an apple tree, but more usually lower and crooked, with a rough bark, spreading arms and branches far abroad. The leaves are a little like those of the apple tree, but thicker, broader, and fuller of veins, and whiter on the other side, not dented at all about the edges. The flowers are large and white, sometimes dashed over with a blush. The fruit is yellow being ripe, and covered with a white frieze, or cotton, thick set on the younger, and growing less as they get ripe, bunched out often in some places, some being like an apple, and some a pear, of a strong scent, and not durable to keep, and is sour, harsh, and of an unpleasant taste to eat fresh; but being scalded, roasted, baked, or preserved, becometh more pleasant.

Place.—It grows near ponds and water-sides, and is frequent through this land.

Time.—It flowereth not until the leaves be come forth. The fruit is ripe in September or October.

Government and Virtues. — Saturn governs the tree. Quinces when they are green, relieve all sorts of fluxes, and choleric lasks, casting, and whatever needed astriction, more than any way prepared by fire; yet the syrup of the juice, or the conserve, are much conducible, much of the binding quality being consumed by the fire; if a little vinegar be added, it stirreth up a languishing appetite, and relieveth vomiting; some spices being added, it strengtheneth decaying and fainting spirits, and cureth inflammation of the liver, a healthy flow of bile. If for purging, put honey to them instead of sugar; and if more laxative, for choler, rhubarb; for phlegm, turbith; for watery humours, scammony; but if more forcibly to bind, use the unripe quinces, with roses and acacia. To take the crude juice of quinces, is held a preservative against the force of deadly poison; for it hath been found most certainly true, that the very smell of the quince hath taken away all the strength of the poison of white hellebore. If there be need of any outwardly binding and cooling of hot fluxes, the oil of quinces, or other medicines that may be made thereof, are very available to anoint the belly or other parts therewith; it likewise strengthens the stomach and belly, and the sinews that are loosened by sharp humours falling on them, and restraineth immoderate sweatings. The mucilage taken from the seeds of quinces and boiled in a little water, is very good to cool the heat and heal the sore breasts of women. The same with a little sugar, is good to lenify the harshness and hoarseness of the throat, and roughness of the tongue. The cotton or down of quinces boiled and applied to plague sores, healeth them; and laid as a plaster made with wax, it bringeth hair to them that are bald, and keepeth it from falling off if it be ready to shed.

RADISH, or HORSE-RADISH.

THE garden radish is well known.

Description.—The horse radish hath its first leaves that rise before winter about a foot and a half long, much cut in or torn on the edges into many parts, of a dark green colour, with a great rib in the middle; after these have been up a while, others follow, which are greater, rougher, broader, and longer, whole and not divided at first, but only somewhat rougher dented about the edges; the stalks when it beareth flowers, which is seldom, are great, rising up with some few lesser leaves thereon to three or four feet high, spreading at the top many small branches of whitish flowers, four leaves a piece; after which come small pods like those of shepherd's purse, but seldom with any seed in them. The root is great, long, white and rugged, shooting divers heads of leaves, which may be parted for increase, but it doth not creep in the ground, and is of a strong sharp and bitter taste, almost like mustard.

Place.—It is found wild in some places, but is chiefly planted in gardens, and delighteth in moist and shady places.

Time.—It flowereth sometimes in July.

Government and Virtues.—They are both under Mars. The juice of horse-radish given to drink, is very effectual for the scurvy. It killeth worms, being drunk. The root bruised and laid to the place cureth sciatica, joint-ache, or hard swellings of the liver and spleen. The distilled water of the herb and root is more familiar to be taken with a little sugar for all the purposes aforesaid.

Garden radishes are good for such as are troubled with the gravel, stone, or stoppage of urine, if the body be strong that takes them ; you may make the juice of the roots into a syrup if you please, for that use. They purge by urine exceedingly.

RAGWORT.

It is also called St. James' wort, stagger wort, stammer wort, and segrum.

Description.—The greater common ragwort hath many large and long dark green leaves lying on the ground, very much rent on the sides in many places ; from among which rise up sometimes but one, and sometimes two or three square or crested blackish or brownish stalks, three or four feet high, sometimes branched, bearing such like leaves upon them unto the top, where it branches forth into many stalks bearing many flowers, consisting of divers leaves set as a pale or border, with a dark yellow thrum in the middle, which do abide a great while, but at last are turned into down, and with the small blackish grey seed are carried away with the wind. The root is made of many fibres, whereby it is firmly fastened into the ground, and abideth many years.

There is another sort different from the former, as it riseth not so high, the leaves are not so finely jagged, nor of so dark a green colour, but rather somewhat whitish, soft and woolly, and the flowers usually paler.

Place.—They grow wild in pastures and untilled grounds in many places.

Time.—They flower in June and July, and the seed is ripe in August.

Government and Virtues.—Ragwort is under the command of Venus, and cleanseth, digesteth, and discusseth. The decoction of the herb is good to wash the mouth or throat that hath ulcers or sores therein ; and for swellings, hardness, or imposthumes, for it thoroughly cleanseth and healeth them ; as also the quinsy and the king's evil. It helpeth to stay catarrhs, thin rheums, and defluctions from the head into the eyes, nose, or lungs. The juice is found by experience to be very good to heal green wounds, and to cleanse and heal old and filthy ulcers in many parts of the body, as also inward wounds and ulcers ; stayeth the malignity of fretting and running cancers, and hollow fistulas, not suffering them to spread farther. It is also much commended to help aches and pains either in the fleshy parts, or in the nerves and sinews ; as also the sciatica, or pain of the hips or huckle-bone, to bathe the places with the decoction of the herb, or to anoint them with an ointment made of the herb bruised and boiled in old hog's suet, with some mastich, and olibanum in powder added unto it after it is strained forth. In Sussex we call it ragweed.

RATTLE GRASS.

OF this there are two kinds, which I shall speak of, viz. the red and yellow.

Description.—The common red hath sundry reddish, hollow stalks, and sometimes green, rising from the root, lying on the ground, some growing more upright, with many reddish or green leaves set on both sides of a middle rib, finely dented about the edges ; the flowers stand at the tops of the stalks or branches, of a fine purplish red colour, like small gaping hooks, after which come blackish seed in small husks, which lying loose therein will rattle with shaking. The root consists of two or three small whitish strings with fibres.

The common yellow rattle hath seldom above one round

great stalk, rising from the root about half a yard or two feet high, and but few branches thereon, having two long and somewhat broad leaves set at a joint, deeply cut in on the edges, resembling the comb of a cock, broadest next to the stalk and smaller to the end. The flowers grow at the tops of the stalks with some shorter leaves with them, hooded after the same manner that the others are, but of a fair yellow colour, or in some paler and in some more white. The seed is contained in large husks, and being ripe will rattle or make a noise with lying loose in them. The root is small and slender, perishing every year.

Place.—They grow in meadows and woods generally throughout this land.

Time.—They are in flower from midsummer until August be past, sometimes.

Government and Virtues.—Both are under the dominion of the Moon. The red rattle is accounted profitable to heal fistulas and hollow ulcers, and to stay the flux of humours in them, as also the abundance of the courses, or any other flux of blood, being boiled in port wine and drunk.

The yellow rattle, or cock's-comb, is held to be good for those that are troubled with a cough or dimness of sight, if the herb, being boiled with beans and some honey put thereto, be drunk or dropped into the eyes. The whole seed being put into the eyes, draweth forth any skin, dimness or film from the sight, without trouble or pain.

REST HARROW, OR CAMMOCK.

Description.—Common rest harrow riseth up with rough woody twigs, half a yard or a yard high, set at the joints without order, with little roundish leaves, sometimes more than two or three at a place, of a dark green colour, without thorns while they are young; but afterwards armed in sundry places with short and sharp thorns. The flowers come forth at the tops of the twigs and branches, whereof it is full fashioned like peas or broom blossoms, but less, flatter, and somewhat closer, of a faint purplish colour; after which come small pods, containing small, flat, round seed: the root is blackish on the outside, and whitish within, very rough, and hard to break when it is fresh and green, and as hard as a horn when it is dried, thrusting deep into the ground, and spreading, every piece growing again if it be left in the ground.

Place.—It groweth in many places of this land, as well in the arable as waste ground.

Time.—It flowereth about the beginning or middle of July, and the seed is ripe in August.

Government and Virtues.—It is under the dominion of Mars. It is very good to provoke urine when it is stopped, and to break and expel the stone, which the powder of the bark of the root taken in wine performeth effectually. Matthiolus saith, the same helpeth the disease called *hernia carnosa*, the flesh rupture, by taking the said powder for some months together constantly, and that it hath cured some which seemed incurable. The decoction made with vinegar, gargled in the mouth, easeth the tooth-ache, especially when it comes of rheum ; and it is very powerful to open obstructions of the liver and spleen, and other parts. A distilled water, with four pounds of the root first sliced small, and steeped in a gallon of Canary wine, is good for all the purposes aforesaid, and to cleanse the passages of the urine. The powder of the said root made into an electuary, or lozenges with sugar, and also the bark of the fresh roots boiled tender, and afterwards beaten to a conserve with sugar, worketh the like effect. The powder of the root strewed upon the brims of ulcers, or mixed with any other convenient thing, and applied, consumeth the hardness and causeth them to heal the better.

WILD ROCKET.

I SHALL only speak of the common wild rocket.

Description.—The common wild rocket hath longer and narrower leaves, much more divided into slender cuts and jags on both sides the middle ribs than the garden kinds have, of a sad green colour : from among which rise up stalks two or three feet high, sometimes set with the like leaves, but smaller and smaller upwards, branched from the middle into stiff stalks, bearing sundry yellow flowers on them, made of four leaves a-piece, as the others are, which afterwards yield small reddish seed in very small long pods, of a more bitter and hot biting taste than the garden kinds, as the leaves are also.

Place.—It is found wild in many places of this land.

Time.—It flowers about June or July, and the seed is ripe in August.

Government and Virtues.—The wild rockets are forbidden to be used alone, as their sharpness fumeth into the head, causing aches and pains therein, and are less hurtful to hot and choleric persons, for fear of inflaming their blood, and therefore for such we may say a little doth but a little harm, for angry Mars rules them, and he sometimes will be rusty when he meets with fools. The wild rocket is more strong and effectual to increase sperm and venomous qualities, whereunto all the seed is more effectual than the garden kind. It serveth also to help digestion, and provoketh urine exceedingly. The seed is used to cure the biting of serpents, the scorpion, and the shrew mouse, and other poisons, and expelleth worms. The herb boiled or stewed, and some sugar put thereto, relieveth cough in children. The seed taken in drink, taketh away the ill scent of the arm-pits, increaseth milk in nurses, and wasteth the spleen. The seed mixed with honey, and used on the face, cleanseth the skin from morphew, and used with vinegar, taketh away freckles and redness in the face or other parts ; and with the gall of an ox, it removes foul scars, black and blue spots, and the marks of the small pox.

WINTER ROCKET, OR CRESSES.

Description.—Winter rocket, or winter cresses, hath large sad green leaves lying upon the ground, torn or cut in divers parts, somewhat like rocket, or turnip leaves, with smaller pieces next the bottom, and broad at the ends, which so abide all the winter, (if it spring up in autumn, when it is used to be eaten) from among which rise up divers small round stalks full of branches, bearing many small yellow flowers of four leaves a-piece, after which come small pods with reddish seed in them. The root is sowewhat stringy, and perisheth every year.

Place.—It groweth of its own accord in gardens and fields, by the way-sides in divers places.

Time.—It flowereth in May, seedeth in June, and then perisheth.

Government and Virtues.—This is profitable to provoke urine, to help strangury, and expel gravel and stone. It is good for the scurvy, and found to be a singular good wound herb to cleanse inward wounds ; the juice or the decoction being drunk, or outwardly applied to wash foul ulcers and sores, cleansing them by sharpness, and hindering or abating the dead flesh from growing therein, and healing them by its drying quality.

ROSES.

It is needless to give a description of any of these, since both the garden roses and the roses of the briar are well known : And first I shall begin with the garden kinds.

Government and Virtues.—What a pother have authors made with roses ! I shall add, that red roses are under Jupiter, damask under Venus, and white under the Moon. The white and red roses are cooling and drying, and yet the white is taken to exceed the red in both the properties, but is seldom used inwardly in any medicine. The bitterness in roses when they are fresh, especially the juice, purgeth choler and watery humours : but being dried, and the heat which causeth the bitterness being consumed, they have then a binding quality ; those also that are not full blown, do both cool and bind more than those that are full blown, and the white rose more than the red. The decoction of red roses made with wine, is very good for the head-ache, and pains in the eyes, ears, throat, and gums ; as also for the fundament, the lower parts of the belly, and the matrix, being bathed, or put into them. The decoction with the roots remaining in it, is profitably applied to the region of the heart to ease the inflammation therein ; as St. Anthony's fire, and other diseases of the stomach. Being dried and beaten to powder, and taken in steeled wine or water, it stayeth women's courses. The yellow threads in the middle of the roses, being powdered and drunk in the distilled water of quinces, stayeth the courses, and stayeth the defluctions of rheum upon the gums and teeth, preserving them from corruption and fastening them if they be loose, being washed and gargled therewith, and some vinegar of squills added thereto. The heads with the seed being used in powder, or in a decoction, stayeth the lask and spitting of blood. Red roses do strengthen the heart, the stomach, the liver, and the retentive faculty : they mitigate the pains that arise from heat, assuage inflammations, procure rest and sleep, stay whites and reds in women, the gonorrhœa, or running of the reins or fluxes of the belly ; the juice of them doth cleanse the body from choler and phlegm. The husks of the roses, with their beards and nails, are binding and cooling ; and the distilled water of them is good for redness of the eyes, and to stay and dry up the rheums and watering of them.

Of the red roses are usually made many compositions, all serving to sundry good uses, viz. electuary of roses, conserve, both moist and dry, which is more usually called sugar of roses, syrup of dry roses, and honey of roses. The cordial powder called *diarrhoden abbatis,* and *aromatic rosarum.* The distilled water of roses, vinegar of roses, ointment, and oil of roses, and the rose leaves dried, are of very great use and effect.

The electuary is purging, whereof two or three drachms taken by itself in some convenient liquor, is a purge sufficient for a weak constitution, but may be increased to six drachms, according to the strength of the patient. It purgeth choler without trouble, and is good in hot fevers, and pains of the head arising from hot choleric humours, and heat in the eyes, the jaundice also, and joint-aches proceeding of hot humours. The moist conserve is of much use, both binding and cordial ; for until it be about two years old, it is more binding than cordial, and after that, more cordial than binding. Some of the younger conserve taken with mithridate mixed together, is good for those that are troubled with distillations of rheum from the brain to the nose, or the defluctions of rheum into the eyes; as also for fluxes and lasks of the belly ; and being mixed with the powder of mastich, is good for the running of the reins, and for the looseness of humours in the body. The old conserve mixed with aromaticum rosarum, is a very good cordial against faintings, swoonings, weakness and trembling of the heart, strengthens a weak stomach, promotes digestion, stayeth casting, and is a very good preservative in the time of infection. The dry conserve called the sugar of roses, is a very good cordial to strengthen the heart and spirits, and to stay defluctions. The syrup of roses cooleth an over-heated liver, and the blood in agues, comforteth the heart, and resisteth putrefaction and infection, and stayeth lasks and fluxes. Honey of roses is much used in gargles and lotions to wash sores, either in the mouth, throat, or other parts, both to cleanse and heal them, and to stay the fluxes of humours falling upon them. It is also used in clysters to cool and cleanse. The cordial powders, called diarrhoden abbatis, and aromatica rosarum, comfort and strengthen the heart and stomach, procure an appetite, help digestion, stay vomiting, and are very good for those that have slippery bowels, to strengthen them, and to dry up their moisture. Red rose water is well known, and of a familiar use on all occasions, and better than damask rose-water, being cooling and cordial, refreshing, quickening the weak and faint spirits, used either in meats or broths, to wash the temples, or to smell the sweet vapours thereof out of a perfuming pot, or cast into a hot fire shovel. It is also of good use against the redness and inflammations of the eyes, to bathe them therewith, and the temples of the head; as also against pain and ache, for which purpose also vinegar of roses is of much good use, and to procure rest and sleep, if some thereof and rose-water together be used to smell unto, or the nose and temples moistened therewith. The ointment of roses is much used for heat and inflammations in the head, to anoint the forehead and temples, and being mixed with unguentum populneum, to procure rest; it is also used for the heat of the liver, the back and reins, and to cool and heal pushes, wheals, and other red pimples rising in the face or other parts. Oil of roses is not only used by itself to cool any hot swellings or inflammations, and to stay fluxes of humours unto sores, but is also put into ointments and plasters that are cooling and binding, and restraining the flux of humours. The dried leaves of the red roses are used both inwardly and outwardly, as cooling, binding, and cordial, for with them are made both aromaticum rosarum, diarrhoden abbatis, and saccharum rosarum, whose properties are before declared. Rose leaves and mint, heated and applied outwardly to the stomach, stay vomiting, and strengthen a weak stomach ; and applied as a fomentation to the region of the liver and heart, cool and temper them, and quiet the over-hot spirits, and cause rest and sleep.

The syrup of damask roses is both simple and compound, and made with agaric. The simple solutive syrup, is a safe, gentle, and easy medicine, purging choler, taken from one ounce to three or four, yet this is remarkable herein, that the distilled water of this syrup should bind the belly. The syrup with agaric is more strong and effectual, for one ounce thereof by itself will open the body more than the other, and worketh as much on phlegm as choler. The compound syrup is more forcible in working on melancholic humours ; and available against the leprosy, itch, tetters, &c., and the French disease; also honey of roses solutive is made of the same infusions that the syrup is made of, and therefore worketh the same effect, both opening and purging, but is oftener given to phlegmatic and choleric persons, and is more used in clysters than in potions, as the syrup made with sugar is. The conserve and preserved leaves of roses gently open the bowels.

The dried leaves are used to make sweet powders, and fill sweet bags ; they have some purging quality. The fruit of the wild brier, which are called heps, being thoroughly ripe and made into a conserve with sugar, besides the pleasantness of the taste, doth gently bind the belly, and stay defluctions from the head upon the stomach, drying up the moisture thereof, and promoting digestion. The pulp of the heps dried into a hard consistence, like the juice of liquorice, or so dried that it may be made into a powder and taken in drink, stayeth the whites. The briar ball is often used, being made into powder and drunk, to break the stone, and to provoke urine when it is stopped, and to ease and help the colic ; some appoint it to be burnt, and then taken for the same purpose.

ROSA SOLIS, or SUN-DEW

Description.—It hath divers small, round, hollow leaves, greenish, but full of red hairs, which make them seem red, each standing upon his own foot-stalk, reddish, and hairy. The leaves are continually moist in the hottest day, yea, the hotter the sun shines on them, the moister they are, with a sliminess that will rope, as we say, the small hairs always holding this moisture. Among these leaves rise up slender stalks, reddish also, three or four fingers high, bearing small white knobs one above another, which are flowers; after which come heads with small seeds. The root is a few small hairs.

Place.—It groweth usually in bogs and wet places, and sometimes in moist woods.

Time.—It flowereth in June, and then the leaves are fittest to be gathered.

Government and Virtues.—The sun rules it, and it is under the sign Cancer. Rosa Solis is accounted good to help those that have a salt rheum distilling on the lungs, which causeth consumption, and therefore the distilled water in wine is profitable for such to drink, which water will be of a good yellow colour. The same water is held to be good for phthisics, wheezings, shortness of breath, and cough; also to heal ulcers in the lungs; and it comforteth the heart and fainting spirits. The leaves outwardly applied to the skin will raise blisters, which has caused some to think it dangerous to be taken inwardly. There is a drink made thereof with *aqua vitæ* and spices, and without any danger, used in qualms and passions of the heart.

ROSEMARY.

GARDEN rosemary is well known.

Time.—It flowereth in April and May, and sometimes again in August.

Government and Virtues.—The sun claims privilege in it, and it is under the celestial Ram. It is an herb of great use, both for inward and outward diseases, for by the warm and comforting heat thereof, it relieves all cold diseases of the head, stomach, liver, and belly. The decoction in wine removes cold distillations of rheums in the eyes, and other cold diseases of the head and brain, as gidddiness or swimmings, drowsiness or dulness of the mind and senses, the dumb palsy, or loss of speech, the lethargy and falling sickness, to be drunk and the temples bathed therewith. It relieveth pains in the gums and teeth by rheum falling into them, causing a stinking breath. It quickens a weak memory, and the senses. It warms the stomach in all the cold griefs thereof, helpeth both retention of meat and digestion, the decoction or powder being taken in wine. It is a remedy for windiness in the stomach, bowels, and spleen, and expels it powerfully. It helpeth those that are liver grown, by opening the obstructions thereof. It helpeth dim eyes, and procureth clear sight, the flowers thereof being taken all the while it is flowering, every morning, fasting, with bread and salt. Dioscorides and Galen say, that if a decoction be made with water, it will cure the yellow jaundice. The flowers and conserve made of them, are good to comfort the heart, and to expel the contagion of the pestilence : to burn the herb in houses and chambers, correcteth the air in them. The flowers and leaves are a remedy for the whites, if they be daily taken. The dried leaves shred small, and taken in a pipe as tobacco is taken, relieves cough, phthisic, or consumption, by warming and drying 'the thin distillations which cause those diseases. The leaves are much used in bathings ; and made into ointments or oil, are good to warm cold and benumbed joints, sinews, or members. The chemical oil drawn from the leaves and flowers, is a sovereign remedy for all the diseases aforesaid ; to touch the temples and nostrils with two or three drops for all the diseases of the head and brain spoken of before ; as also to take one drop, two, or three, as the case requireth for the inward griefs ; yet it must be done with discretion, for it is very quick and piercing, and therefore very little must be taken at a time. There is also another oil made by insolation in this manner :—Take a quantity of the flowers and put them into a strong glass closely stopped, tie a fine linen cloth over the mouth, and turn the mouth down into another strong glass, which being set in the sun, an oil will distil down into the lower glass, to be preserved as precious for divers uses, both inward and outward, as a sovereign balm to heal the diseases before mentioned, to clear dim sight, and take away spots, marks, and scars in the skin.

RHUBARB, or RAPHONTICK.

THIS is well known to every body.

Description.—At the first appearing out of the ground, it hath a great round brownish head rising from the middle or sides of the root, which openeth into leaves one after another, very much crumpled or folded together at the first, and brownish ; but afterwards it spreadeth itself, and becometh smooth, very large and almost round, every one standing on a brownish stalk of the thickness of a man's thumb when they are grown to their fulness, and most of them two feet and more in length, especially when they grow in moist and good ground ; and the stalk of the leaf, from the bottom thereof to the leaf itself, being also two feet, the breadth thereof from edge to edge, in the broadest place, being also two feet, of a dark green colour, of a fine tart or sourish taste, much more pleasant than the garden or wood sorrel. On strong stalks are white flowers, spreading forth into many branches consisting of five or six small leaves a-piece, after which come brownish seed, like dockseed but larger. The root grows large, with sundry spreading branches, of a dark reddish colour on the outside, with a pale yellow skin under it. The root is purgative, like the foreign, but not so strong.

Place.—It groweth in gardens, flowereth the beginning or middle of June, and the seed is ripe in July.

Time.—The roots that are to be dried and kept all the next year, are not to be taken up before the stalks and leaves be about the middle or end of October, and if they be taken a little before the leaves do spring, or when they are sprung up, the roots will not have so good a colour in them.

I come now to describe that which is called patience, or monk's rhubarb ; and next unto the bastard rhubarb, for one of these may supply in the absence of the other, being not much unlike in their virtues, only more powerful and efficacious than the other ; and lastly, will show you the virtues of all the three sorts.

GARDEN PATIENCE, or MONK'S RHUBARB.

Description.—This is a dock bearing the name of rhubarb for some purging quality therein, and groweth up with large tall stalks set with broad and long fair green leaves, not dented at all. The tops of the stalks being divided into many small branches, bear reddish or purple flowers, and three-square seed like unto other dock. The root is long, great, and yellow, like unto the wild docks, but a little redder ; and if it be a little dried, showeth less store of discoloured veins than the next doth when it is dry.

GREAT ROUND-LEAVED DOCK, or BASTARD RHUBARB.

Description.—This hath large, round, thin, yellowish green leaves, a little waved about the edges, each standing upon a thick and long brownish foot-stalk, from among which riseth up a large stalk two feet high, with some such like leaves growing thereon, but smaller ; at the top whereof stand in a long spike small brownish flowers, which turn into a hard, three-square, shining brown seed. The root groweth great, with many branches of great fibres, yellow on the outside, and pale yellow within, with some discoloured veins like the rhubarb first described, but much less than it, especially when it is dry.

Place and Time.—It grows in gardens, an flowers and seeds at or near the same time the true rhubarb doth, viz. they flower in June, and the seed is ripe in July.

Government and Virtues.—Mars claims predominancy over all those wholesome herbs. A drachm of the dried root of monk's rhubarb, with a scruple of ginger made into powder, and taken fasting in a draught or mess of warm broth, purgeth both choler and phlegm very gently and safely. The seed thereof, on the contrary, doth bind the bowels, and helpeth to stay any sort of lasks or bloody-flux. The distilled water healeth scabs ; also foul ulcerous sores, and to allay the inflammation ; the juice of the leaves or roots, or the decoction of them in vinegar, is used as a most effectual remedy to heal scabs and running sores.

The bastard rhubarb hath all the properties of the monk's rhubarb, but is more effectual for both inward and outward diseases.   The decoction without vinegar, dropped into the ears, taketh away pains ; gargled in the mouth, cures the toothache ; and being drunk healeth the jaundice.   The seed thereof taken, easeth gnawing pains of the stomach, and taketh away the loathing heat.   The root being boiled in wine, cureth the swelling of the throat, and the king's evil.   It is a cure for the stone, provoketh urine and cures the dimness of sight.   The roots of this bastard rhubarb are used in purging diet drinks, with other things, to open the liver, and cleanse and cool the blood.

The properties of the English rhubarb are the same with the former, but much more effectual, and hath all the properties of the true Italian rhubarbs, except as an aperient, it is but half the strength, and therefore a double quantity must be used ; it is not so bitter and astringent.— It purgeth the body of choler and phlegm, being either taken of itself made into powder and drunk in a draught of white wine, or steeped therein all night and taken fasting, or put among other purges as shall be thought convenient, cleansing the stomach, liver, and blood ; opening obstructions, and helping those griefs that come thereof, as the jaundice, dropsy, swelling of the spleen, tertian and daily agues, and pricking pains of the sides ; it stayeth spitting of blood.   The powder taken with cassia dissolved, and washed Venice turpentine, cleanseth the reins and strengtheneth them afterwards, and is very effectual to stay the running of the reins, or gonorrhœa.   It is also given for swellings and pains in the head, for melancholy, it is good for sciatica, gout, and cramp.   The oil also wherein it hath been boiled worketh the like effects, being anointed.   It is used to heal those ulcers that happen therein.   Whey or white wine are the best liquors to steep it in, and thereby worketh more effectually in opening obstructions, and purging the stomach and liver.   Many use a little Indian spikenard as the best corrector thereof.

MEADOW RUE.

Description.—Meadow rue riseth up with a yellow stringy root, much spreading in the ground, shooting forth new sprouts round about, with many green stalks two feet high, crested the length of them, set with joints here and there, and many large leaves upon them, above as well as below, being divided into smaller leaves nicked or dented in the fore part of them, of a red green colour on the upper side, and pale green underneath; towards the top of the stalk there shooteth forth branches, on every one whereof stand two, three, or four small heads or buttons, which, breaking the skin that incloses them, shooteth forth a tuft of pale greenish yellow threads, which falling away, appear small three-cornered pods, containing small, long, and round seed. The plant hath a strong unpleasant scent.

Place.—It groweth in many places of this land, in the borders of moist meadows and ditch-sides.

Time.—It flowereth in July, or August.

Government and Virtues.—Dioscorides saith, that this herb bruised and applied, perfectly healeth old sores, and the distilled water of the herb and flowers doth the like. It is used by some among other pot herbs to open the body and make it soluble; but the roots washed clean and boiled in ale and drunk, provoke to stool more than the leaves, but yet very gently. The root boiled in water, and the places of the body most troubled with vermin and lice washed therewith while it is warm, destroyeth them utterly. In Italy it is used against the plague, and in Saxony against the jaundice, as Camerarius saith.

GARDEN-RUE.

GARDEN RUE is well known.

Government and Virtues.—It is an herb of the Sun, and under Leo. It provoketh urine and women's courses, being taken either in meat or drink. The seed taken in wine, is an antidote against all dangerous medicines or deadly poisons. The leaves taken either by themselves or with figs and walnuts, is called Mithridates' counter poison against the plague, being often taken in meat and drink, it abateth venery, and ability to procreate. A decoction made with dried dill leaves and flowers, easeth pains and torments, to be drunk, and outwardly applied warm to the affected place. The same being drunk helpeth the pains both of the chest and sides, coughs, hardness of breathing, inflammation of the lungs, and tormenting pains of sciatica, and pains in the joints, being anointed or laid to the places ; as also the shaking fits of agues, to take a draught before the fit comes ; being boiled or infused in oil, it is good for colic, and freeth women from the suffocation of the mother, if the share and the parts thereabouts be anointed therewith : it killeth worms, if it be drunk after it is boiled in wine to the half, with a little honey ; it relieveth the gout or pains in the joints, hands, feet or knees, applied thereunto ; and with figs it arrests the dropsy, being bathed therewith ; bruised and put into the nostrils, it stayeth bleeding ; it reduces swelling of the testicles, rue and bay-leaves made into a decoction, and applied by fomenting. It taketh away wheals and pimples, if, being bruised with a few myrtle leaves, it be made up with wax, and applied. It also cureth morphew, and all sorts of warts, if boiled in wine with some pepper and nitre, and the place rubbed therewith ; and with almonds and honey removeth dry scabs, tetter or ringworm. The juice thereof warmed in a pomegranate shell or rind, and dropped into the ears easeth pain. The juice of it and fennel, with a little honey and the gall of a cock put thereto, removes dimness of the sight. An ointment made of the juice, with oil of roses, ceruse, and a little vinegar, and anointed, cureth St. Anthony's fire, and all running sores in the head, and stinking ulcers of the nose or other parts. The antidote used by Mithridates every morning, fasting, to secure himself from any poison or infection, was this : take twenty leaves of rue, a little salt, two walnuts and two figs, beaten together into a mess with twenty juniper berries, the quantity for every day. Another electuary is made thus : take of nitre, pepper, and cummin-seed, of each equal parts ; of the leaves of rue clean picked, as much in weight as all the other three weighed ; beat them well together, and put as much honey as will make it up into an electuary, (first steep the cummin-seed in vinegar twenty-four hours, and then dry it, or rather roast it in a hot fire shovel or in an oven) and it is a remedy for the pains and griefs of the chest or stomach, of the spleen, belly, or sides, by wind or stitches ; of the liver by obstructions, of the reins and bladder by the stopping of urine, and helpeth also to extenuate fat corpulent bodies.

What an infamy is cast upon the ashes of Mithridates. The whole world is beholden to Mithridates for his studies in physic, and he that uses the quantity but of an hazel nut of that receipt every morning, to which his name is adjoined, shall to admiration preserve his body in health, if he do but consider that rue is an herb of the Sun, and under Leo, and gather it and the rest accordingly.

RUPTURE WORT.

Description.—This spreads very many thready branches round about upon the ground, about a span long, divided into many other several parts full of small joints set very thick together, whereat come forth two very small leaves of a French yellow, green coloured branches and all, where groweth forth also a number of exceeding small yellow flowers, scarce to be discerned from the stalks and leaves, which turn into seeds as small as dust. The root is long and small, and deep in the ground. This hath neither smell nor taste at first, but afterwards hath a little astringent taste, without any manifest heat ; yet a little bitter and sharp.

Place.—It groweth in dry, sandy, and rocky places.

Time.—It is fresh and green all the summer.

Government and Virtues.—This herb is Saturn's own, and is a noble anti-venerean. Rupture Wort hath not its name in vain ; for it is found by experience to cure the rupture, not only in children, but also in elder persons if the disease be not too inveterate, by taking a drachm of the powder of the dried herb every day in wine, or a decoction drunk for certain days together. The juice or distilled water of the green herb, taken in the same manner, helpeth all other fluxes either of man or woman ; vomitings also, and the gonorrhœa or running of the reins, being taken any of the ways aforesaid. It benefits those that have the strangury, or are troubled with the stone or gravel in the reins or bladder. It removes stitches in the sides, griping pains of the stomach or belly, the obstructions of the liver, and cureth the yellow jaundice; it kills worms in children. Being outwardly applied, it conglutinateth wounds notably, and helpeth much to stay defluctions of rheum from the head to the eyes, nose, and teeth, being bruised green and bound thereto; or the forehead, temples, or nape of the neck behind, bathed with the decoction of the dried herb. It also drieth up the moisture of fistulous ulcers, or any other that are foul and spreading.

RUSHES.

ALTHOUGH there are many kinds of rushes, yet I shall only here insist upon those which are best known, and most medicinal; as the bulrushes and others of the soft and smooth kinds, which grow in almost every part of this land.

Government and Virtues.—The seed of the soft rushes, saith Dioscorides and Galen, (toasted, saith Pliny) drunk in wine and water, stayeth the lask and women's courses, when too abundant: but it causeth head-ache; it provoketh sleep, but must be given with caution. The root boiled in water to one-third helpeth the cough.

What I have written concerning rushes is to satisfy my countrymen's question: *Are our rushes good for nothing?* Yes, and as good to let them alone as taken. There are remedies enough without them for any disease, and therefore as the old proverb is, I care not a rush for them; or rather, they will do you as much good as if one had given you a rush.

RYE.

THIS is well known, especially to country people, who feed much upon it.

Government and Virtues.—Rye is more digesting than wheat; the bread and leaven thereof ripen and break impostumes, boils, and other swellings; the meal of rye put between a double cloth and moistened with a little vinegar, and heated in a pewter dish set over a chafing dish of coals, and bound fast to the head while it is hot, doth much ease the continual pains in the head. Matthiolus saith that the ashes of rye-straw put into water and steeped therein a day and a night, and the chops of the hands or feet washed therewith, doth heal them.

SAFFRON.

THE herb needs no description, it being known generally where it grows.

Place.—It grows frequently in Walden, in Essex, and in Cambridgeshire, and some other places.

Government and Virtues.—It is an herb of the Sun, and under the Lion, and therefore you need not demand a reason why it strengthens the heart so exceedingly. Let not above ten grains be given at a time, for the sun, which is the fountain of light, may dazzle the eyes and make them blind : a cordial being taken in an immoderate quantity hurts the heart instead of helping it. It quickeneth the brain, for the Sun is exalted in Aries, as he hath his house in Leo. It helps consumptions of the lungs and difficulty of breathing, it is excellent in epidemical diseases, as pestilence, small pox, and measles. It is a notable expulsive medicine and remedy for the yellow jaundice.

SAGE.

Time.—It flowereth in or about July.

Government and Virtues.—Jupiter claims this herb. It is good for diseases of the liver, and to make blood. A decoction of the leaves and branches of sage made and drunk, saith Dioscorides, provokes urine, bringeth down the courses, and causeth the hair to become black. It stayeth the bleeding of wounds, and cleanseth ulcers and sores. A decoction cures itching in the testicles. Agrippa saith, that if women cannot conceive, by reason of the moist slipperiness of their wombs, shall take the juice of sage with a little salt, four days before they company with their husbands, it will help them to conceive, and to retain the birth. Orpheus saith, three spoonfuls of the juice of sage, taken fasting, with a little honey, arrests spitting or vomiting of blood in consumption. These pills are much commended :—Take of spikenard and ginger of each two drachms ; of the seed of sage toasted at the fire, eight drachms ; of long pepper, twelve drachms ; all these being brought into powder, put thereto so much juice of sage as may make them into a mass of pills, taking a drachm of them every morning fasting, and so likewise at night, drinking a little pure water after them. Matthiolus saith, it is very profitable for all pains in the head coming of cold and rheumatic humours ; as also for all pains in the joint, whether inwardly or outwardly, and therefore prevents the falling sickness, the lethargy, such as are dull and heavy of spirits, the palsy, and is of much use in all defluctions of rheum from the head and for diseases of the chest or breast. The leaves of sage and nettles bruised together, and laid upon an imposthume behind the ears, doth assuage it much.

The juice of sage in warm water cureth hoarseness and cough. The leaves steeped in wine, and laid upon the place affected with the palsy, helpeth much if the decoction be drunk ; also sage taken with wormwood is good for the bloody-flux. Pliny saith, it procureth women's courses, and stayeth them when too profuse ; cureth stinging and biting of serpents, and killeth worms in the ears, and in sores. Sage is of excellent use to help the memory, warming and quickening the senses ; and the conserve made of the flowers is used for the same purpose, and for all the former recited diseases. The juice of sage drunk with vinegar hath been of good use in the time of the plague, at all times. Gargles are made with sage, rosemary, honeysuckles and plantain, boiled in wine or water with some honey or alum put thereto, to wash sore mouths and throats, cankers, or the secret parts, as need requireth. And with other hot and comfortable herbs sage is boiled to bathe the body and legs in the summer time, especially to warm cold joints or sinews troubled with the palsy or cramp, and to strengthen the parts. It is very good for stitch or pains in the sides coming of wind, if the place be

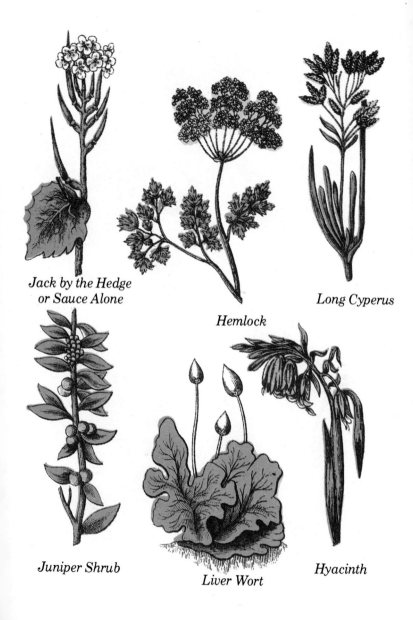

Jack by the Hedge or Sauce Alone

Hemlock

Long Cyperus

Juniper Shrub

Liver Wort

Hyacinth

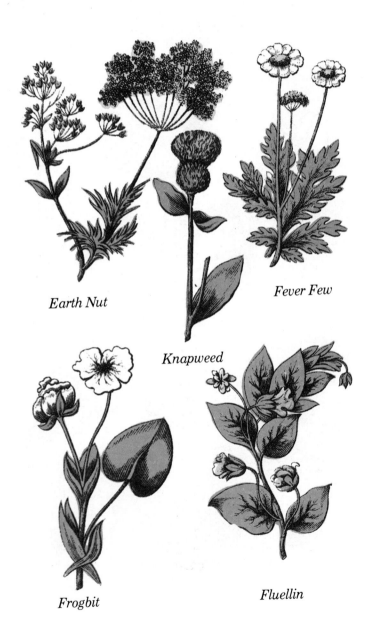

Earth Nut

Fever Few

Knapweed

Frogbit

Fluellin

fomented warm with the decoction in wine, and the herb also after boiling be laid warm thereunto.

WOOD SAGE.

Description.—Wood sage riseth up with square hoary stalks, two feet high at least, with two leaves set at every joint, somewhat like other sage leaves, but smaller, softer, whiter, and rounder, and a little dented about the edges, and smelling somewhat stronger. At the tops of the stalks and branches stand the flowers, on slender-like spikes, turning themselves all one way when they blow, and are of a pale and whitish colour, smaller than sage, but hooded and gaping like them. The seed is blackish and round; four usually seen in a husk together; the root is long and abideth many years.

Place.—It groweth in woods and by wood-sides; as also in divers fields and bye-lanes.

Time.—It flowereth in June, July, and August.

Government and Virtues.—The herb is under Venus. The decoction of the wood sage provoketh urine and the menses. It also provoketh sweat, digesteth humours, and discusseth swellings and nodes in the flesh. The decoction of the green herb made with wine, is a safe and sure remedy for those who by falls, bruises, or blows, suspect some vein to be inwardly broken, to disperse and void the congealed blood, and consolidate the veins. The drink used inwardly and the herb outwardly, is good for such as are inwardly or outwardly bursten, and is found to be a sure remedy for the palsy. The juice of the herb, or the powder thereof dried, is good for moist ulcers and sores in the legs and other parts, to dry them and cause them to heal more speedily. It is no less effectual also in green wounds, to be used upon any occasion.

SOLOMON'S SEAL.

Description.—The common Solomon's seal riseth up with a round stalk half a yard high, bowing or bending down to the ground, set with single leaves one above another, somewhat large, and like the leaves of the lily convally, or May lily, with an eye of bluish upon the green, with some ribs therein, and more yellowish underneath. At the foot of every leaf, almost from the bottom up to the top of the stalk, come forth small, long, white, and hollow pendulous flowers, somewhat like the flowers of May lily, but ending in five long points, two together, at the end of a long foot-stalk, and sometimes but one, and sometimes also two stalks, with flowers at the foot of a leaf, which are without any scent at all, and stand on one side of the stalk. After they are past come in their places small round berries, great at the first, and blackish green, tending to blueness when they are ripe, wherein lie small, white, hard seeds. The root is of the thickness of one's finger or thumb, white and knotted in some places, a flat round circle representing a seal, whereof it took the name, lying along under the upper crust of the earth, and not growing downward.

Place.—It is frequent in Kent and other counties, and it is frequent in gardens.

Time.—It flowereth about May; the root abideth and shooteth anew every year.

Government and Virtues.—Saturn owns the plant. The root of Solomon's seal is found by experience to be available in wounds, hurts, and outward sores, to heal and close up the lips of those that are green, and to dry up and restrain the flux of humours to those that are old. It is very good to stay vomitings and bleedings, and all fluxes, whether whites or reds in women, or the running of the reins in men ; also to knit any joint, which by weakness useth to be out of place, or will not stay in long when it is set ; also, to knit and join broken bones in any part of the body, the roots being bruised and applied to the places ; yea, it hath been found by late experience that the decoction of the root in wine, or the bruised root put into wine or other drink, and after a night's infusion, strained and drunk, hath helped both man and beast whose bones have been broken, which is the most assured refuge of help to people of divers counties of the land that they can have. It is effectual for ruptures and burstings, the decoction in wine, or the powder in broth or drink being inwardly taken, and outwardly applied to the place. The same is also available for outward or inward bruises, falls, or blows, to dispel the congealed blood, and to take away both the pains and the black and blue marks. The same also, or the distilled water of the whole plant, used to the face or other parts of the skin, cleanseth it from morphew, freckles, spots, or marks, leaving the place fresh, fair, and lovely.

SAMPHIRE.

Description.—Rock samphire groweth up with a tender green stalk, about half a yard or two feet high at the most, branching forth almost from the very bottom, and stored with sundry thick, and almost round (somewhat long) leaves, of a deep green colour, sometimes two together, and sometimes more on a stalk, and sappy, and of a pleasant, hot, and spicy taste. At the tops of the stalks and branches stand umbels of white flowers, and after them come large seed bigger than fennel seed, yet somewhat like it. The root is great, white, and long.

Place.—It groweth on the rocks that are often moistened or overflowed with sea-water.

Time.—And it flowereth and seedeth in the end of July and August.

Government and Virtues.—It is an herb of Jupiter, and was in former times used more than now it is ; the more is the pity. It is well known almost to every body, that ill digestions and obstructions are the cause of most diseases which the frail nature of man is subject to ; both which might be remedied .by the frequent use of this herb. If people would have sauce to their meat, they may take some for profit as well as for pleasure. It is a safe herb, very pleasant both to taste and stomach, helpeth digestion, and openeth obstructions of the liver and spleen ; provoketh urine, and helpeth thereby to wash away the gravel and stone engendered in the kidneys or bladder.

SANICLE.

Description.—Ordinary sanicle sendeth forth many great round leaves, standing upon long brownish stalks, every one somewhat deeply cut or divided into five or six parts, and some of these also cut like the leaf of crow's-foot, or dove's-foot, and finely dented about the edges, smooth, and of a dark shining colour, and sometimes reddish about the brims; from among which rise up small, round green stalks, without any joint or leaf thereon saving at the top, where it branches forth into flowers, having a leaf divided into three or four parts at that joint with the flowers, which are small and white, starting out of small, round, greenish yellow heads, many standing together in a tuft, in which afterwards are the seeds contained, which are small round burs, somewhat like the leaves of cleavers, and stick in the same manner upon anything that they touch. The root is composed of many blackish fibres, set together at a little long head, which abideth with green leaves all the winter.

Place.—It is found in many shadowy woods, and other places of this land.

Time.—It flowereth in June, and the seed is ripe shortly after.

Government and Virtues.—This is one of Venus's herbs to cure the wounds or mischiefs Mars inflicteth upon the body of man. It heals green wounds speedily, or any ulcers, imposthumes, or bleedings inward, also tumours in any part of the body; for the decoction or powder in drink taken, and the juice used outwardly, dissipateth the humours; and there is not found any herb that can give such present help either to man or beast when the disease falleth upon the lungs or throat, and to heal up putrid malignant ulcers in the mouth, throat, and privities, by gargling or washing with the decoction of the leaves and roots in water, and a little honey put thereto. It restrains profuse menstruation, and all other fluxes of the blood, either by the mouth, urine, or stool, and lasks of the belly; the ulcerations of the kidneys also, and pains in the bowels and gonorrhœa, or running of the reins, being boiled in wine or water, and drunk. The same also is no less powerful to subdue ruptures or burstings, used both inwardly and outwardly; and it is effectual in binding, restraining, consolidating, warming, drying, and healing, as comfrey, bugle, self-heal, or any other of the vulnerary herbs.

SARACEN'S CONFOUND, or SARACEN'S WOUND-WORT.

Description.—This groweth high, with brownish stalks, and sometimes with green, to a man's height, having narrow green leaves snipped about the edges, like those of the peach-tree or willow leaves, but not of such a white green colour. The tops of the stalks are furnished with many yellow star-like flowers standing in green heads, which when they are fallen and the seed ripe, which is somewhat long, small, and of a brown colour, wrapped in down, is carried away with the wind. The root is composed of fibres set together at a head, which perisheth not in winter, but the stalks dry away, and no leaf appeareth in the winter. The taste is strong and unpleasant, and so is the smell also.

Place.— It groweth in moist and wet grounds by wood-sides, and sometimes in the moist places of shadowy groves, as also the water sides.

Time.—It flowereth in July, and the seed is soon ripe, and carried away with the wind.

Government and Virtues.—Saturn owns the herb, and it is of a sober condition. Among the Germans this wound herb is preferred before all others of the same quality. Being boiled in wine and drunk, it cureth the indisposition of the liver, and freeth the gall from obstructions, whereby it is good for the yellow jaundice, and for the dropsy ; for all inward ulcers of the reins, mouth, or throat, and inward wounds and bruises, likewise for sores in the privy parts ; being steeped in wine, and then distilled, the water thereof drunk, easeth all gawnings in the stomach or other pains of the body, as also the pains of the mother ; and being boiled in water, it cureth continual agues : and the said water, or the simple water of the herb distilled, or the juice or decoction, are very effectual to heal any green wound, or old sore whatsover, cleansing them from corruption, and quickly healing them. Briefly, whatsoever hath been said of bugle or sanicle may be found in this.

SAUCE-ALONE, OR JACK BY THE HEDGE SIDE.

Description.—The lower leaves of this are rounder than those that grow towards the tops of the stalks, and are set singly on the joint, being somewhat round and broad, pointed at the ends, dented also about the edges, resembling nettle leaves for the form, but of a fresher green colour, not rough or pricking : the flowers are white, growing at the tops of the stalks one above another, which being past, follow small round pods, wherein are contained round seed somewhat blackish. The root stringy and thready, perisheth every year after it hath given seed, and raiseth itself again of its own sowing. The plant, or any part thereof being bruised, smelleth of garlic, but more pleasantly, and tasteth hot and sharp, almost like rocket.

Place.—It groweth under walls and by hedge sides, and path-ways in fields in many places.

Time.—It flowereth in June, July, and August.

Government and Virtues.—It is an herb of Mercury. This is eaten by many country people as sauce to their salt fish, and helpeth well to digest the crudities and other corrupt humours engendered thereby. It warmeth the stomach, and causeth digestion. The juice thereof boiled with honey, is accounted to be as good as hedge mustard for cough, to cut and expectorate the tough phlegm. The seed bruised and boiled in wine is a good remedy for the wind colic or the stone, being drunk warm : it is also given to women troubled with the mother, both to drink, and the seed put into a cloth, and applied while it is warm is of singular good nse. The leaves also or the seed boiled is good to be used in clysters to ease the pains of the stone. The green leaves are held to be good to heal the ulcers in the legs.

WINTER AND SUMMER SAVORY.

BOTH these are so well known as inhabitants in our gardens, that they need no description.

Government and Virtues.—Mercury claims the dominion over this herb, neither is there a better remedy against the colic and iliac passion than this herb ; keep it dry by you all the year, if you love yourself and your ease, and it is a hundred pounds to a penny if you do not; keep it dry, make conserves and syrups of it for your use, and take notice, that the summer kind is the best. They are both of them hot and dry, and especially the summer kind, which is both sharp and quick in taste, expelling wind in the stomach and bowels, and is a present help for the rising of the mother procured by wind; provoked urine and women's courses, aud is much commended for women with child to take inwardly, and to smell often unto. It cureth tough phlegm in the chest and lungs, and helpeth to expectorate it the more easily : quickens the dull spirits in a lethargy, the juice thereof being snuffed into the nostrils. The juice dropped into the eyes cleareth a dull sight, if it proceed of thin cold humours distilled from the brain. The juice heated with oil of roses and dropped into the ears easeth them of the noise and singing in them, and of deafness also. Outwardly applied with wheat flour as a poultice, it giveth ease to sciatica and palsied members, heating and warming them, and taketh away their pains. It also taketh away the pain that comes by stinging of becs, wasps, &c.

SAVINE.

To describe a plant so well known is needless, it being nursed up almost in every garden, and abiding green all the winter.

Government and Virtues.—It is under the dominion of Mars, being hot and dry in the third degree, and being of very clean parts, is of a very digesting quality. If you dry the herb into powder, and mix it with honey, it is an excellent remedy to cleanse ulcers and fistulas ; but it hinders them from healing. The same is good to break carbuncles and plague sores ; and cureth the king's evil, being applied to the place. Being spread over a piece of leather, and applied to the navel, it kills worms, helps scabs and itch, running sores, cankers, tetters, and ringworms, and being applied to the place, may haply cure venereal sores. It is always applied *outwardly* never *inwardly.*

THE COMMON WHITE SAXIFRAGE.

Description. —This hath a few small reddish kernels of roots covered with some skins, lying among small blackish fibres, which send forth divers round, faint or yellow green leaves, and greyish underneath, lying above the ground, unevenly dented about the edges, and somewhat hairy, every one upon a little foot-stalk, from whence riseth round, brownish, hairy green stalks two or three feet high, with such like round leaves as grow below, but smaller, and branched at the top, whereon stand pretty large white flowers of five leaves a-piece, with some yellow low threads in the middle, standing in a long, crested, brownish green husk. After the flowers are past, there ariseth sometimes a round hard head, forked at the top, wherein is contained small black seed, but usually they fall away without any seed, and it is the kernels or grains of the root which are usually called the white saxifrage-seed, and so used.

Place. —It groweth in many places of this land, as well in the lowermost as in the upper dry corners of meadows, and grassy sandy places.

Time. —It flowereth in May, and quickly perisheth when any hot weather comes.

Government and Virtues. —It is very effectual to cleanse the reins and bladder, and to dissolve stone therein, and to expel it and the gravel by urine; to relieve the strangury; for which purpose the decoction of the herb or roots in white wine is most usual, or the powder of the small kernelly root, which is called the seed, taken in white wine, or in the same decoction made with white wine is most usual. The distilled water of the whole herb, root, and flowers, is good to be taken. It provoketh also women's courses, and freeth and cleanseth the stomach and lungs from thick and tough phlegm that trouble them. There are not many better medicines to break the stone than this.

BURNET SAXIFRAGE.

Description. —The greatest sort of our English burnet saxifrage groweth up with long stalks of winged leaves set directly opposite one to another on both sides, each being somewhat broad, and a little pointed and dented about the edges, of a sad green colour. At the top of the stalks stand umbels of white flowers, after which come small and blackish seed. The root is long and whitish, abiding long.

Our lesser burnet saxifrage hath much finer leaves than the former, and very small, and set one against another, deeply jagged about the edges, and of the same colour as the former. The umbels of the flowers are white, and the seed very small, and so is the root, being also somewhat hot and quick in taste.

Place.—These grow in moist meadows of this land, and are easy to be found, being well sought for among the grass, wherein many times they lay hid and are scarcely to be discerned.

Time.—They flower about July, and their seed is ripe in August.

Government and Virtues.—They are both of them herbs of the Moon. The saxifrages are as hot as pepper ; and Tragus saith, by his experience, that they are wholesome. They have the same properties the parsleys have, but in provoking urine, and easing the pains thereof, and of the wind and colic, are much more effectual, the roots or seeds being used either in powder or in decoction, or any other way ; and also helpeth pains of the mother, and to procure their courses, and to break and void the stone in the kidneys, to digest cold, viscous, and tough phlegm, and is an especial remedy against all kinds of venom. Castoreum being boiled in the distilled water, is very good for cramps and convulsions. Some make the seeds into comfits, as they do carraway seeds, which is effectual to all the purposes aforesaid. The juice of the herb dropped into the most grievous wounds of the head, drieth up their moisture and healeth them quickly. Some women used the distilled water to take away freckles or spots in the skin or face ; and to drink the same sweetened with sugar for all the purposes aforesaid.

SCABIOUS, (THREE SORTS.)

Description.—Common field scabious groweth up with many hairy, soft, whitish green leaves, some are small, jagged upon the edge, others much rent and torn on the sides, and have threads in them, which upon breaking may be plainly seen; from among which rise up hairy green stalks three or four feet high, and with hairy green leaves on them, but more deeply and finely divided, branched forth a little; at the tops, which are naked and bare of leaves for a good space, stand round heads of flowers of a pale bluish colour, set together in a head, with the outermost whereof are larger than the inward, with many threads also in the middle, flat at the top, as the head with the seed is also. The root is great, white, and thick, growing deep in the ground, and abideth many years. There is another sort of field scabious differing in nothing from the former, but only it is smaller in all respects.

The corn scabious differeth little from the first, but that it is larger in all respects, and the flowers more inclined to purple, and the root runneth not deep into the ground like the first.

Place.—The first groweth usually in meadows. The second in dry fields and other fields. The third in standing corn or fallow fields, and the borders of such fields.

Time.—They flower in June and July, and some abide flowering until it be late in August, and the seed is ripe in the mean time.

Government and Virtues.—Mercury owns the plant. Scabious is very effectual for all coughs, shortness of breath, and all other diseases of the breast and lungs, ripening and digesting cold phlegm and other tough humours, and voideth them by coughing. It ripeneth also all sorts of inward ulcers and imposthumes; pleurisy also, if the decoction of the herb dry or green be made into wine, and drunk for some time together. Three ounces of the clarified juice of scabious taken in the morning fasting, with a drachm of mithridate or Venice treacle, freeth the heart from any infection or pestilence, if after the taking of it the party sweat two hours in bed, and this medicine be repeated if need require. The green herb bruised and applied to any carbuncle or plague-sore, is found to dissolve and break it in three hours' space. The same decoction removeth pains and stitches in the sides. The decoction of the roots taken for forty days together, or a drachm of the powder of them taken at a time in whey, wonderfully cures running and spreading scabs, tetters, ringworms, and the French pox. The juice or decoction drunk, cureth the itch, and its eruptions. The juice also made up into an ointment and used, is effectual for the same purpose. The same also healeth all inward wounds by the drying, cleansing, and healing quality therein ; and a syrup made of the juice and sugar, is very effectual for all the purposes aforesaid, and so is the distilled water of the herb and flowers made in due season, especially to be used when the green herb is not in force to be taken. The decoction of the herb and roots outwardly applied, doth wonderfully subdue all hard or cold swellings in any part of the body, is effectual for shrunk sinews or veins, and healeth green wounds, old sores, and ulcers. The juice of scabious made up with the powder of borax and samphire, cleanseth the skin of the face, and removeth freckles, pimples, morphew and leprosy ; the head washed with the decoction, cleanseth from dandriff, scurf, sores, itch, and the like, used warm. The herb bruised and applied, doth in a short time draw forth any splinter, broken bone, arrow head, or other such like thing lying in the flesh.

SCURVY-GRASS.

Description.—English scurvy-grass hath many thick flat leaves, longer than broad, and sometimes longer and narrower ; smooth on the edges, and sometimes a little waved ; sometimes plain, smooth, and pointed, of a sad green, and sometimes a bluish colour, every one standing alone upon a long foot-stalk, which is brownish or greenish also, from among which rise slender stalks bearing few leaves, but longer and lesser for the most part ; at the tops grow many whitish flowers, with yellow threads in the middle, standing about a green head, which becometh the seed vessel, rather flat when it is ripe ; wherein is contained reddish seed tasting hot. The root has many white strings which stick deeply into the mud, wherein it chiefly delights, yet it will well abide in the more upland and drier ground, and tasteth a little brackish, but not so much so as where it hath the salt water to feed upon.

Place.—It groweth along the Thames side, on the Essex and Kentish shores, from Woolwich round about the sea coast to Dover, Portsmouth, and Bristol, where it is had in plenty ; the other with round leaves groweth in the marshes in Holland, and in Lincolnshire by the sea-side.

Description.—There is also another kind called Dutch Scurvy-grass, which is most known and frequent in gardens, which hath fresh, green, and almost round leaves rising from the ground, not so thick as the former, yet in some rich grounds twice as large as in others, not dented about the edges or hollow in the middle, standing on a long foot-stalk ; from among these rise long, slender stalks, higher than the former, with more white flowers at the tops of them, which turn into small pods, and smaller brownish seeds than the former. The root is white, small, and thready. It hath a very hot, aromatical, and spicy taste.

Time.—It flowereth in April and May, and giveth ripe seed quickly after.

Government and Virtues.—It is an herb of Jupiter. The English scurvy grass is more used for its salt taste, which gently purges and cleanses ; but the Dutch scurvy-grass is of better effect, and chiefly used by those that have the scurvy, and is of singular good effect to cleanse the blood, liver, and spleen, taking the juice in the spring every morning, in a cup of drink. The decoction is good for the same purpose, and openeth obstructions, evacuating cold, clammy, and phlegmatic humours, both from the liver and spleen, and bringing the body to a more lively colour. The juice also helpeth all foul ulcers and sores in the mouth, gargled therewith ; and being used outwardly, cleanseth the skin from spots, marks, or scars that happen therein.

SELF-HEAL : CALLED ALSO PRUNEL, CARPENTER'S HERB, HOOK-HEAL, AND SICKLE-WORT.

Description.— The common self-heal is a small, low, creeping herb, having many small, roundish-pointed leaves like leaves of wild mint, of a dark green colour, without dents on the edges ; from among which rise square hairy stalks scarce a foot high, which spread sometimes into branches with small leaves set thereon up to the tops, where stand brown spiked heads of small brownish leaves like scales and flowers set together, almost like the head of cassidony, which flowers are gaping, and of a bluish purple, or more pale blue, in some places sweet, but not so in others. The roots consist of many fibres downwards, and spreadeth strings also whereby it increaseth. The small stalks, with the leaves creeping on the ground, shoot forth fibres taking hold on the ground, whereby it is made a great tuft in a short time.

Place.—It is found in woods and fields every where.

Time.—It flowereth in May, and sometimes in April.

Government and Virtues.—Here is another herb of Venus, self-heal, whereby, when you are hurt, you may heal yourself ; it is an especial herb for inward and outward wounds. Take it inwardly in syrups for inward wounds ; outwardly in unguents and plasters for outward. As self-heal is like bugle in form, so also in the qualities and virtues, serving for all the purposes whereunto bugle is applied with good success, either inwardly or outwardly ; for inward wounds or ulcers in the body, for bruises or falls, and hurts. If it be combined with bugle, sanicle, and other like woundherbs, it will be more effectual to wash or inject into ulcers in the parts outwardly. Where there is cause to repress the heat or sharpness of humours flowing to any sores, ulcers, inflammations, swellings, and the like, or to stay the flux of blood in any wound or part, this is used with some good success ; as also to cleanse the foulness of sores, and cause them more speedily to heal. It is an especial remedy for all green wounds, to close the lips of them, and to keep the place from further inconveniences. The juice used with oil of roses to anoint the temples and forehead, is very effectual to remove the head-ache, and the same mixed with honey of roses, cleanseth and healeth ulcers in the mouth and throat, and those also in the secret parts. And the proverb of the Germans, French, and others, is verified in this, *that he needeth neither physician nor surgeon that hath self-heal and sanicle to help himself.*

THE SERVICE TREE.

It is so well known in the place where it grows, that it needeth no description.

Time.—It flowereth before the end of May, and the fruit is ripe in October.

Government and Virtues.—Services, when they are mellow, are fit to be taken to stay fluxes, scouring, and casting, yet less than medlars. If they be dried before they be mellow, and kept all the year, they may be used in decoctions for the said purpose, either to drink, or to bathe the parts requiring it; and are profitably used in that manner to stay the bleeding of wounds, and of the mouth or nose, to be applied to the forehead and nape of the neck; and are under the dominion of Saturn.

SHEPHERD'S PURSE.

It is called shepherd's scrip, shepherd's pounce, toywort, pickpurse, and casewort.

Description.—The root is small, white, and perishing every year. The leaves are small and long, of a pale green colour, and deeply cut in on both sides, among which spring up a stalk which is small and round, containing small leaves upon it even to the top. The flowers are white and very small; after which come the little heart-shaped seed-pods.

Place.—They are frequent in this nation, almost by every path-side, and in field furrows.

Time.—They flower all the summer long; nay, some of them are so fruitful that they flower twice a year.

Government and Virtues.—It is under the dominion of Saturn, and of a cold, dry, and binding nature. It helps all fluxes of blood, caused by inward or outward wounds; as also flux of the belly and bloody-flux, spitting and voiding of blood, stops the terms in women; being bound to the wrists of the hands, and the soles of the feet, it cureth the yellow jaundice. The herb being made into a poultice subdues inflammations and St. Anthony's fire. The juice being dropped into the ears, subdues the pains, noise, and matterings thereof. A good ointment may be made of it for all wounds, especially for wounds in the head.

SMALLAGE.

THIS is also very well known, and I shall not trouble the reader with any description of it.

Place.—It groweth naturally in dry and marshy ground; and in gardens.

Time.—It abideth green all the winter, and seedeth in August.

Government and Virtues.—It is an herb of Mercury. Smallage is hotter, drier, and much more medicinal than parsley, for it much more openeth obstructions of the liver and spleen, expectorates thick phlegm, and cleanses the blood. It provoketh urine and women's courses, and is very good against the yellow jaundice, tertian and quartan agues if the juice be taken, but especially made into syrup. The juice also put to honey of roses and barley water, is very good to gargle the mouth and throat of those that have sores and ulcers in them, and will quickly heal them. The same lotion also cleanseth and healeth all other foul ulcers and cankers elsewhere, if they be washed therewith. The seed is especially used to break and expel wind, kill worms, and to sweeten stinking breath. The root is effectual to all the purposes aforesaid, and is held to be stronger in operation than the herb, but especially to open obstructions, and to rid away any ague, if the juice be taken in wine, or the decoction in wine be used.

SOPEWORT, OR BRUISEWORT.

Description.—The root creepeth underground far and near, with many joints therein, of a brown colour on the outside, and yellowish within, shooting forth weak and round stalks full of joints, set with two leaves a-piece at every one of them on the contrary side, which are ribbed like the plantain, and fashioned like the common field white campion leaves, seldom having any branches from the sides of the stalks, but set with flowers at the top, standing in long husks, like the wild campions, made of five leaves a-piece, round at the ends, and dented in the middle, of a rose colour, almost white, sometimes deeper, and sometimes paler, and of a good scent.

Place.—It groweth wild in many low and wet grounds of this land, by brooks and the sides of running waters.

Time.—It flowereth in July, and continueth all August and part of September.

Government and Virtues.—Venus owns it. Country people in divers places bruise the leaves of sopewort, and lay it to their fingers, hands, or legs when they are cut, to heal them. Some make great boast thereof that it is diuretic to provoke urine, and thereby to expel gravel and the stone in the reins or kidneys, and do also account it very good to void hydropical waters ; and extol it as an absolute cure of the French pox, more than sarsaparilla, guiacum, or china can do ; which how true it is, I leave others to judge.

SORREL.

Our ordinary sorrel which grows in gardens, and also wild in fields, is well known.

Government and Virtues.—It is under the dominion of Venus. Sorrel is prevalent in all hot diseases to cool inflammation and heat of blood in agues, pestilential or choleric, or sickness and fainting, arising from heat, and to refresh the overspent spirits with the violence of furious or fiery fits of agues ; to quench thirst, and procure an appetite in fainting or decaying stomachs. It resisteth putrefaction of the blood, killeth worms, and is a cordial to the heart, which the seed doth more effectually, being more drying and binding, and thereby stayeth the hot fluxes of women's courses, or of humours in the bloody-flux, or flux in the stomach. The root also in a decoction, or in powder, is effectual for all the said purposes. Both roots and seed, as well as the herb, are held powerful to resist the poison of the scorpion. The decoction of the roots is a cure for the jaundice and to expel the gravel and stone. The decoction of the flowers made with wine and drunk, cures the black jaundice, as also the inward ulcers of the body and bowels. A syrup made with the juice of sorrel and fumitory, is a sovereign remedy for those sharp humours that cause the itch. The juice with a little vinegar, serveth well to be used outwardly for the same cause, and is also good for tetters, ringworms, &c. It removeth kernels in the throat; and gargled in the mouth cures sores. The leaves wrapped in a colewort leaf and roasted in the embers, and applied to a hard imposthume, blotch, boil, or plague sore, doth ripen and break it. The distilled water of the herb is of much use for all the purposes aforesaid.

WOOD SORREL.

Description.—This groweth upon the ground, having a number of leaves coming from the root, made of three leaves like tre-foil, but broad at the ends and cut in the middle, of a yellowish green colour, every one standing on a long foot-stalk, which at their first coming up are closely folded together to the stalk, but opening themselves afterwards, and are of a fine sour relish, and yielding a juice which will turn red when it is clarified, and maketh a most dainty clear syrup. Among these leaves rise up divers slender, weak foot-stalks with every one of them a flower at the top, consisting of five small-pointed leaves, star-fashion, of a white colour in most places, and in some dashed over with a small show of bluish, on the backside only. After the flowers are past, follow small round heads with small yellow seeds in them. The roots are nothing but small strings fastened to the end of a small long piece; all of them being of a yellowish colour.

Place.—It groweth in many places of our land, in woods and wood sides where they be moist and shadowed, and in other places not too much open to the sun.

Time.—It flowereth in April and May.

Government and Virtues.—Venus owns it. Wood sorrel serveth to all the purposes that the other sorrels do, and is more effectual in hindering putrefaction of the blood, and ulcers in the mouth and body, and to quench thirst, to strengthen a weak stomach, to procure an appetite, to stay vomiting, and very excellent in any contagious fevers. The syrup made of the juice is effectual in all the cases aforesaid, and so is the distilled water of the herb. Sponges or linen cloths wet with the juice, and applied outwardly to any hot swelling or inflammation, doth much cool them.

The juice taken and gargled in the mouth repeatedly, doth wonderfully cure a stinking canker, or ulcers. It is first-rate to heal wounds, or to stay the bleeding of thrusts or stabs in any part of the body.

SOW THISTLE.

Sow Thistles are generally well known.

Place.—They grow in gardens and manured grounds, sometimes by old walls, path-sides of fields, and high-ways.

Government and Virtues.—This and the former are under the influence of Venus. Sow thistles are cooling and somewhat binding, and are very fit to cool a hot stomach and ease the pains thereof. The herb boiled in wine is very helpful to stay the decay of the stomach, and the milk that is taken from the stalks when they are broken, given in drink, is very beneficial to those that are short-winded, and have a wheezing. Pliny saith, that it hath caused the gravel and stone to be voided by urine, and that the eating thereof cures a stinking breath. The decoction of the leaves and stalks causeth abundance of milk in nurses, and their children to be well-coloured. The juice or distilled water is good for all inflammations, wheals, and eruptions or heat in the skin, and itching of the hæmorrhoids. The juice boiled or thorougly heated in a little oil of bitter almonds in the peel of a pomegranate, and dropped into the ears, is a sure remedy for deafness, singing, &c. Three spoonfuls of the juice taken warmed in white wine, and some wine put thereto, causeth women in travail to have so easy and speedy a delivery, that they may be able to walk presently after. It is wonderfully efficacious for women to wash their faces with, to clear the skin and give it lustre.

SOUTHERN WOOD.

Southern Wood needs no description.

Time.—It flowereth in July and August.

Government and Virtues.—It is a gallant Mercurial plant, worthy of more esteem than it hath. Dioscorides saith, that the seed bruised, heated in warm-water, and drunk, is good for plethora, or for the cramp or convulsions of the sinews, sciatica, or difficulty in making water, and bring-ing down women's courses. The same taken in wine is an antidote against all deadly poison, and driveth away serpents and other venomous creatures : also the smell of this herb being burnt doth the same. The oil thereof anointed on the back bone before the fits of the agues come, taketh them away ; it taketh away inflammations in the eyes, if it be put with some part of a roasted quince, and boiled with a few crumbs of bread, and applied. Boiled with barley-meal, it taketh away pimples, pushes, or wheals that arise in the face or other parts of the body. The seed as well as the dried herb is often given to kill worms in children. The herb bruised and laid to, helpeth to draw forth splinters and thorns out of the flesh. The ashes thereof drieth up and healeth old ulcers that are without inflammation, although by the sharpness thereof it putteth them to sore pains. The ashes mingled with old salad oil, restoreth the hair—and cures baldness. Darentes saith, the oil made of southern wood made into an oint-ment, is very effectual to kill lice in the head. The dis-tilled water of the herb is said to help them much that are troubled with the stone, as also for the diseases of the spleen and mother. The Germans commend it for a singu-lar wound-herb, and therefore call it stab-wort. It is held by all writers, ancient and modern, to be more offensive to the stomach than wormwood.

SPIGNEL.

Description.—The roots of common spignel spread much and deep in the ground, many strings or branches growing from one head, which is hairy at the top, of a blackish brown colour on the outside, and white within, smelling well, and of an aromatic taste, from whence arise sundry long stalks of most fine cut leaves like hair, smaller than dill, set thick on both sides of the stalks, and of a good scent. Among these leaves rise up round stiff stalks with a few joints and leaves on them, and at the tops an umbel of pure white flowers ; at the edges sometimes will be seen a show of the reddish bluish colour, especially before they be full blown, and are succeeded by small, round seeds, of a brown colour, divided into two parts, and crusted on the back, as most of the umbelliferous seeds are.

Place.—It groweth wild in Lancashire, Yorkshire, and other northern counties, and in gardens.

Government and Virtues.—It is an herb of Venus. Galen saith, the roots of spignel are available to provoke urine and women's courses; but if too much be taken, it causeth headache. The roots boiled in wine or water, and drunk, is good for strangury and stoppings of urine, the wind, swellings and pains in the stomach, pains of the mother, and all joint-aches. If the powder of the root be mixed with honey, and the same taken as an electuary, it breaketh tough phlegm, and drieth up the rheum that falleth on the lungs. The roots are very effectual against the stinging or biting of any venomous creature, and is one of the ingredients in Mithridate, and other antidotes of the same.

SPLEENWORT, or CETERACH.

Description.—The smooth spleenwort, from a black, thready, and bushy root, sendeth forth many long single leaves cut in on both sides into round dents almost to the middle, which is not so hard as that of polypody, each division being not always set opposite unto the other, but between each, smooth, and of a light green on the upper side, and a dark yellowish roughness on the back, folding or rolling itself inward at the first spring up.

Place.—It groweth as well upon stone walls as moist and shadowy places, about Bristol and other western parts plentifully; as also in Berkshire, Kent, and elsewhere, and abideth green all the winter.

Government and Virtues.—Saturn owns it. It is generally used against infirmities of the spleen; it is good for the strangury, and wasteth the stone in the bladder, and is good against the yellow jaundice and the hiccup. Matthiolus saith, that if a drachm of the dust, that is on the backsides of the leaves be mixed with half a drachm of amber in powder, and taken with the juice of purslain or plantain, it cures running of the reins speedily, and that the herb and roots being boiled and taken, cureth melancholy diseases. Camerarius saith, that the distilled water being drunk, is very effectual against the stone in the reins and bladder; and that the lye that is made of the ashes being drunk for some time, cureth splenetic persons. It is used in outward remedies for the same purpose.

STAR THISTLE.

Description.—A common star thistle hath divers narrow leaves lying next the ground, cut on the edges deeply into many parts, soft or a little woolly, all over green, among which rise up weak stalks parted into many branches, all lying down to the ground, that it seemeth a pretty bush, set with the like divided leaves up to the top, where severally do stand small whitish green heads set with sharp pricks which are yellowish; out of the middle whereof riseth the flowers, composed of many small reddish purple threads; and in the heads after the flowers are past, come small, whitish round seed, the root is small, long and woody, perishing every year, and rising again from its seed.

Place.—It grows on heaths, waste land, &c.

Time.—It flowereth early, and seedeth in July, sometimes in August.

Government and Virtues.—This, and almost all thistles, are under Mars. The seed of this star thistle made into powder, and drunk in wine, provoketh urine, and helpeth to break the stone and driveth it forth. The root in powder given in wine and drunk, is good against the plague and pestilence, and drunk in the morning fasting for some time, is very profitable for a fistula in any part of the body. Baptista Sardas doth much commend the distilled water, being drunk, to open obstructions of the liver, and cleanse the blood from corrupted humours, and is profitable against the quotidian or tertian ague.

STRAWBERRIES.

Time.—They flower in May ordinarily, and the fruit is ripe shortly after.

Government and Virtues.—Venus owns the herb. Strawberries, when they are green, are cool and dry, but when they are ripe, they are cool and moist: the berries are excellent to cool the liver, the blood, and the spleen, or an hot choleric stomach ; to refresh and comfort the fainting spirits, and quench thirst ; they are good also for other inflammations ; yet it is not amiss to refrain from them in a fever, lest by their putrifying in the stomach they increase the fits. The leaves and roots boiled in wine and water, and drunk, likewise cool the liver and blood, and assuage, all inflammations in the reins and bladder, provoke urine, and allay the heat and sharpness thereof. The same also being drunk, stayeth the bloody-flux, and women's courses, and reduces the swelling of the spleen. The water of the berries carefully distilled, is a sovereign remedy and cordial in the panting and beating of the heart, and is good for the yellow jaundice. The juice dropped into foul ulcers or washed therewith, or the decoction of the herb and root doth wonderfully cleanse and help to cure them. Lotions and gargles for sore mouths, or ulcers therein, or in the privy parts, are made with the leaves and roots, which is also good to fasten loose teeth, and to heal foul spongy gums. It helpeth to stay catarrhs, or defluctions of rheum in the mouth, throat, teeth, or eyes. The juice or water is very good for hot and red inflamed eyes, if dropped into them, or they be bathed therewith. It is also of excellent property for all pushes, wheals, and other breakings forth of hot and sharp humours in the face and hands, and other parts of the body, to bathe them therewith, and to take away any redness in the face, or spots in the face, or spots, or other deformities in the skin, and to make it clear and smooth. Some use this medicine :—Take so many strawberries as you shall think fitting, and put them into a distillatory, or body of glass fit for them, which being closed, set it in a bed of horse-dung for your use. It is an excellent water for inflamed eyes, and to take away a film or skin that beginneth to grow over them, and for such other defects in them, as may be remedied by any outward medicine.

SUCCORY.

Description.—The garden succory hath longer and narrower leaves than the endive, and more cut in or torn on the edges, and the root abideth many years. It beareth also blue flowers like endive, and the seed is hardly distinguished from the seed of the smooth, or ordinary endive.

The wild succory hath divers long leaves lying on the ground, very much cut in or torn on the edges, on both sides even to the middle rib, ending in a point ; sometimes it hath a rib down the middle of the leaves from among which riseth up a hard, round, woody stalk, spreading into many branches, set with smaller and lesser divided leaves on them up to the tops, where stand the flowers, which are like the garden kind, as the seed is also ; (only take notice that the flowers of the garden kind are gone in on a sunny day, they being so cold that they are not able to bear the beams of the sun, and therefore more delight in the shade,) the root is white, but more hard and woody than the garden kind. The whole plant is exceeding bitter.

Place.—This groweth in waste, untilled, and barren fields. The other in gardens.

Government and Virtues.—It is an herb of Jupiter. Garden succory, as it is more dry and less cold than endive, so it openeth more. A handful of the leaves or roots, boiled in wine or water, and a draught drunk fasting, driveth forth choleric and phlegmatic humours, openeth obstructions of the liver, gall and spleen ; cureth the yellow jaundice, the heat of the reins, and of the urine ; the dropsy also, and those that have an evil disposition in their bodies by reason of long sickness, evil diet, &c. which the Greeks call cachexy. A decoction made with wine, and drunk, is very effectual against lingering agues; and a drachm of the seed in powder drunk in wine, before the fit of the ague, helpeth to drive it away. The distilled water of the herb and flowers hath the like properties, and is especially good for hot stomachs, and also in agues of long continuance ; for swoonings and passions of the heart, for the heat and headache in children, and for the blood and liver. The said water, or the juice, or the bruised leaves applied outwardly, allay swellings, inflammation, St. Anthony's fire, pushes, wheals, and pimples, especially used with a little vinegar, as also to wash pestiferous sores.

The said water is very effectual for sore eyes that are inflamed with redness, and for nurses' breasts that are pained by the abundance of milk.

The wild succory, as it is more bitter, is more strengthening to the stomach and liver.

STONE-CROP, PRICK-MADAM, or SMALL HOUSE-LEEK.

Description.—It groweth with divers trailing branches upon the ground, set with many thick, flat, roundish, whitish green leaves, pointed at the ends. The flowers stand many of them together somewhat loosely. The roots are small, and run creeping under ground.

Place.—It groweth upon stone walls and mud walls, upon tiles of houses, and pent houses, and amongst rubbish and in other gravelly places.

Time.—It flowereth in June and July, and the leaves are green all the winter.

Government and Virtues.—It is under the dominion of the Moon, cold in quality, and something binding, and therefore very good to stay defluctions, especially such as fall upon the eyes. It stops bleeding both inward and outward, cures cancers and all fretting sores and ulcers. It abates the heat of choler, thereby preventing diseases arising from choleric humours. It expels poison, resisteth pestilential fevers, and is very good for tertian agues ; you may drink the decoction of it for all the foregoing infirmities. It is so harmless an herb, you can scarce use it amiss. Being bruised and applied to the place, it cures the king's evil, and any other knots or kernels in the flesh ; as also the piles.

ENGLISH TOBACCO.

Description.—This riseth up with a round thick stalk, about two feet high, whereon grow thick, flat, green leaves, somewhat round-pointed also, and not dented about the edges. The stalk branches forth, and beareth at the tops divers flowers set on great husks, like the other, but nothing so large : scarce standing above the brims of the husks, round-pointed also, and of a greenish yellow colour.

The seed that followeth is not so bright, but larger, contained in like great heads. The roots are neither so great nor so woody : it perisheth every winter, but riseth generally of its own sowing.

Place.—This came from some part of Brazil, as it is thought, and is more familiar in our country than any of the other sorts ; early giving ripe seed, which the others seldom do.

Time.—It flowereth from June sometimes to the end of August, and the seed ripeneth in the meantime.

Government and Virtues.—It is a martial plant. It is found by good experience to be available to expectorate tough phlegm from the stomach, chest and lungs. The juice thereof made into a syrup, or the distilled water of the herb drunk with some sugar, or the smoke taken by a pipe as is usual, helpeth to expel worms, and to ease the pains in the head, or megrim, and the griping pains in the bowels. It is profitable for those that are troubled with the stone in the kidneys, both to ease the pains by provoking urine, and also to expel gravel and the stone engendered therein, and hath been found very effectual to expel wind, and other humours, which cause the strangling of the mother. The seed is very effectual for tooth-ache, and the ashes of the burnt herb to cleanse the gums, and make the teeth white. The herb bruised and applied to the place affected with scrofula, cures it in nine or ten days. Monardus saith, it is a counter-poison against the biting of any venomous creature, the herb also being outwardly applied to the hurt place. The distilled water is given with some sugar before the fit of an ague, to lessen it and take it away by two or three times using. The distilled liquor is good to use in cramps, aches, gout and sciatica, and to heal itches, scabs, and running ulcers, cancers, and all foul sores. The juice is also good for all the said griefs, and to kill lice in children's heads. The green herb bruised and applied to any green wounds, cureth any fresh wound or cut whatsoever ; and the juice put into old sores, both cleanseth and healeth them. There is also made hereof a singular good salve to help imposthumes, hard tumours, and other swellings by blows and falls.

THE TAMARISK TREE.

IT is so well known in the places where it grows, that it needeth no description.

Time.—It flowereth about the end of May, or in June, and the seed is ripe and blown away in the beginning of September.

Government and Virtues.—A gallant Saturnine herb it is. The root, leaves, young branches, or bark boiled in wine, and drunk, stays the bleeding of the hæmorrhoidal veins, spitting of blood, the too abounding of women's courses, jaundice, colic, and the biting of all venomous serpents, except the asp; and outwardly applied, is very powerful against the hardness of the spleen, the tooth-ache, pains in the ears, and red and watering eyes. The decoction with honey is good to stop gangrenes and fretting ulcers, and to wash those that are subject to lice. Alpinus and Veslingus affirm that the Egyptians do with good success use the wood of it to cure the French disease, as others do with *lignum vitœ* or guiacum; and give it to those who have the leprosy, scabs, ulcers, or the like. Its ashes quickly heal blisters raised by burnings or scaldings. It helps the dropsy arising from the hardness of the spleen, and therefore to drink out of cups made of the wood is good for splenetic persons. It is also helpful for melancholy and the black jaundice that ariseth therefrom.

GARDEN TANSY.

GARDEN Tansy is so well known that it needeth no description.

Time.—It flowereth in June and July.

Government and Virtues.—Venus was minded to please women with child by this herb, for there grows not a herb fitter for their use than this is; it is just as though it were cut out for the purpose. This herb bruised and applied to the navel, stays miscarriages; I know no herb like it for that use: boiled in ordinary beer, and the decoction drunk, doth the like; and if her womb be not so as she would have it, this decoction will make it so. It consumes the phlegmatic humours, the cold and moist constitution, that winter most usually affects the body with, and that is the reason for eating tansies in spring. For want of eating this herb in spring, people are sickly in summer; and that makes work for the physician. Boil it in wine and drink the decoction—it will work the same effect. The decoction of the common tansy, or the juice drunk in wine, is a singular remedy for all the griefs that come by stopping of the urine, helpeth the strangury, and those that have weak reins and kidneys. It is also very profitable to expel wind from the stomach or bowels, to procure women's courses, and expel windiness in the matrix, if it be bruised and often smelled unto, as also applied to the lower part of the belly. It is also very profitable for such women as are given to miscarry in child bearing, to cause them to go out their full time; it is used also against the stone in the reins, especially in men. The herb fried with eggs (as it is the custom in spring-time) which is called a tansy, helpeth to digest and carry downwards those bad humours that trouble the stomach. The seed given to children destroys worms, and the juice in drink is as effectual. Being boiled in oil, it is good for the sinews shrunk by cramps, or pained with colds, if applied.

WILD TANSY, OR SILVER WEED.

This is an herb so well known, that it needeth no description.

Place.—It groweth almost in every place

Time.—It flowereth in June and July.

Government and Virtues.—It is under the government of Venus. Wild tansy stayeth the lask, and all fluxes of blood, which some say it will do, if the green herb be worn in the shoes, so it be next the skin; and it is true enough that it will stop the terms if worn so, and the whites too for aught I know; it stayeth also spitting or vomiting of blood. The powder of the herb taken in some of the distilled water, stayeth the whites, and especially if a little coral and ivory in powder be put to it. It is also commended to help children that have a rupture, being boiled in water and salt; it easeth the griping pains of the bowels, and is good for sciatica and joint aches. The same boiled in vinegar, with honey and alum, and gargled in the mouth, easeth the tooth-ache, fasteneth loose teeth, healeth the gums that are sore, and settleth the palate of the mouth in its place when it is fallen down. It cleanseth and healeth ulcers in the mouth or secret parts, and is very good for inward wounds, and to close the lips of green wounds, and to heal corrupt running sores in the legs or elsewhere. Being bruised and applied to the soles of the feet and hand wrists, it wonderfully cooleth the hot fits of the agues, be they ever so violent. The distilled water cleanseth the skin from all discolourings therein, as morphew, sun-burnings, &c., as also pimples, freckles, and the like, and dropped into the eyes, or cloths wet therein and applied taketh away the heat and inflammations in them.

THISTLES.

Of these there are many kinds growing here in England, which are so well known that they need no description. Their difference is easily known by the places where they grow, viz.,

Place.—Some grow in fields, some in meadows, and some among the corn; others on heaths, greens, and waste grounds in many places.

Time.—They flower in July and August, and their seed is ripe quickly after.

Government and Virtues.—Mars rules it, it is such a prickly business. All these thistles are good to provoke urine, and to mend the stinking smell thereof; as also to mend the rank smell of the arm-pits, or the whole body; being boiled in wine and drunk, they are said to cure a stinking breath, and to strengthen the stomach. Pliny saith, that the juice bathed on the place will cause the hair to grow.

THE MELANCHOLY THISTLE.

Description.—It riseth up with tender, single, hoary, green stalks, bearing thereon four or five green leaves, dented about the edges; the points thereof are little or nothing prickly, and at the top one head, yet sometimes from the bosom of the uppermost leaves there shooteth forth another small head, scaly and prickly, with many reddish thrums or threads in the middle, which being gathered fresh, will keep the colour, and fade not from the stalk for a long time, while it perfects the seed, which is of a mean size, lying in the down. The root hath many strings fastened to the head, which is blackish, and perisheth not.

There is another sort little differing from the former, but that the leaves are more green above, and more hoary underneath, and the stalk, being two feet high, beareth but one scaly head, with threads and seeds as the former.

Place.—They grow in moist meadows.

Time.—They flower about July or August, and their seed ripeneth shortly after.

Government and Virtues.—It is under Capricorn, and therefore under both Saturn and Mars; one rids melancholy by sympathy, and the other by antipathy. Their virtues are but few, but those not to be despised : for the decoction of the thistle in wine being drunk, expels superfluous melancholy out of the body, and makes a man as merry as a cricket ; for melancholy is sure to produce care, fear, sadness, despair, envy, &c., but religion teaches us to wait upon God's providence, and cast our care upon him that careth for us. What a fine thing were it if men and women could live so ! and yet seven years' care and fear makes a man never the wiser, nor a farthing richer. Dioscorides saith, the root borne about one doth the like, and removes all diseases of melancholy. Modern writers laugh at him ; *Let them laugh that win ;* my opinion is, that it is the best remedy against all melancholy diseases that grows.

OUR LADY'S THISTLE.

Description.—Our lady's thistle hath divers very large and broad leaves lying on the ground, cut in and dented on the edges, of a white green shining colour, wherein are many lines and streaks of a milk-white colour running all over and set with many hard and stiff prickles all about, among which riseth up one or more strong, round, and prickly stalks, set full of the like leaves up to the top, where at the end of every branch comes forth a great prickly thistle-like head, strongly armed with prickles, and with bright purple thrums rising out of the middle. After they are past, the seed groweth in the said heads lying in soft white down, which is somewhat in the ground, and many strings and fibres fastened thereunto. All the plant is bitter in taste.

Place.—It is frequent on the banks of almost every ditch.

Time.—It flowereth and seedeth in June, July, and August.

Government and Virtues.—Our lady's thistle is under Jupiter, and thought to be as effectual as carduus benedictus for agues, and to prevent and cure the infection of the plague; as also to open obstructions of the liver and spleen, and thereby is good against the jaundice. It provoketh urine, breaketh and expelleth the stone, and is good for the dropsy. It is effectual also for pains in the sides, and many other inward pains and gripings. The seed and distilled water are held powerful for all the purposes aforesaid, and besides, it is often applied outwardly with cloths or sponges, to the region of the liver, to cool the distemper thereof, and to the region of the heart, against swoonings and passions of it. It cleanseth the blood exceedingly; and in spring, if you please to boil the tender plant (but cut off the prickles) it will change your blood as the season changeth, and that is the way to be safe.

THE WOOLLEN, OR COTTON THISTLE.

Description.—This hath many large leaves lying upon the ground, somewhat cut in and as it were crumpled on the edges, of a green colour on the upper side, but covered over with a long hairy wool or cotton down, set with very sharp pricks; from the middle of whose heads of flowers come forth many purplish crimson threads, and sometimes white. The seed that followeth in those white downy heads is somewhat large and round, resembling the seed of lady thistle, but paler. The root is great and thick, spreading much, yet usually dieth after seed-time.

Place.—It groweth on ditch banks, in corn fields, and highways, and in gardens.

Government and Virtues.—It is a plant of Mars. Dioscorides and Pliny write, that the leaves and roots taken in drink, help those that have a crick in their neck, that they cannot turn it, unless they turn their whole body. Galen saith, that the roots and leaves are good for such as have their bodies drawn together by some spasm or convulsion, or other infirmities ; as the rickets in children, being a disease that hindereth their growth by binding their nerves, ligaments, and whole structure of their body.

THE FULLER'S THISTLE, OR TEAZLE.

IT needs no description.

The wild teazle is like the former, but that the prickles are small, soft, and upright, not hooked or stiff, and the flowers of this are of a fine bluish, or pale carnation colour, but that of the manured kind, whitish.

Place.—The first groweth, being sown in gardens or fields for the use of cloth-workers : the other near ditches and rills of water.

Time.—They flower in July, and are ripe in the end of August.

Government and Virtues.—It is an herb of Venus. Dioscorides saith that the roots bruised and boiled in wine till thick, and kept in a brazen vessel, and after spread as a salve and applied to the fundament, doth heal the cleft thereof, cankers and fistulas therein, also taketh away warts and wens. The juice of the leaves dropped into the ears, killeth worms. The distilled water of the leaves dropped into the eyes, taketh away redness and mists that hinder the sight, and is often used by women to preserve their beauty, and to take away redness and inflammations, and other heats and discolourings.

TREACLE MUSTARD.

Description.—It riseth with a hard round stalk about a foot high, parted into some branches, having soft green leaves long and narrow, set thereon, waved, but not cut into the edges, broadest towards the ends, somewhat round pointed ; the flowers are white that grow at the tops of the branches, spike fashion, one above another ; after

which come round pouches parted in the middle with a
furrow, having one blackish brown seed on either side,
somewhat sharp in taste, and smelling of garlic, especially
in the fields where it is natural, but not much in gardens.
The roots are small and thready, perishing every year.
[*Government and Virtues* afterwards.] *Akin to this is*
MITHRIDATE MUSTARD.

Description. — This groweth higher than the former,
spreading more and higher branches, whose leaves are
smaller and narrower, sometimes unevenly dented about
the edges. The flowers are small and white, growing on
long branches, with much smaller and rounder vessels
after them, and are parted in the same manner, having
smaller brown seeds than the former, and sharper in taste.
The root perisheth after seed-time, but abideth the first
winter after springing.

Place.—They grow in many places by river sides, under
hedges.

Time.—They flower and seed from May to August.

Government and Virtues.—Both are herbs of Mars. The
mustards are said to purge the body both upwards and
downwards, and taken in *moderation*, they promote
menstruation. It breaketh inward imposthumes, being
taken inwardly ; and used in clysters cureth sciatica.
The seed applied doth the same. It is an especial ingredient unto mithridate and treacle, being of itself an antidote, resisting poison, venom, and putrefaction. It is
available in many cases for which the common mustard is
used, but somewhat weaker.

THE BLACK THORN, OR SLOE-BUSH.

IT is so well known, that it needeth no description.

Place.—It groweth in every county, in the hedges and
borders of fields.

Time.—It flowereth in April, and sometimes in March,
but the fruit ripeneth after all other plums, and is not fit
to be eaten until the autumn frosts mellow them.

Government and Virtues.—All the parts of the sloe-bush
are binding, cooling, and dry, and all affectual to stay
bleeding at the nose and mouth, or any other part ; the

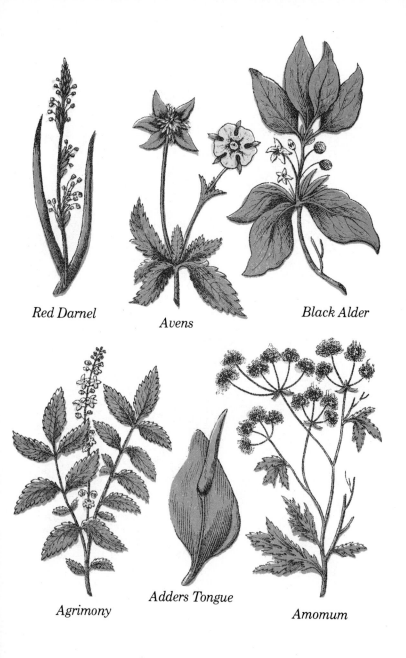

Red Darnel

Avens

Black Alder

Agrimony

Adders Tongue

Amomum

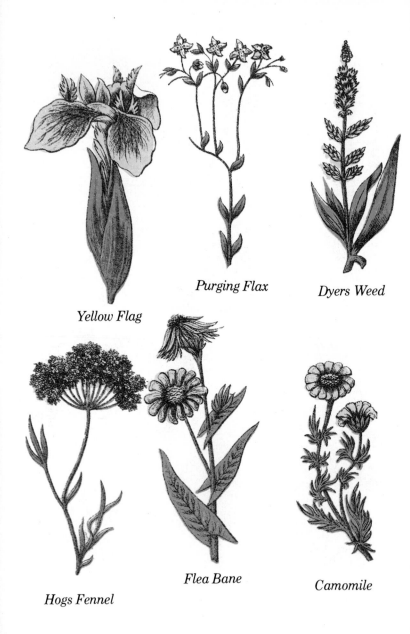

Purging Flax

Dyers Weed

Yellow Flag

Flea Bane

Camomile

Hogs Fennel

lask of the belly or stomach, or bloody flux ; profuse
menstruation, easeth pains in the bowels, and sides, that
come by overmuch scouring, to drink the decoction of the
bark of the roots, or more usually the decoction of the
berries, either fresh or dried. The conserve also is of very
much use, and more familiarly taken for the purpose aforesaid. But the distilled water of the flowers first steeped
in sack for a night, and drawn therefrom, by the heat of
the Balneum Anglico, a bath is a most certain remedy,
tried and approved, to ease all manner of gnawings in the
stomach, the sides and bowels, or any griping pains in any
of them. The leaves are good to make lotions to gargle
the mouth and throat, wherein are swelling sores, or
kernels ; to stay the defluction of rheum to the eyes, or
other parts ; and to cool the heat and inflammations of
them, and ease hot pains of the head, to bathe the forehead
and temples therewith. The simple distilled water of the
flowers is very effectual for the said purposes, and also
the condensed juice of the sloes. The distilled water of
the green berries is used also for the said effects.

THOROUGH WAX, or THOROUGH LEAP.

Description.—Common thorough wax has a straight round
stalk two feet high, whose lower leaves being of a bluish
colour, are smaller and narrower than those up higher, and
stand close thereto, not compassing it ; but as they grow
higher they do more encompass the stalks, until it wholly
passes through them, branching towards the top into many
parts, where the leaves grow smaller again, every one
standing singly, and never two at a joint.   The flowers
are small and yellow, standing in tufts at the heads of the
branches ; the seed is blackish, many thickly thrust
together. The root is small, long, and woody, perishing
every year, after seed-time, and rising again plentifully of
its own sowing.

Place.—It is found growing in many corn-fields and
pasture grounds in this land.

Time.—It flowereth in July, and the seed is ripe in
August.

Government and Virtues.—Both this and the former are

S

under Saturn. Thorough wax is good for all sorts of
bruises and wounds either inward or outward ; and old
ulcers and sores if the decoction of the herb with water
and wine be drunk, and the place washed therewith, or
the juice of the green herb bruised or boiled, either by
itself or with other herbs, in oil or hog's lard, to be made
into an ointment to serve all the year.   The decoction of
the herb, or powder of the dried herb taken inwardly, and
the same or the leaves bruised and applied outwardly, is
very good for ruptures, especially in children before they
are too old.   It being applied with a little flour and wax
to children's navels that stick out, it reduces them.

THYME.

THIS herb is well known.

Government and Virtues.—It is a noble strengthener of
the lungs, as notable a one as grows : nor is there a better
remedy growing for hooping-cough.   It purgeth the body
of phlegm, and is an excellent remedy for shortness of
breath.   It kills worms and being a notable herb of Venus
provokes the terms, and gives safe and speedy delivery to
women in travail.   It is so harmless you need not fear the
use of it.   An ointment made of it takes away hot swellings, warts, sciatica and dulness of sight, and takes away
pains and hardness of the spleen.   'Tis excellent for those
that are troubled with the gout ; as also to anoint swollen
testicles.   It easeth pains in the loins and hips.   The herb
taken any way inwardly comforts the stomach, and expels
wind.

WILD THYME, OR MOTHER-OF-THYME.

WILD THYME also is so well known that it needeth no
description.

Place.—It may be found commonly on commons, and
other barren places throughout this nation.

Government and Virtues.—It is under the dominion of
Venus, and under the sign Aries, and therefore chiefly appropriated to the head.   It provoketh urine and the terms
and easeth griping pains, cramps, ruptures, and inflammation of the liver.   If you make a vinegar of the herb, as

vinegar of roses is made, and anoint the head with it, it presently stops the pains thereof. It is very good to be given either in phrenzy or lethargy, although they are two contrary diseases. It relieves spitting and voiding of blood, coughing, and vomiting; it comforts and strengthens the head, stomach, reins, and womb; expels wind, and breaks the stone.

TORMENTIL, OR SEPTFOIL.

Description.—This hath reddish, slender, weak branches rising from the root, lying on the ground, rather leaning than standing upright, with many short leaves that stand closer to the stalks than cinque-foil (to which this is very like) with the foot-stalk compassing the branches in several places; but those that grow to the ground are set upon long foot-stalks, each whereof are like the leaves of cinquefoil, but somewhat longer, and less dented about the edges, many of them divided but into five leaves, but most of them into seven, whence it is called septfoil: yet some may have six and some eight, according to the fertility of the soil. At the tops of the branches stand small yellow flowers consisting of five leaves, like those of cinque foil, but smaller. The root is smaller than bistort, rather thick, but blacker without and not so red within, yet sometimes a little crooked, having blackish fibres thereat.

Place.—It groweth in woods and shadowy places, in the open country, about the borders of fields in many places of this land, and in every broom-field.

Time.—It flowereth all the summer long.

Government and Virtues.—This is a gallant herb of the Sun. Tormentil is most excellent to stay all fluxes of blood or humours, whether at nose, mouth or belly. The juice of the herb and root, or the decoction thereof, taken with some Venice treacle, and the person laid to sweat, expels any venom or poison, or the plague, fever, or other contagious diseases, as the pox, measles, &c. for it is an ingredient in all antidotes or counter-poisons. Andreas Valesus is of opinion, that the decoction of this root is no less effectual than guiacum or China: and it is not unlikely, because it resisteth putrefaction. The root taken inwardly is most effectual to help any flux of the belly, stomach, spleen or blood ; and the juice wonderfully opens obstructions of the spleen and lungs, and cureth yellow jaundice. The powder or decoction drunk, or to sit thereon as a bath, is an assured remedy against abortion, if it proceed from the over-flexibility or weakness of the inward retentive faculty ; as also a plaster made therewith and vinegar applied to the reins of the back, doth much help not only this, but also those that cannot hold their water, the powder being taken in the juice of plantain, and is commended against worms in children. It is very powerful in ruptures as also for bruises and falls, to be used as well outwardly as inwardly. The root hereof made up with pellitory of Spain and alum, and put into a hollow tooth, not only assuageth the pain, but stayeth the flux of humours which causeth it. Tormentil is no less effectual and powerful a remedy against outward wounds, sores and hurts, than for inward, and is therefore a special ingredient to be used in wound drinks, lotion, and injections, for corrupt sores and ulcers of the mouth, or other parts of the body. The juice or powder of the roots put in ointments, plasters, and such things that are applied to wounds or sores, is very effectual, as the juice of the leaves and the root bruised and applied to the throat or jaws, healeth the king's evil, and easeth the pains of sciatica ; the same used with a little vinegar is a special remedy for running sores of the head or other parts ; scabs also and the itch, or any such eruptions in the skin, proceeding of salt and sharp humours. It is also effectual for the piles, if they be washed or bathed therewith, or with the distilled water of the herbs and roots. It is found also helpful to dry up any sharp rheum that distilleth from the head into the eyes, causing redness, pain, waterings, itching, or the like, if a little prepared tutty, or white amber, be used with the distilled water thereof. It restrains the whites and reds, both to drink it, or inject it with a syringe.

TURNSOLE, OR HELIOTROPIUM.

Description.— The greater turnsole riseth with one upright stalk about a foot high or more, dividing itself almost from the bottom into divers small branches of a hoary colour; at each joint of the stalk and branches grow small broad leaves, somewhat white and hoary. At the tops of the stalks and branches stand small white flowers consisting of four, and sometimes of five leaves, set in order one above another, upon a small crooked spike, which turneth inwards like a bowed finger, opening by degrees as the flowers blow open; after which in their place come forth cornered seed, four for the most part standing together: the root is small and thready, perishing every year, and the seed shedding every year, raiseth it again the next spring.

Place.—It groweth in gardens, and flowereth and seedeth with us, it is a foreign plant, in Spain and France, it grows plentifully.

Government and Virtues.—It is an herb of the Sun, and a good one too. Dioscorides saith, that a good handful of that which is called the great turnsole, boiled in water and drunk, purgeth both choler and phlegm; and boiled with cummin, cureth the stone in the reins, kidneys, or bladder, provoketh urine and women's courses, and causeth an easy and speedy delivery in child-birth. The leaves bruised and applied to places pained with the gout, or that have been out of joint and newly set, and full of pain, give much ease; the seed and juice of the leaves also being rubbed with a little salt upon warts or wens, and other kernels in the face, or eye-lids, or in any part of the body, will by often using, take them away.

MEADOW TREFOIL, or HONEYSUCKLES.

It is well known, especially by the name of honey-suckles, white and red.

Place.—They grow almost every where in this land.

Government and Virtues.—Mercury hath the dominion over the common sorts. Dodoneds saith, the leaves and flowers are good to ease the griping pains of the gout, the herb being boiled and used in a clyster. If the herb be made into a poultice, and applied to inflammations, it will ease them. The juice dropped into the eyes, is a familiar medicine with many country people to take away the pin and web, as they call it, in the eyes ; it also allayeth the heat and bloodshooting of them. Country people in many parts drink the juice against the biting of an adder ; and having boiled the herb in water, they first wash the place with the decoction, and then lay some of the herb also to the hurt place. The herb also boiled in hog's lard, and so made into an ointment, is good to apply to the biting of any venomous creature. The herb also bruised and heated between tiles, and applied to the share, causeth them to make water who had it stopped before. It is held to be good for wounds. The decoction of the herb and flowers, with the seed and root taken for some time, restraineth the whites. The seed and flowers boiled in water, and after made into a poultice with some oil, and applied, helpeth hard swellings and imposthumes.

HEART TREFOIL.

BESIDES the ordinary sort of trefoil, here are two more remarkable, and one of which may be probably called heart trefoil, not only because the leaf is triangular, like the heart of man, but because each leaf contains the perfect icon of a heart, and that in its proper colours, viz. a flesh colour.

Place.—It groweth in Kent, Essex, and in the marshes near the sea.

Government and Virtues.—It is under the dominion of the Sun, and if it were used it would be found as great a strengthener of the heart, and cherisher of the vital spirits as any that grows ; relieving the body against faintings and swoonings, fortifying it against poison and pestilence, and defending the heart against the noisome vapours of the spleen.

PEARL TREFOIL.

IT differs not from the common sort, save only in this one particular, it hath a white spot on the leaf like a pearl. It is particularly under the dominion of the Moon, and its icon showeth that it is of singular virtue against the pearl, or pin and web in the eyes.

TUTSAN, OR PARK LEAVES.

Description.—It hath brownish, shining, round stalks, crested the length thereof, rising two, and sometimes three feet high, branching forth from the bottom, having divers joints, and at each of them two fair large leaves standing, of a dark bluish green colour on the upper side, and of a yellowish green underneath, turning reddish towards autumn. At the top of the stalks stand large yellow flowers, and heads with seed, which, being greenish at the first, and then reddish, turn a blackish purple colour when they are ripe, with small brownish seed within them ; they yield a reddish juice or liquor somewhat resinous, of a harsh styptic taste, like the leaves and flowers, although much less, but do not yield such a clear claret wine colour as some say it doth. The root is brownish, somewhat great, hard, and woody, spreading well in the ground.

Place.—It groweth in many woods, groves, and woody grounds, as parks and forests, and by hedge sides, in many places of this land.

Time.—It flowereth later than St. John's or St. Peter's-wort.

Government and Virtues.—It is an herb of Saturn, and a most noble antivenereal. Tutsan purgeth choleric humours, as St. Peter's-wort is said to do, for therein it worketh the same effects, both to cure sciatica and gout, and to heal burnings by fire ; it stayeth all the bleedings of wounds, if either the green herb be bruised or the powder of the dry be applied thereto. It hath been accounted, and certainly it is, a sovereign herb to heal either wounds or sores, outwardly or inwardly, and therefore always used in drinks, lotions, balms, ointments, or any other sorts of green wounds, old ulcers, or sores, in all which the continual experience of former ages hath confirmed the use thereof to be wonderfully good, though it is not so much in use now as when physicians and surgeons were so wise as to use herbs more than they now do.

GARDEN VALERIAN.

Description.—This hath a thick, short, greyish root, lying above ground, shooting forth on all other sides small pieces of roots, which have all of them many long fibres under them in the ground, whereby it draweth nourishment. From the head of these roots spring up many green leaves, which at first are rather broad and long, without any division in them, or dented on the edges; but those that rise up after are more divided on each side, some to the middle rib, being winged, made of many leaves together on a stalk, and those upon a stalk more divided, but smaller towards the top than below; the stalk riseth to be a yard high, sometimes branched at the top, with many small whitish flowers, sometimes dashed over at the edges with a pale purplish colour, which passing away, is followed by small brownish white seed, that is easily carried away with the wind. The root smelleth more strong than either leaf or flower, and is of more use in medicines.

Place.—It is generally kept with us in gardens.

Time.—It flowereth in June and July, and continueth flowering until the frost pulls it down.

Government and Virtues.—This is under the influence of Mercury. Dioscorides saith, that the garden valerian hath a warming faculty, and that being dried and given to drink, it provoketh urine, and cureth strangury. The decoction taken doth the like also, and taketh away pains of the sides, provoketh the courses, and is used in antidotes. Pliny saith, that the powder of the root given in drink, or the decoction taken, benefits all stoppings and strangling in any part of the body, whether they proceed from pains in the chest or sides, and taketh them away. The root of valerian boiled with liquorice, raisins, and aniseed, is very good for those that are short-winded, and have a cough, and causeth them to expectorate tough phlegm easily. It is given to those that are bitten or stung by any venomou creature, being boiled in wine. It is a special remedy against the plague, the decoction being drunk, and the root being used to smell of. It wonderfully expels wind. The green herb with the root taken fresh, being bruised and applied to the head, taketh away pains and prickings, stayeth rheum and thin distillations, and being boiled in white wine, and a drop thereof put into the eyes, taketh away dimness of sight or pin and web. It is of excellent property to heal inward sores or wounds, and also for out-ward hurts or wounds, and drawing away splinters or thorns out of the flesh.

VERVAIN.

Description.—The common vervain hath rather long, broad leaves next the ground, deeply gashed about the edges, and some only deeply dented, or cut all alike, of a blackish green colour on the upper side, somewhat greyish under. The stalk is square, branched into several parts, rising about two feet high, especially if you reckon the long spike of flowers at the tops of them, which are set on all sides one above another, and sometimes two or three together, being small and gaping, of a blue colour and white intermixed; after which come small round seed, in small long heads. The root is small and long, but of no use.

Place.—It groweth generally underneath hedges and by way-sides, and on waste grounds.

Time.—It flowereth in July, and the seed is ripe shortly after.

Government and Virtues.—This is an herb of Venus, and is first-rate to strengthen and remedy all the cold griefs of the womb, as plantain doth the hot. Vervain is hot and dry, opening obstructions, cleansing and healing. It cur-eth yellow jaundice, dropsy, and gout; it killeth worms, and causeth a good colour in the face and body, strength-eneth and correcteth the diseases of the stomach, liver, and spleen; allays cough, wheezings, and shortness of breath, and the defects of the reins and bladder, expelling gravel and stone. It is held to be good against the plague, and both tertian and quartan agues. It healeth all wounds both inward and outward, stayeth bleedings, and used with honey, healeth ulcers, and fistulas in the legs or other parts of the body; as also those ulcers that happen in the mouth; or used with lard, it allayeth swellings and pains of the secret parts; it is valuable for the piles; applied with some oil of roses and vinegar to the forehead and temples, it easeth the inveterate aches of the head, and is good for those that are frantic. The leaves bruised, or the juice of them mixed with some vinegar, doth wonderfully cleanse the skin, and taketh away morphews, freckles, fistulas, and other such like inflammations and deformities of the skin in any part of the body. The distilled water of the herb when it is in full strength dropped into the eyes, cleanseth them from films, clouds, or mists that darken the sight, and wonderfully strengthens the optic nerves; the said water is very powerful in all the diseases aforesaid, either inward or outward, whether they be old sores or green wounds.

THE VINE.

THE leaves of the English vine being boiled, make a good lotion for sore mouths; being boiled with barley meal into a poultice, it cools inflammations of wounds; the dropping of the vine when it is cut in the spring, which country people call tears, being boiled in a syrup with sugar and taken inwardly, is excellent to stay pregnant women's longings after every thing they see. The decoction of vine leaves in white wine doth the like; also the tears of the vine drunk two or three spoonfuls at a time, breaks the stone in the bladder. This is a very good remedy, and it is discreetly done to kill a vine to cure a man, but the salt of the leaves is held to be better. The ashes of the burnt branches will make teeth that are as black as a coal to be as white as snow, if you but every morning rub them with it. It is a gallant tree of the Sun, very sympathetic with the body of man, and that is the reason spirits of wine is the greatest cordial of any obtained from vegetables.

VIOLETS.

BOTH the garden and wild are so well known that they need uo description.

Time.—They flower until the end of July, but are best in March and the beginning of April.

Government and Virtues.—They are a fine pleasing plant of Venus, of a mild nature, no way hurtful. All the violets are cold and moist while they are fresh and green, and are used to cool any heat of the body, either inwardly or outwardly, as inflammations in the eyes, in the matrix or fundament, in imposthumes also and hot swellings, to drink the decoction of the leaves and flowers made with water and wine, or to apply them poultice-wise to the grieved places : it likewise easeth pains in the head caused through want of sleep ; or any other pains arising of heat, applied in the same manner, or with oil of roses. A drachm weight of the dried leaves or flowers of violets, but the leaves more strongly, doth purge the body of choleric humours, and assuageth the heat, being taken in a draught of wine or any other drink ; the powder of the purple leaves of the flowers only picked and dried and drunk in water, is said to cure the quinsy and the falling sickness, especially in the beginning of the disease. The flowers of the white violets ripen and dissolve swellings. The herb or flowers while they are fresh, or the flowers when dry, are effectual in the pleurisy, and all diseases of the lungs, to lenify the sharpness of hot rheums, and the hoarseness of the throat, the heat and sharpness of urine, and all the pains of the back, or reins and bladder. It is good also for the liver and jaundice, and all hot agues, to cool the liver and quench the thirst ; but the syrup of violets is of most use and of better effect, being taken in some convenient liquor ; and if a little of the juice or syrup of lemons be put to it, or a few drops of acetic acid, it is made the more powerful to cool the heat and quench the thirst, and it giveth to the drink a claret wine colour, and a fine tart relish, pleasing the taste. Violets taken or made up with honey, do more cleanse and cool, and with sugar, contrary-wise. The dried flowers of violets are accounted among the cordial drinks, powders and other medicines, especially where cooling cordials are necessary. The green leaves are used with other herbs to make plasters and poultices for inflammations and swellings, and to ease all pains whatsoever, arising of heat, and for the piles also, being fried with yolks of eggs and applied thereto.

VIPER'S BUGLOSS.

Description.—This hath many long rough leaves lying on the ground, from among which rise hard round stalks, very rough, as if they were thick set with prickles or hairs, whereon are set such like rough, hairy, or prickly sad green leaves, rather narrow ; the middle rib being for the most part white. The flowers stand at the top of the stalk branched forth in many long spiked leaves of flowers, bowing or turning like the turnsole, all opening or turning for the most part on the one side, which are long and hollow, turning up the brims a little, of a purplish violet colour in them that are fully blown, but more reddish while they are in the bud, as also upon their withering ; but in some places of a paler purple colour, with a long pointel in the middle, feathered or parted at the top. The seeds growing to be ripe are blackish, cornered and pointed somewhat like the head of a viper. The root is great and blackish, and woolly when it groweth towards seed-time, and perisheth in the winter. There is another sort differing from the former only in this, it beareth white flowers.

Place.—The first groweth wild almost every where. That with the white flowers about the walls of ruins.

Time.—They flower in summer, and their seed is ripe quickly after.

Government and Virtues.—It is a most gallant herb of the Sun ; it is a pity it is no more in use than it is. It is an especial remedy against the biting of the viper, and all other venomous beasts ; and against poison or poisonous herbs. Dioscorides and others say, that whosoever shall take of the herb or root before they be bitten, shall not be hurt by the poison of any serpent. The root or seed is effectual to comfort the heart, and to expel melancholy ; it tempers the blood, and allayeth hot fits of agues. The seed drunk in wine, procureth abundance of milk in women's breasts. The same also being taken, easeth pains in the loins, back and kidneys. The distilled water of the herb, when it is in flower, or its chief strength, is excellent to be applied inwardly or outwardly for all the purposes aforesaid. There is a syrup made hereof very effectual for comforting the heart, and banishing melancholy.

WALL-FLOWERS, OR WINTER GILLIFLOWERS.

Description.—The common single wall-flowers, which grow wild abroad, have sundry small, long, narrow, dark green leaves, set without order upon small, round, whitish woody stalks, which bear at the top single yellow flowers one above another, bearing four leaves a-piece, and of a very sweet scent; after which come long pods containing a reddish seed. The roots are white, hard, and thready.

Place.—It groweth upon church walls and old walls of many houses, and other stone walls. The other sort in gardens only.

Time.—All the single kinds flower many times in the end of autumn; and if the winter be mild, all the winter long, but especially in the months of February, March, and April, until the heat of the spring do spend them.

Government and Virtues.—The Moon rules them. Galen in his book of simple medicines saith, that the yellow wall-flowers work more powerfully than any of the other kinds, and are of more use in physic. It cleanseth the blood, and freeth the liver and reins from obstructions, provoketh women's courses, and is good for the spleen; it stayeth inflammations and swellings, strengtheneth any weak part, or out of joint; cleanseth the eyes from mistiness or films upon them, and it cleanseth filthy ulcers in the mouth, or any other part, and is a remedy for the gout, and all aches and pains in the joints and sinews. A conserve made of the flowers, is used as a remedy both for the apoplexy and palsy.

THE WALNUT-TREE.

Time.—It blossometh early before the leaves come forth, and the fruit is ripe in September.

Government and Virtues.—This is also a plant of the Sun. Let the fruit of it be gathered accordingly, which you shall find to be of most virtue while they are green, before they have shells. The bark of the tree doth bind and dry very much, and the leaves are much of the same temperature; but the leaves when they are older, are heating and drying in the second degree, and harder of digestion than when they are fresh, which, by reason of their sweetness are more pleasing and better digested in the stomach; and taken with sweet wine, they move the belly downwards, but being old, they grieve the stomach : and in hot bodies cause the choler to abound, and the head-ache, and are an enemy to those that have a cough ; but they are less hurtful to those that have a colder stomach, and are said to kill broad worms. If they be taken with onions, salt, and honey, they cure the biting of a mad dog, or the venom or infectious poison of any beast, &c.

Caias Pompeius found in the treasury of Mithridates, king of Pontus, when he was overthrown, a scroll of his own hand-writing, containing a medicine against poison or infection, which is this :—Take two dry walnuts and as many good figs, and twenty leaves of rue, bruised and beaten together with two or three corns of salt, and twenty juniper berries, which taken every morning, fasting, preserveth from danger of poison and infection that day it is taken. The juice of the other green husk boiled with honey, is an excellent gargle for a sore mouth, or the heat and inflammations in the throat and stomach. The kernels, when they grow old, are more oily, and therefore not fit to be eaten, but are then used to heal the wounds of the sinews, gangrenes, and carbuncles. The said kernels being burned, are then very astringent, and will stay lasks and women's courses, being taken in wine ; and stay the falling of the hair, and make it fair, being anointed with oil and wine. The green husks will do the like being used in the same manner. The kernels beaten with rue and wine, being applied, helpeth the quinsy ; and bruised with rue and wine, and applied to the ears, easeth the pains and inflammations of them. A piece of the green husk put into a hollow tooth easeth pain. The oil that is pressed out of the kernels, is very profitable taken inwardly like oil of almonds, to help the colic and to expel wind very effectually ; an ounce or two thereof may be taken at any time. The young green nuts taken before they be half ripe and preserved with sugar, are of good use to those that have weak stomachs, or defluctions thereon. The distilled water of the green husks before they be half ripe, is of excellent use to cool the heat of agues, being drunk an ounce or two at a time ; as also to resist the infection of the plague, if some of the same be also applied to the sores thereof. The same also cooleth the heat of green wounds and old ulcers, and healeth them, being bathed therewith. The distilled water of the green husks being ripe, when they are shelled from the nuts, and drunk with a little vinegar, is good for the plague, so as before the taking thereof a vein is opened. The said water is very good against the quinsy, being gargled and bathed, and wonderfully relieves deafness and noise, and other pains in the ears. The distilled water of the young green leaves in the end of May, performeth a singular cure on running ulcers and sores, to be bathed with wet clothes or sponges applied to them every morning.

WELD, WOLD, or DYER'S WEED.

THE common kind groweth bushing with many leaves, long, narrow, and flat upon the ground, of a dark bluish green colour, somewhat like woad, but not so large, a little crumpled and round-pointed, which do so abide the first year ; and the next spring, from among them rise up divers round stalks two or three feet high, beset with many such like leaves thereon, but smaller and shooting forth small branches, which with the stalks carry many small yellow flowers in a long spiked head at the top of them : where afterwards come the seed, which is small and black, inclosed in heads that are divided at the tops into four parts. The root is long, white, and thick, abiding the winter. The herb changeth to be yellow after it hath been in flower awhile.

Place.—It groweth every where by the way-sides, in moist grounds as well as dry, in corners of fields and bye-lanes, and sometimes all over the field.

Time.—It flowereth about June.

Government and Virtues.—Matthiolus saith, that the root hereof cureth tough phlegm, digesteth raw phlegm, thinneth gross humours, dissolveth hard tumours, and openeth obstructions. Some highly commend it against the biting of venomous creatures, to be taken inwardly and applied outwardly to the place ; as also for the plague or pestilence. Some persons bruise the herb, and lay it to cuts or wounds to heal them.

WHEAT.

Government and Virtues.—It is under Venus. Dioscorides saith, that to eat the corns of green wheat is hurtful to the stomach, and breedeth worms. Pliny saith that the corns of wheat roasted in an iron pan and eaten, are a present remedy for those that are chilled with cold. The oil pressed from wheat between two thick plates of iron or copper heated, healeth tetters or ringworms being used warm ; and by it Galen saith he hath known many to be cured. Matthiolus commendeth the same to be put into hollow ulcers to heal them, and it is good for chops in the hands or feet, and to make rugged skin smooth. The green corns of wheat being chewed and applied to the place bitten by a mad dog, heal it : slices of wheat bread soaked in red rose water, and applied to the eyes that are hot, red, and inflamed, or blood-shot, relieveth them. Hot bread applied for an hour at times for three days together, perfectly healeth the kernels in the throat, commonly called the king's evil. The flower of wheat mixed with the juice of henbane, stayeth the flux of humours in the joints being laid thereon. The said meal boiled in vinegar is good for shrinking of the sinews, saith Pliny ; and mixed with vinegar, and boiled together, removes freckles, pimples, and spots on the face. Wheat flour mixed with the yoke of an egg, honey, and turpentine, doth draw, cleanse, and heal any boil, plague-sore, or foul ulcer. The bran of wheat meal steeped in vinegar, and bound in a linen cloth and rubbed on the places that have the scurf, morphew, scabs, or leprosy, will take them away, the body being first purged and prepared. The decoction of the bran of wheat or barley, is of good use to bathe a rupture, and the said bran boiled in good vinegar and applied to swollen breasts, stayeth all inflammations. It cures the bitings of vipers (which I take to be no other than our English adder) and all other venomous creatures. The leaves of wheat meal applied with salt, take away hardness of the skin, warts, and hard knots in the flesh. Wafers put in water and drunk, stayeth lasks and bloody-flux, and are profitably used both inwardly and outwardly for ruptures in children.

Boiled in water to a thick jelly, and taken, it stayeth spitting of blood : and boiled with mint and butter, it cures hoarseness.

THE WILLOW TREE.

Government and Virtues.—The Moon owns it.   Both the leaves, bark and the seed are used to staunch bleeding of wounds at the mouth and nose, spitting of blood, and other fluxes of blood and to stay vomiting and provocation thereunto, if the decoction of them in wine be drunk.   It helpeth also to stay thin, hot, sharp, distillations from the head upon the lungs, causing a consumption.   The leaves bruised with some pepper and drunk in wine, cures windy colic.   The leaves bruised and boiled in wine, subdues lust in man or woman ;   the seed has also the same effect. Water that is gathered from the willow when it flowereth, the bark being slit and a vessel fitting to receive it, is very good for redness and dimness of sight, or films that grow over the eyes, and stayeth the rheums that fall into them ; it cures the stoppage of urine, if it be drunk, and clears the face and skin from spots and discolourings.   Galen saith, the flowers have an admirable faculty in drying up humours, being a medicine without any sharpness or corrosion ;   you may boil them in white wine and drink freely. The bark works the same effects if used in the same manner, and the tree hath always a mark upon it, though not always flowers ;   the burnt ashes being mixed with vinegar taketh away warts, corns, and superfluous flesh, being applied to the place.   The decoction of the leaves or bark in wine takes away scurf and dandriff by washing the place with it.   It is a fine cooling tree, the boughs of which are very convenient to be placed in the chamber of one sick of a fever.

WOAD.

Description.—It hath divers large leaves, long and rather broad, like those of the great plantain, but larger, thicker and of a greenish colour, inclining to blue.   From among which leaves riseth up a stalk three or four feet high, with divers leaves set thereon ;   the higher the stalk riseth the

T

smaller are the leaves; at the top it spreadeth divers branches, at the end of which appear very pretty little yellow flowers, and after they pass away like all other flowers of the field, come husks long and flat; in form they resemble a tongue, in colour they are black, and they hang bobbing downwards. The seed contained within these husks, if it be a little chewed, gives an azure colour. The root is white and long.

Place.—It is sowed in fields to dye with, and it is cut three times in a year.

Time.—It flowers in June, but it is long after before the seed is ripe.

Government and Virtues.—It is a cold and dry plant of Saturn. Some people affirm the plant to be destructive to bees, and fluxes them. I should rather think, unless bees be contrary to other creatures, it possesseth them with the contrary disease, the herb being exceeding dry and binding. But if any bees be diseased thereby, the cure is, to set urine by them, but set it in a vessel that they cannot drown themselves, which may be remedied if you put pieces of cork in. The herb is so drying and binding that it is not fit to be given inwardly. An ointment made thereof stauncheth bleeding. A plaster made thereof and applied to the region of the spleen which lies on the left side, takes away the hardness and pains thereof. The ointment is excellent in such ulcers as abound with moisture and takes away the corroding and fretting humours. It cools inflammation, quencheth St. Anthony's fire, and stayeth defluctions of the blood to any part of the body.

WOODBINE, OR HONEY-SUCKLES.

It is a plant well known by almost every one.

Time.—They flower in June, and the fruit is ripe in August.

Government and Virtues.—Honey-suckles are cleansing, consuming, and digesting, and therefore no way fit for inflammations. Take a leaf and chew it in your mouth, and you will quickly find it likelier to cause a sore mouth and throat than cure it. If it be not good for this, what is it good for? It is good for something, for God and nature made nothing in vain. It is an herb of Mercury, and appropriated to the lungs; the celestial Crab claims dominion over it, neither is it a foe to the Lion; if the lungs be afflicted by Jupiter, this is your cure. It is fitting a conserve made of the flowers should be kept in every gentlewoman's house; I know no better cure for the asthma than this: besides it takes away the evil of the spleen, provokes urine, procures speedy delivery of women in travail, relieves cramps, convulsions, and palsies, and whatsoever griefs come of cold or obstructed perspiration; if you make use of it as an ointment, it will clear the skin of morphew, freckles, and sunburnings, or whatever else discolours it, and then the maids will love it. Authors say, the flowers are of more effect than the leaves, and that is true: but they say the seeds are least effectual of all. But there is a vital spirit in every seed to beget its like; there is a greater heat in the seed than any other part of the plant; and heat is the mother of action.

WORMWOOD.

THREE wormwoods grow in this land: I shall describe First, SEA WORMWOOD.—It hath many names, viz.— seriphian, santonieon, belchion, narbinense, hentonicon, and twenty more which I shall not blot paper withal.

The seed of this wormwood is usually given to children for worms. Of all wormwoods that grow here, this is the weakest. The herb is good for something, beause God made nothing in vain.

The seed of the common wormwood is far more powerful than the seed of this to expel worms. The seraphian wormwood is the weakest, and haply may prove fittest for weak bodies. Let such as are strong take the common wormwood, for the others will do but little good. Again, near the sea many people live, and seraphian grows near them, and therefore is more fitting for their bodies because nourished by the same air.

It is known to all that know any thing in the course of nature, that the liver delights in sweet things; if so, it abhors bitter; then if your liver be weak, it is none of the wisest things to plague it with an enemy. If the liver be

weak a consumption follows. Would you know the reason? It is this; a man's flesh is repaired by blood, by a
third concoction, which transmutes the blood into flesh.
The liver makes blood, and if it be so weakened that it
makes not enough, the flesh wasteth; and why must flesh
always be renewed? Because God, when he made the
creation, made one part of it in continual dependency upon
another. And why did he do so? Because himself only is
permanent to teach us, that we should not fix our affections upon what is transitory, but what endures for ever.
The result of this is, if the liver be weak and cannot make
blood enough, the seriphian, which is the weakest of wormwoods, is better than the best.

Place.—It grows in England by the sea-side.

Description.—It starts up out of the earth with many
round, woody, hairy stalks from one root. Its height is
four feet, or three at least. The leaves in longitude are
long, in latitude narrow, in colour white, in form hoary,
in similitude like southern wood, only broader and longer;
in taste rather salt than bitter, because it grows near the
salt water. At the joints with the leaves towards the
tops, it bears little yellow flowers. The root lies deep and
is woody.

COMMON WORMWOOD I shall not describe, for every boy
that can eat an egg knows it.

ROMAN WORMWOOD : The stalks are slender, and shorter
than the common wormwood by one foot at least; the
leaves are more finely cut and divided than they are, but
somewhat smaller; both leaves and stalks are hoary, the
flowers of a pale yellow colour; it is altogether like the
common wormwood save only in size, for it is smaller; in
taste, for it is not so bitter; in smell, for it is spicy.

Place.—It groweth on the tops of mountains, there it is
natural, but usually cultivated in gardens for the use of
the apothecaries in London.

Time.—All wormwoods usually flower in August, a little
sooner or later.

Government and Virtues.—Wormwood is an herb of Mars.
What delights in martial places is a martial herb; and
wormwood delights in martial places, (for about forges and

iron works you may gather a cart-load of it) *ergo*, it is a martial herb. It is hot and dry in the first degree, viz., just as hot as your blood, and no hotter. It remedies the evils choler can inflict on the body of man by sympathy. It helps the evils Venus and the wanton boy produce, by antipathy ; and it doth something else besides. It cleanseth the body of choler. It provokes urine, helps surfeits, or swellings in the belly ; it causeth appetite to meat, because Mars rules the attractive faculty in man. The sun never shone upon a better herb than this is for the yellow jaundice. Take of the flowers of wormwood, rosemary, and black-thorn, of each a like quantity, half that quantity of saffron ; boil this in Rhenish wine, but put it not into saffron till it is almost boiled ; this is the way to keep a man's body in health, appointed by Camerarius, in his book entitled *Hortus Medicus*, and it is a good one too. Wormwood provokes the terms.

If one is injured by eating mushrooms, wormwood, an herb of Mars, cures him, because Mars is exalted in Capricorn, the house of Saturn, and this it doth by sympathy as it doth the other by antipathy. Wheals, pushes, black and blue spots coming either by bruises or beatings, wormwood, an herb of Mars, relieves, because Mars will give you a plaster. Mars eradicates all diseases in the throat by his herbs, of which wormwood is one, and sends them to Egypt on an errand never to return more, this is done by antipathy. The eyes are under the Luminaries ; the right eye of a man and the left eye of a woman, the Sun claims dominion over ; the left eye of a man and the right eye of a woman are privileges of the Moon ; wormwood cures both ; what belongs to the Sun by sympathy, because he is exalted in his house ; but what belongs to the Moon by antipathy, because he hath his fall in her's. Suppose a man to be bitten or stung by a martial creature, a wasp, a hornet, or a scorpion, wormwood, an herb of Mars, giveth you a present cure ; then Mars, choleric as he is, hath learned that patience to pass by your evil speeches of him, and tells you, by my pen, that he gives you no affliction, but he gives you a cure ; you need not run to Apollo, nor Æsculapius ; and if he was so choleric as you make him to be, he would have drawn his sword in anger, to see the ill condition of those people that can spy his vices and not his virtues. Wormwood cures the itch, and scabs, and taken inwardly and applied outwardly as a wash, makes the face fair. It is good for colic. It will kill moths, if laid among clothes. It is a specific remedy for melancholy, as it rectifies the liver and spleen. It expels worms and is a specific for the ague, by drinkiug the decoction in the morning.

YARROW, CALLED NOSE-BLEED, MILFOIL, AND THOUSAND-LEAF.

Description.—It hath many long leaves spread upon the ground, finely cut, and divided into many small parts ; its flowers are white, but not all of a whiteness, and stayed in knots, upon divers green stalks which rise from among the leaves.

Place.—It is frequent in all pastures.

Time.—It flowereth late, even at the end of August.

Government and Virtues.—It is under the influence of Venus. An ointment of them cures wounds, and is most fit for such as have inflammations ; it stops the terms, being boiled in white wine, and the decoction drunk ; as also the bloody flux ; the ointment of it is not only good for green wounds, but also for ulcers and fistulas, especially such as abound with moisture ; it stays the shedding of the hair, the head being bathed with the decoction of it ; inwardly taken it improves the retentive faculty of the stomach ; it cures the running of the reins, and the whites, and helps such as cannot hold their water ; and the leaves chewed in the mouth easeth the tooth-ache ; and these virtues being put together, show the herb to be drying and binding. Achilles is supposed to be the first that left the virtues of it to posterity, having learned them of his master, Chiro, the Centaur : and certainly a very profitable herb it is in cramps, and therefore called Miltaris. The decoction is excellent for colds in the head, influenza, &c. It is a substitute for tobacco, or both may be mixed.

DIRECTIONS FOR GATHERING

LEAVES, ROOTS, BARKS, SEEDS, &C.

LEAVES OF HERBS, OR TREES.

1. Of leaves choose only such as are green and full of juice ; pick them carefully, and cast away such as are declining.

2.—Note what places they most delight to grow in, and gather them there ; for betony that grows in the shade is far better than that growing in the sun because it delights in the shade ; so also such herbs as delight to grow near the water, should be gathered near it, though haply you may find some of them upon dry ground. The treatise will inform you where every herb delights to grow.

3. The leaves of such herbs as run up to seed are not so good when they are in flower as before, (some few excepted, the leaves of which are seldom or never used) in such cases, if through ignorance they were not known, or through negligence forgotten, you had better take the top and the flowers than the leaf.

4. Dry them well in the sun, and not in the shade ; for if the sun draw away the virtues of the herb, it must needs do the like by hay, by the same rule, which the experience of every country farmer will explode for a notable piece of nonsense.

5. Such as are astrologers, I advise ; let the planet that governs the herb be angular, and the stronger the better ; if they can, in herbs of Saturn, let Saturn be in the ascendant ; in the herb of Mars, let Mars be in the Mid-heaven, for in those houses they delight ; let the Moon apply to them by good aspect, and let her not be in the houses of her enemies ; if you cannot well stay till she apply to them, let her apply to a planet of the same triplicity ; if you cannot wait that time neither, let her be with a fixed star of their nature

6. Having well dried them, put them up in brown paper, sewing the paper up like a sack, and press them not too hard together, and keep them in a dry place near the fire.

7. As for the duration of dried herbs, a just time cannot be given, let authors prate at their pleasure ; for,

1st. Such as grow upon dry grounds will keep better than such as grow on moist.

2dly. Such herbs as are full of juice will not keep so long as such as are drier.

3dly. Such herbs as are well dried, will keep longer than such as are slack dried. Yet you may know when they are corrupted by their loss of colour, or smell, or both : and, if they be corrupted, reason will tell you that they must needs corrupt the bodies of those people that take them.

8. Gather all leaves in the hour of that planet that governs them.

Of Flowers.

1. The flower, which is the beauty of the plant, and of none of the least use in physic, groweth yearly, and is to be gathered when it is in its prime.

2. As for the time of gathering them, let the planetary hour, and the plant they come off be observed, as we showed you in the foregoing chapter : as for the time of the day, let it be when the sun shines upon them, that so they may be dry : for if you gather either flowers or herbs when they are wet or dewy, they will not keep.

3. Dry them well in the sun, and keep them in papers near the fire, as I showed you in the foregoing chapter.

4. So long as they retain the smell and colour, they are good ; either of them being gone, so is their virtue also.

Of Seeds.

1. The seed is that part of the plant which is endowed with a vital faculty to bring forth its like, and it contains potentially the whole plant in it.

2. As for the place, let them be gathered from the place where they most delight to grow.

3. Let them be full ripe when they are gathered, and

forget not the celestial harmony before mentioned ; for I have found by experience that their virtues are twice as great at such times as others : "There is an appointed time for every thing under the sun."

4. When you have gathered them, dry them a little, and but a very little, in the sun before you lay them up.

5. You need not be so careful of keeping them so near the fire as the other before mentioned, because they are fuller of spirit, and therefore not so subject to corrupt.

6. As for the time of their duration, it is palpable they will keep a good many years ; yet they are best the first year, and this I make appear by a good argument. They will grow soonest the first year they be set, therefore then they are in their prime ; and it is an easy matter to renew them yearly.

Of Roots.

1. Of roots choose neither such as are rotten or worm-eaten, but proper in their taste, colour, and smell, such as exceed neither in softness nor hardness.

Give me leave to be a little critical against the vulgar received opinion, which is, that the sap falls down into the root in the autumn, and rises in the spring, as men go to bed at night and rise in the morning ; and this idle talk of untruth is so grounded in the heads, not only of the vulgar but also of the learned, that a man cannot drive it out by reason. I pray, let such sap-mongers answer me this argument : If the sap fall into the roots in the fall of the leaf, and lies there all the winter, then must the root grow only in the winter. But the root grows not at all in winter, as experience teacheth, but only in summer ; therefore if you set an apple kernel in the spring, you shall find the root grow to a pretty size in the summer, and be not a whit bigger next spring. What doth the sap do in the root all that while ? Prick straws ? 'Tis as rotten as a post.

The truth is, when the sun declines from the tropic of Cancer, the sap begins to congeal both in root and branch : when he touches the tropic of Capricorn, and ascends to us-ward, it begins to wax thin again, and by degrees, as it congealed.

3. The drier time you gather the roots in, the better they are, for they have the less excrementitious moisture in them.

4. Such roots as are soft, your best way is to dry in the sun, or else hang them in the chimney corner upon a string ; as for such as are hard, you may dry them anywhere.

5. Such roots as are great, will keep longer than such as are small ; yet most of them will keep all the year.

6. Such roots as are soft, it is your best way to keep them always near the fire, and take this general rule for it. If in winter time you find any of your herbs, roots, or flowers begin to be moist, as many times you shall (for it is your best way to look to them once a month) dry them by a very gentle fire, or, if you can, with conveniency, keep them near the fire, you may save yourself the trouble.

7. It is in vain to dry roots that may commonly be had, as parsley, fennel, plantain, &c., but gather them only for present need.

Of Barks.

1. Barks, which physicians use in medicine, are of these sorts : of fruits, of roots, of boughs.

2. The barks of fruits are to be taken when the fruit is full ripe, as oranges, lemons, &c., but because I have nothing to do with exotics here, I pass them without any more words.

3. The bark of trees are best gathered in the spring, if of oak or such great trees ; because then they come easier off, and so you may dry them if you please ; but the best way is to gather all barks only for present use.

4. As for the bark of roots, 'tis thus to be gotten : Take the roots of such herbs as have a pith in them, as parsley, fennel, &c., slit them in the middle, and when you have taken out the pith, which you may easily do, that which remains is called, though improperly, the bark, and indeed is only to be used.

OF JUICES.

1. Juices are to be pressed out of herbs when they are young and tender, out of some stalks, and tender tops of herbs and plants, and also out of some flowers.

2. Having gathered the herb, if you would preserve the juice of it when it is very dry (for otherwise the juice will not be worth a button) bruise it well in a stone mortar with a wooden pestle, then having put it into a canvass bag, the herb I mean, not the mortar, for that will give but little juice, press it hard in a press, then take the juice and clarify it.

3. The manner of clarifying it is this : Put it into a pipkin or skillet, or some such thing, and set it over the fire ; and when the scum ariseth take it off ; let it stand over the fire till no more scum arise ; when you have your juice clarified, cast away the scum as a thing of no use.

4. When you have thus clarified it, you have two ways to preserve it all the year.

1st. When it is cold put it into a glass, and put so much oil on it as will cover it to the thickness of two fingers ; the oil will swim at the top, and so keep the air from coming to putrify it. When you intend to use it, pour it into a porringer, and if any oil come out with it, you may easily skim it off with a spoon, and put the juice you do not use into the glass again, it will quickly sink under the oil.

2nd. The second way is a little more difficult, and the juice of fruits is usually preserved this way. When you have clarified it, boil it over the fire, till being cold it be of the thickness of honey. This is most commonly used for diseases of the mouth, and is called roba and saba.

HOW TO MAKE AND KEEP ALL NECESSARY COMPOUNDS.

Of Distilled Waters.

HITHERTO we have spoken of medicines which consist in their own nature, which authors vulgarly call Simples, though something improperly ; for in truth, nothing is simple but pure elements ; all things else are compounded of them. We come now to treat of the artificial medicines, in the form of which, because we must begin somewhere, we shall place distilled waters ; in which consider,

1. Waters are distilled of herbs, of flowers, of fruits, and of roots.

2. We speak not of strong waters, but of cold, as being to act Galen's part, and not Paracelsus's.

3. The herbs ought to be distilled when they are in the greatest vigour, and so ought the flowers also.

4. The vulgar way of distillations which people use because they know no better, is in a pewter still; and although distilled waters are the weakest of artificial medicines, and good for little but mixtures of other medicines, yet they are weaker by many degrees than they would be were they distilled in sand. If I thought it not impossible to teach you the way of distilling in sand, I would attempt it.

5. When you have distilled your water, put it into a glass covered over with a paper pricked full of holes, so that the excrementitious and fiery vapours may exhale, which cause that settling in distilled waters called the mother, which corrupt them, then cover it close and keep it for use.

6. Stopping distilled waters with a cork makes them musty, and so does paper if it but touch the water; it is best to stop them with a bladder, being first put in water, and bound over the top of the glass.

Such cold waters as are distilled in a pewter still, (if well kept) will endure a year; such as are distilled in sand, as they are twice as strong, so they endure twice as long.

OF SYRUPS.

1. A Syrup is a medicine of a liquid form, composed of infusion, decoction, and juice. And

1st. For the more graceful taste.

2dly. For the better keeping of it; with a certain quantity of honey or sugar hereafter mentioned, boiled to the thickness of new honey.

2. You see at the first view that this aphorism divides itself into three branches, which deserves severally to be treated of, viz.,

  1. Syrups made by infusion.
  2. Syrups made by decoction.
  3. Syrups made by juice.

Of each of these, for your instruction's sake, kind countrymen and women, I speak a word or two apart.

1st. Syrups made by infusion are usually made of flowers, and of such flowers as soon loose their colour and strength by boiling, as roses, violets, peach-flowers, &c. My translation of the London Dispensatory will instruct you in the rest. They are thus made : Having picked your flowers clean, to every pound of them, add three pounds, or three pints, which you will, for it is all one, of spring water, made boiling hot ; but first put your flowers into a pewter pot with a cover, and pour the water on them ; then shutting the pot let it stand by the fire to keep hot twelve hours, and strain it out ; (in such syrups as purge, as damask roses, peach-flowers, &c., the usual, and indeed the best way, is to repeat this infusion, adding fresh flowers to the same liquor divers times, so that it may be stronger) having strained it out, put the infusion into a pewter bason, or an earthren one well glazed, and to every pint of it add two pounds of sugar, which being only melted over the fire without being boiled, and then skimmed will produce you the syrup you desire.

2dly. Syrups made by decoction are usually made of compounds, yet may any simple herb be thus converted into syrup. Take the herb, roots or flowers you would make into a syrup, and bruise a little ; then boil it in a convenient quantity of spring water ; the more water you boil it in the weaker it will be ; a handful of the herb or root is a convenient quantity for a pint of water ; boil it till half the water be consumed, then let it stand till it be almost cold, and strain it through a woollen cloth, letting it run out at leisure, without pressing. To every pint of this decoction add one pound of sugar, and boil it over the fire till it comes to a syrup, which you may know if you now and then cool a little of it with a spoon ; skim it all the while it boils, and when it is sufficiently boiled, while it is hot strain it again through a piece of woollen cloth, but press it not. Thus you have the syrup perfected.

3dly. Syrups made of juice are usually made of such herbs as are full of juice, and indeed they are better made into a syrup this way than any other ; the operation is thus : having beaten the herb in a stone mortar with a wooden pestle, press out the juice and clarify it, as you are taught in the juices ; then let the juice boil away till about a quarter of it be consumed ; to a pint of this add a pound of sugar, and boil it to a syrup, always skimming it, and when it is boiled enough, strain it through a woollen cloth, as we taught you before, and keep it for your use.

3. If you make a syrup of roots, that are anything hard, as parsley, fennel, and grass roots, &c., when you have bruised them, lay them to steep in that water that you intend to boil them, hot, so will the virtues the better come out.

4. Keep your syrups either in glasses or stone pots, and stop them not with cork or bladder, unless you would have the glass break and the syrup lost, only bind paper about the mouth.

All syrups, if well made, will continue a year with some advantage ; yet such as are made by infusion keep shortest.

Of Juleps.

1. Juleps were first invented, as I suppose, in Arabia, and my reason is, because the word julep is an Arabic word.

2. It signifies only a pleasant potion, as is vulgarly used by such as are sick and want help, or such as are in health, and want no money to quench their thirst.

3. Now-a-day it is commonly used,
1. To prepare the body for purgation.
2. To open obstructions and the pores.
3. To digest tough humours.
4. To qualify hot distempers, &c.

4. Simples, juleps, (for I have nothing to say to compounds here) are thus made : Take a pint of such distilled water as conduces to the cure of your distemper, which this treatise will plentifully furnish you with, to which add two ounces of syrup conducing to the same effect ; (I shall give you rules for it in the next chapter) mix them together and drink a draught of it at your pleasure. If you love tart things, add ten drops of oil of vitrol to your pint, and shake it together, and it will have a fine grateful taste.

5. All juleps are made for present use, and therefore it is in vain to speak of their duration.

Of Decoctions.

1. All the difference between decoctions, and syrups made by decoction, is this ; syrups are made to keep, decoctions only for present use ; for you can hardly keep a decoction a week at any time ; if the weather be hot, you cannot keep it half so long.

2. Decoctions are made of leaves, roots, flowers, seeds, fruit, or barks, conducing to the cure of the disease you make them for, and are made in the same manner as we showed you in syrups.

3. Decoctions made with wine last longer than such as are made with water ; and if you take your decoction to cleanse the passage of the urine or open obstructions, your best way is to make it with white wine instead of water, because this is penetrating.

4. Decoctions are of the most use in such diseases as lie in the passage of the body, as the stomach, bowels, kidneys, passage of urine and bladder, because decoctions pass quicker to those places than any other form of medicine.

5. If you will sweeten your decoction with sugar, or any syrup fit for the occasion you take it for, which is better, you may, and no harm.

6. If in a decoction you boil both roots, herbs, flowers and seed together, let the roots boil a good while first, because they retain their virtues longest ; then the next in order by the same rule, viz. 1. the barks. 2. the herbs. 3. the seeds. 4. the flowers. 5. the spices, if you put any in, because then the virtues come soonest out.

7. Such things as by boiling cause sliminess to a decoction, as figs, quince-seed, linseed, &c. your best way is, after you have bruised them, to tie them up in a linen rag, as you tie up calf's brains, and so boil them.

8. Keep all decoctions in a glass close stopped, and the cooler place you keep them in the longer they will last ere they be sour.

Lastly. The usual dose to be given at one time is two,

three four, or five ounces, according to the age and strength of the patient, the season of the year, the strength of the medicine, and the quality of the disease.

OF OILS.

1. OLIVE OIL, which is commonly known by the name of salad oil, I suppose, because it is usually eaten with salads by them that love it; if it be pressed out of ripe olives, according to Galen, is temperate, and exceeds in no one quality.

2. Of oils, some are simple, and some are compound.

3. Simple oils are such as are made of fruits or seeds by expression, as oil of sweet or bitter almonds, linseed and rape seed oil, &c. of which see in my dispensatory.

4. Compound oils are made of oil of olives, and other simples, fragrant herbs, flowers, roots, &c.

5. The way of making them is this: having bruised the herbs or flowers you make your oil of, put them into an earthen pot, and to two or three handsful of them pour a pint of oil, cover the pot with a paper, set it in the sun about a fortnight or so, according as the sun is in hotness; then having warmed it very well by the fire, press out the herb, &c. very hard in a press, and add as many more herbs to the same oil; bruise the herbs (I mean not the oil) in like manner, set them in the sun as before; the oftener you repeat this, the stronger your oil will be; at last, when you conceive it strong enough, boil both oil and herbs together, till the juice be consumed, which you may know by its leaving its bubbling, and the herbs will be crisp; then strain it while it is hot, and keep it in a stone or glass vessel for your use.

6. As for chemical oils, I have nothing to say here.

7. The general use of these oils is for pains in the limbs, roughness in the skin, the itch, &c. as also for ointments and plasters,

8. If you have occasion to use it for wounds or ulcers, in two ounces of oil, dissolve half an ounce of turpentine, the heat of the fire will quickly do it; for oil itself is offensive to wounds, and the turpentine qualifies it.

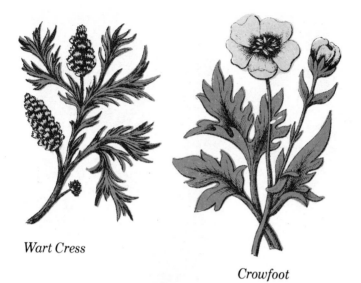

Wart Cress

Crowfoot

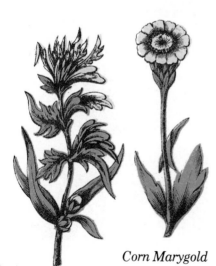

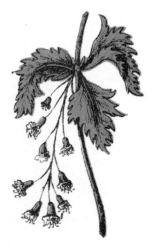

Corn Marygold

Cow Wheat

Black Currant

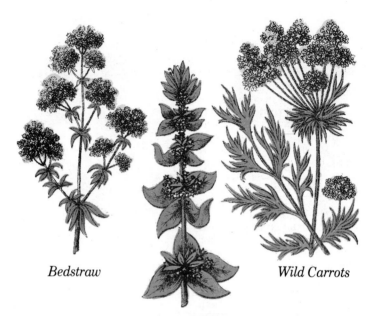

Bedstraw

Cross Wort

Wild Carrots

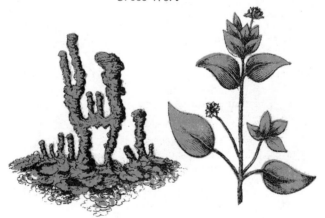

Cup Moss

Chickweed

Of Electuaries

I WILL give but one general way of making them up : as for ingredients you may vary them as you please, and as you find occasion, by the last chapter.

1. That you may make electuries when you need them, it is requisite that you keep always herbs, roots, flowers, &c. ready dried in your house, that so you may be in readiness to beat them into a powder when you need them.

2. It is better to keep them whole than beaten ; for being beaten, they are more subject to lose their strength, because the air soon penetrates them.

3. If they be not dry enough to beat into powder when you need them, dry them by a gentle fire till they are so.

4. Having beaten them, sift them through a fine tiffany sieve, that no great pieces may be found in your electuary.

5. To one ounce of your powder add three ounces of clarified honey ; this quantity I hold to be sufficient. If you would make more or less electuary, vary your proportion accordingly.

6. Mix them well together in a mortar, and take this for a truth, you cannot mix them too much.

7. The way to clarify honey, is to set it over the fire in a convenient vessel till the scum arise, and when the scum is taken off it is clarified.

8. The usual dose of cordial electuaries is from half a drachm to two drachms ; of purging electuaries, from half an ounce to an ounce.

9. The manner of keeping them is in a pot.

10. The time of taking them is either in a morning fasting, and fasting an hour after them ; or at night going to bed, three or four hours after supper.

Of Conserves.

THE way of making conserves is two-fold ; one of herbs and flowers, and the other of fruits.

2. Conserves of herbs and flowers are thus made ; if you thus make your conserve of herbs, as of scurvy grass, wormwood, rue, and the like, take only the leaves, and the tender tops (for you may beat your heart out before you

U

can beat the stalks small) and having beaten them, weigh them, and to every pound of them add three pounds of sugar ; you cannot beat them too much.

3. Conserves of fruits, as barberries, sloes, and the like, are thus made : first scald the fruit, then rub the pulp through a thick hair sieve made for that purpose, called a pulping sieve : you may do it for a need with the back of a spoon, then take this pulp thus drawn and add to it its weight of sugar, and no more ; put it into a pewter vessel and over a charcoal fire : stir it up and down till the sugar be melted, and your conserve is made.

4. Thus you have the way of making conserves ; the way of keeping them is in earthern pots.

5. The dose is usually the quantity of a nutmeg at a time, morning and evening, or (unless they are purging) when you please.

6. Of conserves, some keep many years, as conserve of roses ; others but a year, as conserve of borage, bugloss, cowslips, and the like.

7. Have a care of the working of some conserves presently after they are made ; look to them once a day, and stir them about. Conserves of borage, bugloss, and wormwood, have an excellent faculty at that sport.

8. You may know when your conserves are almost spoiled by this ; you shall find a hard crust at the top with little holes in it as though worms had been eating them.

Of Preserves.

Of preserves are sundry sorts, and the operation of all being somewhat different, we shall handle them all apart. These are preserved with sugar.

1. Flowers.
2. Fruits.
3. Roots.
4. Barks.

1. Flowers are very seldom preserved ; I never saw any that I remember save only cowslip flowers, and that was a great fashion in Sussex when I was a boy. It is thus done. Take a flat glass, we call them jar-glasses, strew on a laying of fine sugar, on that a laying of flowers, and on

that another laying of sugar, on that another laying of flowers, so do till your glass be full ; then tie it over with a paper, and in a little time you shall have very excellent and pleasant preserves.

There is another way of preserving flowers, namely, with vinegar and salt, as they pickle capers and broom buds ; but as I have little skill in it myself, I cannot teach you.

2. Fruits, as quinces and the like, are preserved two different ways.

1st. Boil them well in water, and then pulp them through a sieve, as we showed you before ; then with the like quantity of sugar boil the water they were boiled in into a syrup, viz. a pound of sugar to a pint of liquor ; to every pound of this syrup add four ounces of the pulp, then boil it with a very gentle fire to their right consistence, which you may easily know if you drop a little of syrup on a trencher ; if it be enough, it will not stick to your fingers when it is cold.

2nd. Another way to preserve fruits is this : First pare off the rind, then cut them in halves and take out the core, and boil them in water till they are soft ; if you know when beef is enough you may easily know when they are, then boil the water with its like weight of sugar into a syrup ; put the syrup into a pot, and put the boiled fruit as whole as you left it when you cut it into it, and let it remain till you have occasion to use it.

3. Roots are thus preserved : First scrape them very clean, and cleanse them from the pith, if they have any, for some roots have not, as eringo and the like : boil them in water till they be soft, as we showed you before in the fruits : then boil the water you boiled the root in into a syrup as showed yon before, then keep the root whole in the syrup till you use them.

4. As for barks, we have but few come to our hands to be done, and of those the few that I can remember, are oranges, lemons, citrons, and the outer barks of walnuts which grow without-side the shell, for the shells themselves would make but scurvy preserves ; these are they I can remember, if there be any more put them into the number

The way of preserving these is not all one in authors, for some are bitter, some are hot ; such as are bitter, say authors, must be soaked in warm water, oftentimes changing till the bitter taste be fled ; but I do not like this way, and my reason is this, because I doubt when their bitterness is gone so is their virtue also ; I shall then prescribe one common way, the same with the former, viz. first boil them whole till they be soft, then make a syrup with sugar and the liquor you boil them in, and keep the barks in the syrup.

5. They are kept in glasses or in glazed pots.

6. The preserved flowers will keep a year, if you can forbear eating them ; the roots and barks much longer.

7. This art was plainly and first invented for delicacy, yet came afterwards to be of excellent use in physic ; for,

1st. Hereby medicines are made pleasant for sick and squeamish stomachs, which would else loath them.

2nd. Hereby they are preserved from decaying a long time.

Of Lohocks.

1. That which the Arabians call lohocks, and the Greeks eclegmia, the Latins call linctus, and in plain English signifies nothing else but a thing to be licked up.

2. Their first invention was to prevent and remedy afflictions of the breast and lungs, to cleanse the lungs of phlegm, and make it fit to be cast out.

3. They are in body thicker than a syrup, and not so thick as an electuary.

4. The manner of taking them is often to take a little with liquorice stick, and let it go down at leisure.

5. They are easily thus made : Make a decoction of pectoral herbs, and the treatise will furnish you with enough, and when you have strained it with twice its weight of honey or sugar, boil it to a lohock ; if you are molested with much phlegm, honey is much better than sugar, and if you add a little vinegar to it you will do well ; if not, I hold sugar to be better than honey.

6. It is kept in pots, and may be kept a year and longer.

7. It is excellent for roughness of the wind-pipe, in-

flammations and ulcers of the lungs, difficulty of breathing, asthmas, coughs, and distillations of humours.

OF OINTMENTS.

1. VARIOUS are the ways of making ointments, which authors have left to posterity, and which I shall omit, and quote one which is easiest to be made, and therefore most beneficial to people that are ignorant in physic, for whose sake I write this. It is thus done :

Bruise those herbs, flowers, or roots, you will make an ointment of, and to two handfuls of your bruised herbs add a pound of hog's lard dried, or cleansed from the skins, beat them very well together in a stone mortar with a wooden pestle, then put it into a stone pot, (the herb and grease I mean, not the mortar) cover it with a paper, and set it either in the sun or some other warm place, three, four, or five days, that it may melt; then take it out and boil it a little, and whilst it is hot strain it out, pressing it out very hard in a press ; to this lard add as many more herbs as before, let them stand in like manner as long, then boil them as you did the former. If you think your ointment not strong enough, you may do it the third and fourth time ; yet this I will tell you, the fuller of juice the herbs are, the sooner will your ointment be strong : the last time you boil it, boil it so long till your herbs be crisp, and the juice consumed, then strain it, pressing it hard in a press, and to every pound of ointment add two ounces of turpentine and as much wax, because grease is offensive to wounds as well as oil.

2. Ointments are vulgarly known to be kept in pots, and will last above a year, sometimes above two years.

OF PLASTERS.

1. THE Greeks made their plasters of divers simples, and put metals into most of them, if not all; for having reduced their metals into powder, they mixed them with that fatty substance whereof the rest of the plaster consisted whilst it was yet hot, continually stirring it up and down lest it should sink to the bottom ; so they continually stirred it till it was stiff; then they made it up into

rolls, which when they needed for use, they could melt it by the fire again.

2. The Arabians made up theirs with oil and fat, which needeth not so long boiling,

3. The Greeks' emplasters consisted of these ingredients, metals, stones, divers sorts of earth, fœces, juices, liquors, seeds, roots, excrements of creatures, wax, rosin, and gums.

Of Poultices.

Poultices are those kind of things which the Latins call *cataplasmata*, and our learned fellows, that if they can read English, that's all, call them cataplasms, because 'tis a crabbed word few understand ; it is indeed a very fine kind of medicine to ripen sores.

2. They are made of herbs and roots fitted for the disease aforesaid, being chopped small and boiled in water to a jelly ; then adding a little barley meal, or meal of lupins, and a little oil or rough sweet suet, which I hold to be better, spread upon a cloth and applied to the grieved place.

3. Their use is to ease pains, to break sores, to cool inflammations, to dissolve hardness, to ease the spleen, to concoct humours, and dissipate swellings.

4. I beseech you take this caution along with you : Use no poultices, if you can help it, that are of an healing nature, before you have first cleansed the body because they are subject to draw the humours to them from every part of the body.

Of Troches.

1. The Latins call them *placentula*, or little cakes, and the Greeks *prochikois*, *kukliscoi*, and *artiscoi ;* they are usually little round flat cakes, or you make make them square if you will.

2. Their first invention was, that powders being so kept might resist the intermission of air, and so endure pure longer.

3. Besides, they are easier carried in the pockets of such as travail ; as any man, for example, is forced to travail whose stomach is too cool, or at least not so hot as it should

be, which is more proper, for the stomach is never cold till a man be dead : in such a case it is better to carry troches of wormwood or galangal, in a paper in his pocket, than to take a gallipot along with him.

4. They are made thus : At night when you go to bed, take two drachms of fine gum tragacanth ; put it into a gallipot, and put half a quarter of a pint of any distilled water fitting for the purpose you would make your troches for to cover it, and the next morning you shall find it such a jelly as the physicians call mucilage : with this you may (with a little pains taken) make a powder into a paste, and that paste into cakes called troches.

5. Having made them, dry them in the shade, and keep them in the pot for your use.

Of Pills.

1. They are called *pilulæ*, because they resemble little balls ; the Greeks call them *catapolia*.

2. It is the opinion of modern physicians, that this way of making medicines was invented only to deceive the palate, that so by swallowing them whole, the bitterness of the medicine might not be perceived, or at least it might not be insufferable ; and indeed most of their pills, though not all, are very bitter.

3. I am of clean contrary opinion to this. I rather think they were done up in this hard form that so they might be the longer digesting ; and my opinion is grounded upon reason too, not upon fancy or hearsay. The first invention of pills was to purge the head ; now, as I told you before, such infirmities as lie near the passages were best removed by decoctions, because they pass to the grieved parts soonest ; so here, if the infirmity lies in the head or any other remote part, the best way is to use pills, because they are longer in digestion, and therefore better able to call the offending humours to them.

4. If I should tell you here a long tale of medicines working by sympathy and antipathy, you would not understand a word of it ; they that are set to make physicians may find it in the treatise. All modern physicians know not what belongs to a sympathetical cure, no more than a

cuckoo what belongs to flats and sharps in music, but follow the vulgar road, and call it a hidden quality, because it is hidden from the eyes of dunces, and indeed none but astrologers can give a reason for it ; and physic without reason is like a pudding without fat.

5. The way to make pills is very easy, for with the help of a pestal and mortar, and a little diligence, you may make any powder into pills, either with syrup or the jelly I told you before.

THE WAY OF MIXING MEDICINES ACCORDING TO THE CAUSE OF THE DISEASE, AND PART OF THE BODY AFFLICTED.

THIS being the key of the work, I shall be very particular. I shall address myself

1. To the vulgar.

2. To such as study astrology ; or such as study physic astrologically.

1st. To the vulgar. Kind souls, I am sorry it hath been your hard mishap to have been so long trained in such Egyptian darkness, even darkness which to your sorrow may be felt. The vulgar road of physic is not my practice) and I am therefore the more unfit to give you advice. I have now published a little book, (Galen's Art of Physic, which will fully instruct you, not only in the knowledge of your own bodies, but also in fit medicines to remedy each part of it when afflicted ; in the mean season take these few rules to stay your stomachs.

1. With the disease regard the cause, and the part of the body afflicted ; for example, suppose a woman to be subject to miscarry through wind, thus do :

(1.) Look for abortion in the table of diseases, and you shall be directed by that how many herbs prevent miscarriage.

(2.) Look for wind in the same table and you shall see how many of these herbs expel wind.

These are the herbs medicinal for your grief.

2. In all diseases strengthen the part of the body afflicted.

3. In mixed diseases there lies some difficulty, for some-

times two parts of the body are afflicted with contrary humours, as sometimes the liver is afflicted with choler and
water, as when a man hath had the dropsy and yellow
jaundice ; and this is usually mortal.

In the former, suppose the brain to be too cold and
moist, and the liver to be hot and dry ; thus do :

1. Keep your head outwardly warm.

2. Accustom yourself to the smell of hot herbs.

3. Take a pill that heats the head at night going to bed.

4. In the morning take a decoction that cools the liver,
or that quickly passeth the stomach, and is at the liver immediately.

You must not think, courteous people, that I can spend
time to give you examples of all diseases. These are enough
to let you see so much light as you without art are able to
receive. If I should set you to look at the sun, I should
dazzle your eyes and make you blind.

2dly. To such as study astrology, (who are the only men
I know that are fit to study physic—physic, without astrology, being like a lamp without oil) you are the men I exceedingly respect, and such documents as my brain can
give you at present, being absent from my study, I shall
give you.

1. Fortify the body with herbs of the nature of the Lord
of the Ascendant, 'tis no matter whether he be a Fortune
or Infortune in this case.

2. Let your medicine be something anti-pathetical to the
Lord of the Sixth.

3. Let your medicine be something of the nature of his
sign ascending.

4. If the Lord of the Tenth be strong, make use of his
medicines.

5. If this cannot well be, make use of the medicines of
the Light of Time.

6. Be sure always to fortify the grieved part of the body
by sympathetical remedies.

7. Regard the heart, keep that upon the wheels, beause
the sun is the foundation of life, and therefore those universal remedies *Aarum Potabile*, and the Philosopher's
stone cure all diseases by fortifying the heart.

DEFINITION OF TERMS.

AGARIC.—A mushroom, fungus.
ALEMBIC.—A still.
ANTIDOTE.—Preservation against sickness or poison.
ASTRICTION.—A binding, or contraction.
ASTRINGENT.—Binding.
ATTENUATE.—To make thin, or lean.
BLAIN.—Boil or blister.
BOT.—A small worm.
CACHEXY.—Bad habit of body.
CANKER.—Any that corrupts or consumes.
CASTING.—Vomiting.
CEPHALIC.—Pertaining to the head.
CERUSE.—White lead.
CHILBLAINS.—Frosted hands or feet.
CHOLER.—Excess of bile, producing anger, &c.
CHRONIC.—Relating to time, abiding.
CRICK.—A spasm, or cramp, crooked.
DECOCTION.—Preparation by boiling.
DEFLUXION.—A flowing down.
DIARRHŒA.—A lax, looseness of bowels.
DISCUSS.—To disperse.
DIVERS.—Various, several.
DISURY.—Difficulty of voiding urine.
ELECTUARY.—Medicine mixed with treacle, or preserves.
ERYSIPELAS.—St. Anthony's fire, or inflammation of the skin.
EXPECTORATE.—To cough up.
FLATULENCY.—Windiness in the stomach, or bowels.
FUNDAMENT.—Lower part, or seat of the body.
GANGRENE.—Dying of, mortification.
HÆMORRHOIDS.—Piles.
HERMODACTYLE.—A root.
HYDROPIC.—Dropsical.
HYPOCHONDRIAC.—Affected with melancholy.
IMPOSTHUME.—Abscess, gathering.
ICON.—An image.
KIBE.—Chap in the heel.
LASK.—Diarrhœa, lax, looseness of the bowels.
LETHARGY.—drowsiness, stupor.
LEY, OR LYE.—Water alkalized with wood ashes.

LUMBAR.—Relating to the loins.
MAW.—The stomach.
MEGRIM.—Vertigo, dizziness.
MENSES.—Women's monthly courses.
MENSTRUATION.—Ditto.
MITHRIDATE.—An antidote, mustard.
MOLLIFY.—To soften.
MORPHEW.—Scurf on the face.
MOTHER.—Womb.
MUMPS.—Swelling of the glands of the neck.
MUSCATEL.—A kind of wine.
PESSARY.—Supporter for the vagina, or womb.
PLETHORA.—Fulness of blood, or humours
PHTHISIS.—A wasting of the lungs.
POLYPUS.—Formation of flesh in the nose.
PUSHES.—Pustules, effect of a thrust.
PUSTULE.—A small swelling, pimple.
PUTREFACTION.—Rottenness, corruption.
RECTUM.—Last gut of the entrails, near the fundament.
REINS.—Kidneys, loins.
RHEUMS.—Thin serous fluid from the mucous glands.
ST. ANTHONY'S FIRE.—Erysipelas, inflammation of the skin.
SATURNINE.—Gloomy, heavy, sad.
SCIATICA.—Rheumatism in the hip joint.
SPLEEN.—Milt on the left side, the seat of melancholy.
SPLENETIC.—One troubled with the spleen.
STRANGURY.—Painful, difficult discharge of urine.
SUPPOSITORY.—A thick clyster.
TENT.—A roll of lint for wound or sore.
TESTICLE.—A stone, a gland that secretes seminal fluid.
THRUM.—Stamen of a flower.
TURBITH.—Bark of the root of turpethun.
TUTTY.—Oxide of zinc.

A TABLE

SHOWING THE TEMPERAMENT OF ALL THE HERBS.

The letter t *signifies Temperate. The Figures* 1, 2, 3, *and* 4 *are Degrees from the Medium.*

	Hot.	Dry.	Cold.	Moist.		Hot.	Dry.	Cold.	Moist.
Acanthus	-	-	2	2	Bifoil	-	1	1	-
Adders Tongue	t	2	-	-	Bilberries	1	1	-	-
Agrimony	2	2	-	-	Birch Tree	-	-	2	2
Agrimony, Water	2	2	-	-	Birds Foot	-	1	1	-
Alder Tree. Black	-	-	t	1	Bishops Weed	3	3	-	-
Alder Tree, Common	-	-	2	2	Bistort	t	3	-	-
Alexander	3	3	-	-	Black Hellebore	-	2	4	-
Alkanet	-	-	t	2	Black Thorn	-	2	2	-
All Heal	3	3	-	-	Blites	-	1	1	-
Amaranthus	-	2	2	-	Blue Bottle	-	2	2	-
Anemone	2	2	-	-	Borage	-	-	t	2
Angelica	2	2	-	-	Bramble	-	3	1	-
Archangel	-	-	1	1	Briony	3	3	-	-
Arrach, Garden	-	-	3	3	Brook Lime	2	2	-	-
Arrach, Wild	-	-	3	3	Broom	2	2	-	-
Arssmart	4	4	-	-	Bucks Horn Plantain	-	2	2	-
Artichokes	2	-	-	2	Bucks Horn	-	2	2	-
Asarabacca	3	3	-	-	Bugle	1	-	-	1
Ash-Tree	2	2	-	-	Burdock	1	1	-	-
Asparagus	t	-	-	-	Burnet	t	1	-	-
Avens	2	2	-	-	Burnet Saxifrage	3	3	-	-
Balm	2	2	-	-	Butchers Broom	2	1	-	-
Barberry	1	1	-	-	Butter Bur	2	2	-	-
Barley	-	1	1	-	Cabbages	t	1	-	-
Bastard Rhubarb	2	2	-	-	Calamint	3	3	-	-
Bay-Tree	3	3	-	-	Caltrops, Water	-	-	3	3
Bazil, Garden	3	-	-	3	Camomile	2	2	-	-
Beans	-	1	1	-	Campion Wild	-	3	3	-
Beans, French	-	1	1	-	Carduus Benedictus	2	2	-	-
Bed Straw, Ladies	1	1	-	-	Carraway	3	3	-	-
Beech Tree	-	1	1	-	Carrots, Wild	-	-	t	1
Beets	2	2	-	-	Celandine, Great	3	3	-	-
Betony, Water	2	-	-	2	Celandine, Lesser	2	2	-	-
Betony, Wood	2	2	-	-	Centaury, Small	3	3	-	-

	H	D	C	M		H	D	C	M
Cherry–Tree	2	–	–	2	Fever Few	2	3	–	–
Cherries, Winter	2	–	–	2	Fig Tree	2	2	–	–
Chervil	1	–	–	1	Fig Wort	4	4	–	–
Chestnut Tree	2	2	–	–	Fillependula	2	–	–	2
Chestnuts, Earth	·	–	3	3	Flax Weed	t	3	–	–
Chick-pease	1	–	–	1	Flea Wort	–	–	2	t
Chickweed	–	–	3	3	Flower de Luce	2	2	–	–
Cinquefoil	t	–	–	–	Fluellin	–	–	2	2
Cives	4	4	–	–	Fox Gloves	2	2	–	–
Clary, Garden	–	–	1	1	French Mercury	3	3	–	–
Clary, Wild	–	–	1	1	Fuller's Thistle	–	–	t	1
Cleavers	–	–	1	1	Fumatory	–	1	1	–
Clowns Wound Wort	–	2	2	–	Furze Bush	3	3	–	–
Cocks Head	2	–	–	2	Garden Patience	2	2	–	–
Colewort, Sea	t	1	–	–	Garden Tansy	2	3	–	–
Colts Foot	1	–	–	1	Garden Valerian	2	2	–	–
Columbines	2	–	–	2	Garlic	4	4	–	–
Comfrey	–	3	3	–	Gentian	3	2	–	–
Coral Wort	–	–	2	2	Germander	3	3	–	–
Costmary	2	2	–	–	Gilliflowers	t	–	–	–
Cowslips	t	–	–	–	Golden Maiden Hair	2	2	–	–
Crabs Claw	–	–	1	1	Golden Rod	2	–	–	2
Cress, Black	3	3	–	–	Gooseberry Bush	–	2	2	–
Cresses, Sciatica	–	2	2	–	Gout Wort	2	2	–	–
Cress, Water	3	3	–	–	Grass Polly	–	–	1	1
Croswort	–	2	2	–	Gromwell	2	2	–	–
Crowfoot	3	3	–	–	Ground Ivy	1	1	–	–
Cuckoo Pint	3	3	–	–	Ground Pine	2	3	–	–
Cucumbers	–	–	1	2	Garden Rue	3	4	–	–
Cudweed	2	–	–	2	Groundsell	2	2	–	–
Daises	–	–	1	2	Hart's Tongue	–	1	1	–
Dandelion	t	1	–	–	Hawthorn	3	3	–	–
Darnel	–	2	2	–	Hawk Weed	–	2	2	–
Devils Bit	2	2	–	–	Hazel Nut	t	1	–	–
Dill	3	2	–	–	Hearts Ease	–	–	1	2
Dock	t	3	–	–	Heart Trefoil	3	3	–	–
Dog Mercury	1	1	–	–	Hedge Hyssop	3	3	–	–
Dog's Grass	t	–	–	–	Hedge Mustard	2	2	–	–
Dove's Foot	2	2	–	–	Hemlock	–	3	4	–
Dragons	4	4	–	–	Hemp	–	1	1	–
Duck Weed	–	–	3	3	Henbane	–	1	4	–
Elecampane	3	3	–	–	Herb Robert	2	–	–	2
Elm Tree	–	2	2	–	Herb True-Love	–	–	t	1
Endive	–	2	2	–	Holly Holm	2	2	–	–
English Tobacco	2	2	–	–	Honeysuckle	–	1	1	–
Eryngo	2	–	–	2	Hops	2	2	–	–
Eyebright	3	3	–	–	Horehound	2	3	–	–
Fennel	2	1	–	–	Horsetail	–	2	2	–
Fennel, Hog's	2	1	–	–	Hound's Tongue	–	2	2	–
Fern, Male	2	2	–	–	Houseleek	–	–	3	t
Fern, Water	–	1	1	–	Hyssop	t	2	–	–

	H	D	C	M		H	D	C	M
Ivy	2	2	–	–	Parsnip	1	1	–	–
Juniper Bush	3	1	–	–	Peach Tree	–	–	2	2
Kidney Wort	–	–	t	1	Pear Tree	–	–	t	1
Knap Weed	–	3	3	–	Pearl Trefoil	–	–	2	2
Knot Grass	–	2	2	–	Pellitory of Spain	3	3	–	–
Ladies Mantle	2	2	–	–	Pellitory of the Wall	2	2	–	–
Ladies Smock	3	3	–	–	Pennyroyal	3	3	–	–
Lady's Thistle	2	2	–	–	Peony	2	2	–	–
Lavender	3	3	–	–	Pepperwort	4	3	–	–
Lavender Cotton	3	3	–	–	Periwinkle	2	1	–	–
Lettuce	–	1	3	–	Pimpernel	3	3	–	–
Lilly of the Valley	1	1	–	–	Primroses	1	1	–	–
Liquorice	t	–	–	▲	Plaintain	–	2	2	–
Liverwort	–	1	1	–	Plums	.	–	1	1
Loosestrife	–	1	1	–	Pollypody	t	1	–	–
Lovage	1	1	–	–	Poplar Tree	–	–	1	1
Lung Wort	–	1	1	–	Poppy	–	–	4	2
Madder	–	1	1	1	Privet	–	1	1	–
Mallows	–	.	t	–	Purslane	–	–	3	2
Maple Tree	t	–	–	–	Queen of the meadow	2	2	–	–
Marigold	1	1	–	–	Quince Tree	–	2	1	–
Masterwort	3	3	–	–	Radish	3	2	–	–
Meadow Rue	3	3	–	–	Ragwort	2	2	–	–
Medlar	–	3	3	–	Rattle Grass	–	–	1	1
Melancholy Thistle	2	2	–	–	Rest Harrow	3	3	–	–
Mellilot	1	1	–	–	Rhubarb	2	2	–	–
Mint	3	3	–	–	Rocket	3	3	–	–
Miseltoe	2	2	–	–	Rosa Solis	4	4	–	–
Mithridate Mustard	3	3	–	–	Rosemary	3	3	–	–
Moneywort	–	1	1	–	Roses	t	2	–	–
Moonwort	–	1	1	–	Rupture Wort	–	2	1	–
Mosses	–	2	1	–	Rye	–	1	1	–
Motherwort	2	2	–	–	Saffron	2	2	–	–
Mouse Ear	2	2	–	–	Sage	2	3	–	–
Mugwort	1	2	–	–	Samphire	2	–	–	2
Mulberry Tree	–	1	1	–	Sanicle	2	3	–	–
Mullein	t	1	–	–	Saracens Confound	–	2	2	–
Mustard	4	4	–	–	Sauce Alone	4	4	–	–
Nailwort	2	2	–	–	Savine	3	3	–	–
Nep	2	2	–	–	Savory	2	2	–	–
Nettles	2	2	–	–	Scabious	2	2	–	–
Nightshade	–	4	4	–	Scurvy Grass	3	3	–	–
Oak, The	–	3	1	–	Self Heal	1	1	–	–
Oats	–	1	1	–	Service Tree	–	1	1	–
One Blade	1	1	–	–	Shepherd's Purse	–	3	3	–
Onions	4	4	–	–	Silver Weed	2	3	–	–
Orchis	1	1	–	–	Smallage	–	2	2	–
Orpine	–	2	2	–	Soapwort	2	2	–	–
Parsley	3	2	–	–	Solomon's Seal	1	1	–	–
Parsley, Macedonian	2	2	–	–	Sorrel	1	1	–	–
Parsley Pert	2	2	–	–	Southern Wood	1	1	–	–

	H	D	C	M		H	D	C	M
Sow Thistle	–	–	2	1	Vipers Bugloss	–	–	t	2
Spignel	3	2	–	–	Wall Flowers	t	–	–	–
Spleen Wort	1	2	–	–	Wallnut Tree	3	3	–	–
St. John's Wort	2	2	–	–	Wall Rue	1	1	–	–
St. Peter's Wort	2	2	–	–	Water Flag	4	4	–	–
Star Thistle	2	2	–	–	Water Lily	–	3	3	–
Stinking Gladwin	3	3	–	–	Wheat	1	t	–	–
Stone Crop	–	2	2	–	White Lilies	–	–	2	2
Strawberries	–	–	1	1	White Saxifrage	2	2	–	–
Succory	1	1	–	–	Wild Majoram	2	2	–	–
Sweet Marjoram	3	3	–	–	Wild Thyme	2	2	–	–
Tamarisk Tree	3	3	–	–	Willow Tree	–	2	2	–
Thistle, Cotton	2	2	–	–	Winter Green	–	3	2	–
Thorough Wax	–	2	2	–	Winter Rocket	3	3	–	–
Thyme	2	3	–	–	Woad	–	3	3	–
Tormental	3	3	–	–	Wold	2	2	–	–
Treacle Mustard	3	3	–	–	Woodbine	1	1	–	–
Turnsole	3	3	–	–	Wood Sage	2	2	–	–
Tutsan	–	2	2	–	Wood Sorrel	–	2	1	–
Vervain	t	2	–	–	Woollen Thistle	3	3	–	–
Vine, The	–	3	1	–	Wormwood	1	1	–	–
Violets	–	–	1	1	Yarrow	–	2	1	–

DISEASES CURED BY THE HERBS

DESCRIBED IN THIS HERBAL.

☞ *In some cases the Disease may not fall on the page stated; but by referring to the preceding or the following page, it will probably be found.*

INDEX TO THE HERBS,

AND THE

NAMES OF THE PLANETS WHICH GOVERN THEM.

WILLIAM NICHOLSON AND SONS, PRINTERS, WAKEFIELD.